W0050842

Paediatric Neoplasia

Current Histopathology

Consultant Editor
Professor G. Austin Gresham, TD, ScD, MD, FRCPath.
Emeritus Professor of Morbid Anatomy and Histopathology,
University of Cambridge

Volume Twenty-two

PAEDIATRIC NEOPLASIA

by
S. VARIEND
Department of Histopathology
Sheffield Children's Hospital
Western Bank
Sheffield, UK

SPRINGER-SCIENCE+BUSINESS MEDIA, B.V.

A catalogue record for this book is available from the
British Library.

ISBN 978-94-010-4986-3   ISBN 978-94-011-2224-5 (eBook)
DOI 10.1007/978-94-011-2224-5

Copyright

© 1993 by S. Variend

Originally published by Kluwer Academic Publishers in

All rights reserved. No part of this publication may be
reproduced, stored in a retrieval system, or transmitted
in any form or by any means, electronic, mechanical,
photocopying, recording or otherwise, without prior
permission from the publishers,
Springer-Science+Business Media, B.V.

Typeset and originated by Speedlith Photo Litho Ltd.,
Stretford, Manchester M32 0JT

Contents

Current Histopathology Series

Consultant Editor's Note

At the present time books on morbid anatomy and histopathology can be divided into two broad groups: extensive textbooks often written primarily for students and monographs on research topics.

This takes no account of the fact that the vast majority of pathologists are involved in an essentially practical field of general diagnostic pathology providing an important service to their clinical colleagues. Many of these pathologists are expected to cover a broad range of disciplines and even those who remain solely within the field of histopathology usually have single and sole responsibility within the hospital for all this work. They may often have no colleagues in the same department. In the field of histopathology, no less than in other medical fields, there have been extensive and recent advances, not only in new histochemical techniques but also in the type of specimen provided by new surgical procedures.

There is a great need for the provision of appropriate information for this group. This need has been defined in the following terms:

1. It should be aimed at the general clinical pathologist or histopathologist with existing practical training, but should have value for the trainee pathologist.

2. It should concentrate on the practical aspects of histopathology taking account of the new techniques which should be within the compass of the worker in a unit with reasonable facilities.

3. New types of material, e.g. those derived from endoscopic biopsy should be covered fully.

4. There should be an adequate number of illustrations on each subject to demonstrate the variation in appearance that is encountered.

5. Colour illustrations should be used wherever they aid recognition.

Paediatric pathology is a rapidly expanding subject. The establishment of posts in paediatric and neonatal pathology in the regions has gone some way to meet this challenge. However, general histopathologists are faced with the problems of diagnosing paediatric neoplasia from time to time. This atlas provides a comprehensive account of paediatric neoplasms which will be of considerable help to the general pathologist and clinician involved with paediatric neoplasia.

G. A. Gresham

Introduction

Cancer is an important cause of death within the first 15 years of life. Many childhood cancers are fundamentally different from those arising in adults by virtue of pathogenesis, behaviour and response to therapy. One of the great success stories of recent years has been the dramatic improvement in survival of children with many different types of cancer. This has been made possible largely through the development and implementation of multimodality treatment regimes, as well as increasingly accurate histological categorization.

A number of ancillary methods for the microscopic diagnosis of tumours is now available as part of an expanding repertoire. This includes immunohistochemistry, enzyme histochemistry, electron microscopy and cytogenetics. Molecular biological techniques are likely to promote our understanding of the biology of many childhood tumours; they have already proved extremely effective in enhancing prognostic assessment and promise to play an important part in determining the initial choice of optimal therapy. However, the opportunity to apply this methodology has been, to some extent, limited by the increasing trend towards smaller biopsy samples submitted for diagnosis and also a tendency to procure material after the commencement of therapy. The pathologist should, however, regard such developments as a challenge rather than an obstacle.

The present work focuses specifically on tumours likely to be encountered in childhood but the list of tumours covered is by no means exhaustive and those related to the central nervous system, skeletal system, haemopoietic system, skin and salivary tissue are not formally included. Information relevant to these structures may be found in many of the existing organ-orientated texts, as well as past (and future) editions in this Series.

Despite the implementation of modern methodologies, a small core of childhood neoplasia persistently defies diagnostic categorization: knowledge of its existence should continue to prompt the development of newer diagnostic strategies. Many cooperative studies in Europe (International Society of Paediatric Oncology, United Kingdom Childhood Cancer Study Group) and United States of America (National Wilms' Tumor Study Group and the Intergroup Rhabdomyosarcoma Study) have played an important role in assembling valuable data concerning some of the less common neoplasms. Such sources of information, as well as those produced by large repositories of material (e.g. The American Armed Forces Institute of Pathology), are widely utilized throughout the text.

Paediatric neoplasia is a field which is evolving fast on several different fronts, and, against this backdrop, the accompanying text can only provide a 'snapshot' account. Some insight into related issues, such as histogenesis, differential diagnosis and prognosis, is also provided, but no detailed account of epidemiology or oncogenesis, issues essentially outside the scope of this work. This project is essentially designed as a diagnostic aid for histopathologists embroiled from time to time with problems concerning childhood tumours, although it is hoped that postgraduate students of general and paediatric pathology will also find sanctuary among its pages. References have been chosen judiciously to reflect current thought and, so far as possible, recent reviews have been extensively used.

ACKNOWLEDGEMENTS

Many colleagues have contributed material for the preparation of microphotographs and, in this regard, I am very much indebted to Professor J. Berry (Bristol), Dr Gillian Batcup (Leeds), Dr Shirley Hill (Sheffield), Dr G. Cullity (Perth, Australia), Dr C. Sinclair-Smith (Cape Town), Dr J. Rapola (Helsinki), Dr R. Jaffe (Pittsburgh), Dr J.E. Haas (Seattle), Dr Claudie Scheiner (Marseille), Dr J. Briner (Zürich), Dr J.N. Cox (Geneva), Dr K.A. Shakoor (Karachi), Dr J. Goepel (Sheffield), Dr A. Malcolm (Newcastle), Mr A.M. Potter (Sheffield) and Dr. A. Gibson (Glasgow).

I would also like to express gratitude to many of my immediate clinical colleagues who have assisted through discussion and the provision of clinical material. I am especially indebted to the X-ray Department of the Sheffield Children's Hospital for allowing me to include the radiographs. The technical staff of the Histopathology Department have been unstinting in their support

Primary hepatic tumours are rare in children. They present a wide spectrum of benign and malignant entities that take origin from the mesenchymal and epithelial structures of the organ (Table 1.1). Many of the diagnostic categories are strongly age related and, among the malignant tumours, prognosis is often strongly linked to tumour type. The most common benign liver tumours are haemangiomas and hamartomas, both of mesenchymal origin[1]. In Western countries, hepatoblastoma is one of the least common malignant neoplasms in the paediatric population, but, at the same time, it is the most common primary malignant tumour of the liver in childhood[2].

Table 1.1 Primary hepatic tumours

Malignant epithelial	Hepatoblastoma Hepatocellular carcinoma
Malignant mesenchymal	Undifferentiated (embryonal) sarcoma Rhabdomyosarcoma
Benign epithelial	Focal nodular hyperplasia Adenoma
Benign mesenchymal	Mesenchymal hamartoma Haemangioendothelioma

HEPATOBLASTOMA

The incidence of hepatoblastoma among children in the UK is about 1 in 100 000, amounting to some eight cases a year[3]. Children under 5 years old are usually affected and there are about twice as many males as females[4]. About half of Gonzalez-Crussi's series[5] was aged less than one year at diagnosis. The tumour is rarely present at birth[2]. An upper abdominal mass or an enlarging abdomen is the most common presenting symptom[2]. Anorexia, weight loss and pain are also frequent. Icterus is rarely seen.

The tumour is associated with a number of unusual clinical associations (Table 1.2). Familial adenomatous polyposis has been reported to occur with an unexpectedly high incidence on the maternal side of hepatoblastoma patients[9] and among long-term survivors of hepatoblastoma[10].

Table 1.2 Hepatoblastoma – clinical associations

Hemihypertrophy[4]
Beckwith–Wiedemann syndrome[6]
Isosexual precocity[4]
Thrombocytosis[4]
Osteopenia[4]
Familial hepatoblastoma[7,8]
Familial adenomatous polyposis[9,10]

Complete surgical resection remains the cornerstone of treatment. Serum alpha-fetoprotein is raised in the great majority of cases and is a valuable biochemical marker to aid diagnosis and monitor disease; however, less-differentiated histological subtypes are less likely to be associated with alpha-fetoprotein production[11]. (Yolk sac carcinoma, another alpha-fetoprotein producing tumour, rarely arises in the liver.) Hepatic angiography usually shows a hypervascular pattern (Figure 1.1) and the technique is useful for assessing the location and extent of the tumour. The right lobe of the liver is involved in 60–65% of cases. The neoplasm is usually a single well-circumscribed mass confined to one lobe of the liver. Rarely, multiple nodules are present. A pseudocapsule is common and the external surface is generally nodular. The cut surface is typically variegate with bulging lobules of variable size (Figure 1.2). Colour and consistency are also variable, often punctuated with areas of necrosis[4,11]. The tumour is not associated with cirrhosis.

Histological subtypes (Table 1.3)

Accurate identification of histological subtypes is dependent upon adequate sampling and the availability of sufficient and suitable material for histological assessment[12]. There seems little doubt that lack of uniformity of diagnostic criteria has led to difficulty in comparing data from different studies[12].

Table 1.3 Histological subtypes of hepatoblastoma

Epithelial
  Fetal
  Embryonal
  Macrotrabecular
  Small cell undifferentiated ('anaplastic')
Epithelial/mesenchymal (mixed)

Fetal subtype

In this subtype, the tumour cells are arranged in slender cords, usually two cell layers thick, separated by sinusoids[13,14] (Figure 1.3). Mitoses are infrequent. Vessels resembling central veins are present but portal triads and bile ducts are absent. Canaliculi with or without bile may be present. Foci of extramedullary haemopoiesis (immature myeloid, erythroid elements and megakaryocytes) are common (Figure 1.4). Tumour cell cytoplasm is often vacuolated due to the content of fat and glycogen (Figure 1.4). Some studies insist on a pure fetal pattern for inclusion in this subtype[12].

Embryonal subtype

Compared with the fetal pattern, tumour cells of this subtype lack cohesion and there is a higher nucleocytoplasmic ratio (Figure 1.5). Nuclei are larger with a coarser chromatin pattern. Nucleoli are prominent and mitoses are more frequent[14].

Acini with distinct luminal borders and pseudorosette-like tubular structures recapitulate some of the features of embryonic liver. This histological pattern is reminiscent of the liver of embryos before the sixth week of gestation[5].

Embryonal and fetal patterns often coexist (Figure 1.6) and transition between fetal and embryonal patterns is often seen. In an analysis of 105 hepatoblastomas, no pure embryonal pattern was encountered[12]. Lakes of red blood cells, so-called pelioid foci, are frequently found associated with embryonal histology (Figure 1.7)[4]. Foci of extramedullary haemopoiesis may also be seen in association with this subtype[12].

Macrotrabecular subtype

In this variant, tumour cells are arranged in broad trabeculae, 10, 20 or more cells thick (Figure 1.8)[5]. The cells

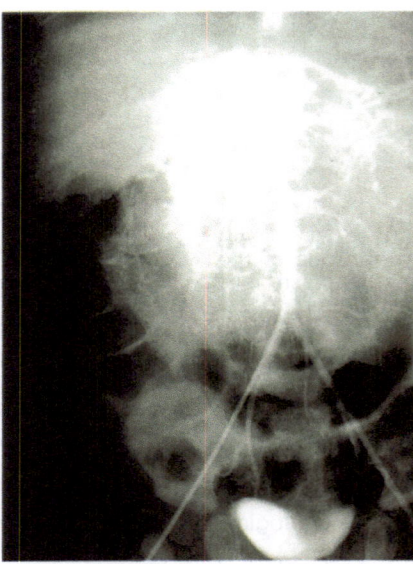

Fig. 1.1 Marked vascularity typical of hepatoblastoma is demonstrated on hepatic angiography. The patient was a 7-month-old girl who had a tumour involving the right lobe of liver

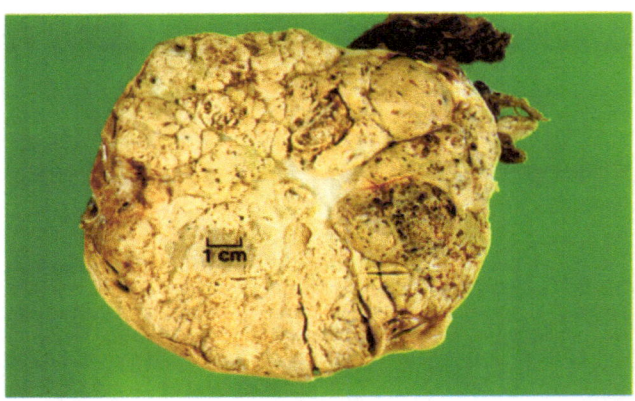

Fig. 1.2 Fetal hepatoblastoma shows a characteristic well-circumscribed lobulated appearance on the cut surface. The specimen measured 13 × 11 × 6 cm and weighed 477 g. Same case as in Figure 1.1

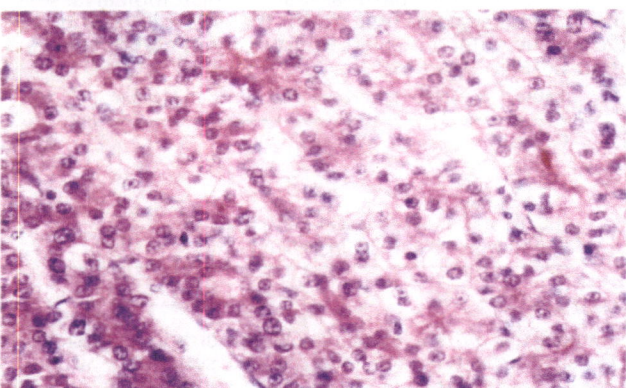

Fig. 1.3 Fetal hepatoblastoma shows tumour cells arranged in cords, generally two layers thick. The nucleocytoplasmic ratio of the tumour cells is low and mitoses are infrequent. H&E × 300

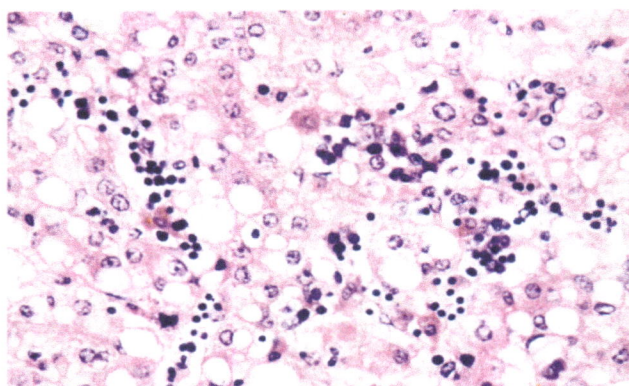

Fig. 1.4 Extramedullary haemopoiesis is striking in this microscopic field of fetal hepatoblastoma. H&E × 300

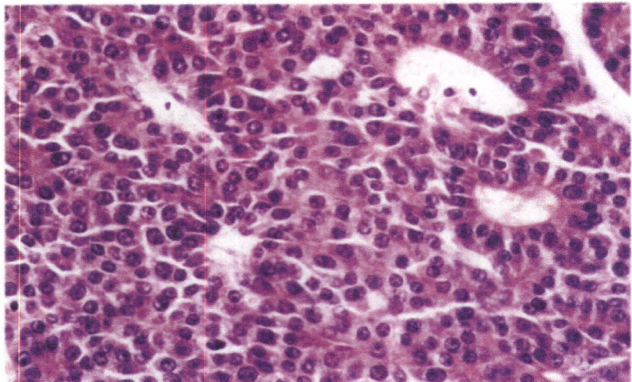

Fig. 1.5 Cords of tumour cells from embryonal hepatoblastoma display a high nucleocytoplasmic ratio. The nuclear chromatin is coarser and nucleoli more conspicuous, compared with the fetal pattern. A rosette/glandular arrangement is prominent. H&E × 300

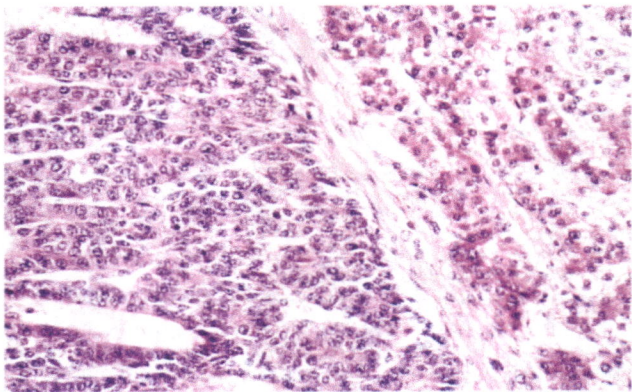

Fig. 1.6 A delicate fibrous septum divides this area of hepatoblastoma into embryonal pattern (left) and fetal pattern (right). H&E × 185

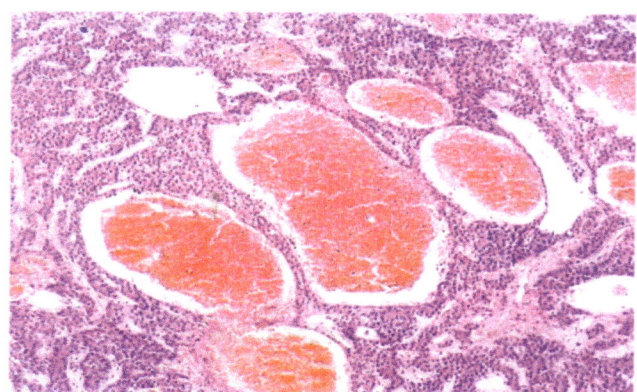

Fig. 1.7 A pelioid picture comprising lakes of red blood cells is often seen in association with an embryonal pattern of hepatoblastoma. H&E × 75

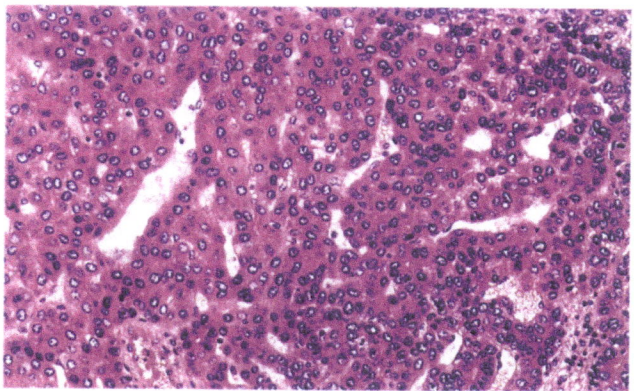

Fig. 1.8 A macrotrabecular pattern is demonstrated here; the tumour cells are arranged typically in broad trabeculae. This pattern may be difficult to separate from hepatocellular carcinoma. H&E × 300

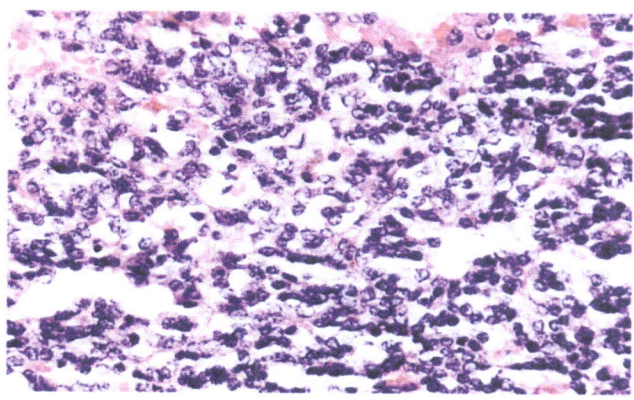

Fig. 1.9 Small-cell undifferentiated (anaplastic) hepatoblastoma is composed of cells that are small round-to-oval with scant cytoplasm. The differential diagnosis should include other undifferentiated small-cell tumours. H&E × 300

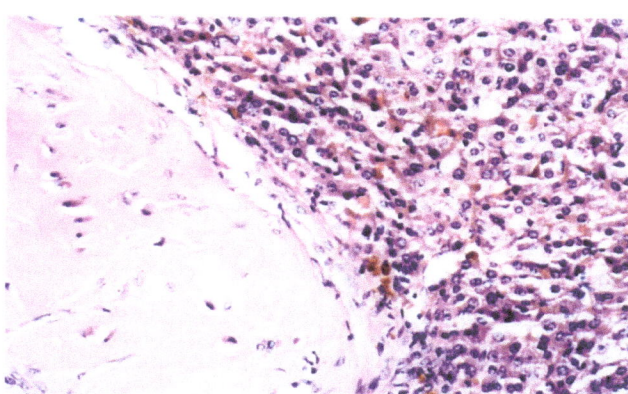

Fig. 1.10 Fetal hepatoblastoma of mixed pattern shows conspicuous osteoid formation. Definitive surgery was preceded by liver biopsy and chemotherapy. H&E × 75

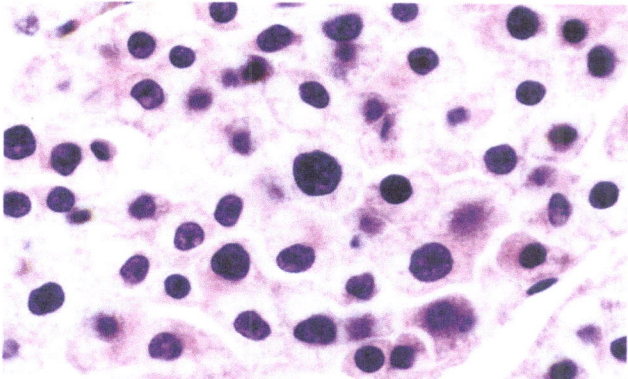

Fig. 1.11 High magnification view of hepatocellular carcinoma showing relatively large cells with high nucleocytoplasmic ratio and nuclear pleomorphism. H&E × 750

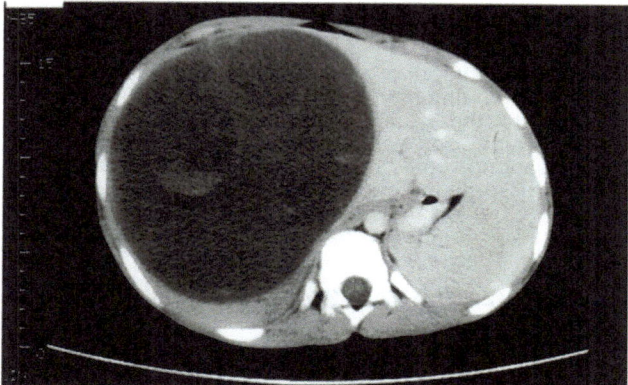

Fig. 1.12 A computerized tomogram of an undifferentiated (embryonal) sarcoma of the liver showing an echolucent mass in the right lobe

making up the trabeculae may have features of fetal or embryonal histology. Tumour cells are occasionally larger than the cells of the adjacent normal hepatocytes and distinction from hepatocellular carcinoma may be difficult. This pattern tends to occur in the very young patient. The distribution of this subtype has been variously reported as 3%[12] and 10%[13].

Small cell undifferentiated ('anaplastic')

This histological subtype of hepatoblastoma is the least differentiated[14–16]. The term 'anaplastic' is best avoided as this refers to a specific feature of Wilms' tumour. The pattern may occur in 'pure' form or as a component in one of the other subtypes. In order to qualify, the cellular pattern should occupy more than 50% of the cross-sectional area of representative sections. In its 'pure' form, this cellular pattern is very rare; the distribution of the subtype in various reports has been 8%[5], 6%[3], and 3%[12].

Cells are usually round or oval with scant cytoplasm and small vesicular nuclei (Figure 1.9), although a spindle pattern may be present. The differential diagnosis includes undifferentiated small-cell tumours: neuroblastoma, non-Hodgkin's lymphoma and embryonal rhabdomyosarcoma[15]. The diagnosis may be especially difficult when limited amounts of tissue are available for examination. The tumour has a propensity to infiltrate around and incorporate normal bile ducts.

Mixed epithelial–mesenchymal hepatoblastoma

Tumours comprising epithelial and mesenchymal components are traditionally referred to as mixed hepatoblastomas[14]. The mesenchymal component is represented by hyaline material resembling osteoid or an immature spindle stroma; it does not include mature supporting stroma, blood vessels and haemopoeitic tissue. Osteoid-like material is present in 20–30% of all hepatoblastomas (Figure 1.10). Rarely present are immature cartilage and skeletal muscle. The immature spindle stroma may merge with the mature supporting stroma and even with embryonal epithelium. The epithelial component may be any of the subtypes, but most mixed hepatoblastomas contain fetal and embryonal patterns[12]. Squamous epithelium is present in up to 20% of cases of mixed hepatoblastoma[17].

Several blocks may need to be examined before the mesenchymal element is apparent. Published data differ widely as to the incidence of mixed tumours, some claiming the presence of mesenchyme in all hepatoblastomas if diligently sought[11]. Osteoid is also encountered in the metastases from mixed hepatoblastomas[4,5].

TERATOID HEPATOBLASTOMA

This hepatic tumour is rare and, histologically, is characterized by multiple lines of tissue differention[12,18]. In addition to the usual components of hepatoblastoma (mesenchymal and epithelial), also revealed are melanocytes, ganglion cells, mature cartilage, skeletal muscle and an assortment of epithelia arranged as tubules or cysts[12,18]. The distinction between such cases and true teratomas of the liver may be subtle (see Chapter 9).

CYTOGENETIC ANALYSIS AND FLOW CYTOMETRY

Four consecutive mixed hepatoblastomas have been reported[19] to show trisomy for all or part of chromosome 2 and trisomy for chromosome 20. Flow cytometry for DNA analysis on nineteen tumours showed that 5 were DNA diploid, 11 were DNA aneuploid, and 3 had uninterpretable histograms[12]. In the latter study, DNA ploidy did not correlate with stage or histological subtype.

PROGNOSTIC FACTORS IN HEPATOBLASTOMA

Complete resection (Stage 1) seems to offer the best chance for survival[12]. The fetal pattern has been reported to confer a good prognosis[5,11,13], but others have challenged this view[12]. Mixed hepatoblastoma seems to be a good prognostic parameter[12], whereas the macrotrabecular[12,15] and the small cell undifferentiated pattern[12,13,15] are linked to aggressive tumour behaviour. On the other hand, the number of tumours with these histological subtypes may be too small to warrant a firm conclusion[12,15]. DNA ploidy does not seem to be a prognostic determinant in hepatoblastoma[12].

HEPATOCELLULAR CARCINOMA

Compared with hepatoblastoma, the potential for tumour resectability in hepatocellular carcinoma is low and, consequently, the prospects for survival are poor[20]. Hence, there is considerable importance in making the distinction between these two tumours.

In western countries it is the second most common hepatic malignancy in the first two decades of life[20], being superseded by hepatoblastoma. Hepatocellular carcinoma is uncommon under the age of 5 years and, in common with the adult type, there is predominance among males. Abdominal swelling in association with pain is the usual clinical presentation[20] and systemic manifestations are common. The serum alpha-fetoprotein is increased in about 80% of patients.

Pseudoencapsulation is less conspicuous when compared with hepatoblastoma. Both hepatic lobes are involved frequently, either diffusely or multifocally, reducing the prospects for complete surgical resection. The average weight of the surgical specimen was found[20] to be 949 g. Macroscopic features include haemorrhage and necrosis, and bile-staining of the tumour is often present. Complete surgical resection is achieved in less than 30% of cases.

Histologically, hepatocellular carcinoma is distinguished from hepatoblastoma in that the tumour cells are larger than normal hepatocytes (Figure 1.11)[14]; other features include nuclear pleomorphism, nucleolar prominence and the presence of tumour giant cells. Extramedullary haemopoiesis is almost never found, and the invasion of small blood vessels by tumour is common. The microscopic picture is indistinguishable from that of hepatocellular carcinoma arising in adults. In most childhood cases, however, there is no accompanying cirrhosis; in Lack et al.'s series[20] cirrhosis was present in 16% of cases. Hepatocellular carcinomas may include areas that are histologically indistinguishable from hepatoblastoma and, in such cases, precise categorization may be impossible. In this event the overall cellular features should be considered in evaluating prognosis.

The tumour is recognized to complicate a number of primary diseases such as Type I glycogenosis (glucose-6-phosphatase deficiency), tyrosinaemia, intrahepatic and extrahepatic biliary atresia, α_1-antitrypsin deficiency, 'giant cell hepatitis' and Wilson's disease[11].

Among patients with the chronic form of tyrosinaemia, Weinberg et al.[21] recorded a 37% incidence of hepatocellular carcinoma. The incidence is maximal between 4 and 5 years of disease, although long periods may supervene before the onset of the neoplasm. The histology of these tumours is no different from those unassociated with metabolic disease. Cirrhosis appears to be present in all cases. The incidence of hepatocellular carcinoma in chronic tyrosinaemia exceeds the incidence of hepatocellular carcinoma associated with cirrhosis without tyrosinaemia. This suggests that factors other than cirrhosis may be operative in the induction of the tumour[21]. The incidence of tumour seems to be unaffected by dietary manipulation, but prospects for survival have been considerably improved since the introduction of liver transplantation for such patients[22].

Hepatocellular carcinoma developing in association with Fanconi's anaemia may be related to the underlying condition or to the administration of androgens[23]. Fanconi's anaemia is also associated with the development of hepatic adenomas and their histological distinction from hepatocellular carcinoma may be difficult[23].

There is a well-recognized association between hepatocellular carcinoma and hepatitis B virus. This is especially so in developing countries[24] where there is a high carrier rate for the virus. The association extends both to adults and children. The lower incubation period between the onset of infection and tumour development in children may be related to congenital infection from vertical transmission of the virus by the mother. In hepatitis B endemic areas, hepatocellular carcinoma may be more common in children than hepatoblastoma[25].

The fibrolamellar carcinoma is a distinct but rare variant of hepatocellular carcinoma[26]. Microscopically, it is characterized by plump cells with abundant granular deeply eosinophilic cytoplasm separated by bands of collagen. Of the 19 cases reviewed by Berman *et al.*[26] three patients were less than 20 years of age. Compared with conventional hepatocellular carcinoma the prognosis is generally more favourable. The serum alpha-fetoprotein is normal in the majority of patients. This variant seems to be unassociated with cirrhosis, hepatitis B virus, glycogen storage disease or tyrosinaemia[26]. With the naked eye, there is often a close resemblance to focal nodular hyperplasia[11].

UNDIFFERENTIATED (EMBRYONAL) SARCOMA OF THE LIVER (UNDIFFERENTIATED SARCOMA OF THE LIVER; MALIGNANT MESENCHYMOMA; EMBRYONAL SARCOMA)

This is a rare but highly aggressive hepatic tumour that usually affects children between the ages of 6 and 10 years[27]. Adults are rarely involved. The lesion comprises 13% of all hepatic tumours encountered in the paediatric age[11]; it is the fourth most common primary tumour of the liver in childhood, preceded by hepatoblastoma, haemangioendothelioma and hepatocellular carcinoma[28]. The neoplasm arises with equal frequency in boys and girls[27] and the right lobe of the liver is more commonly affected (75–80%). An abdominal mass with pain and fever is the usual presentation. The serum level of alpha-fetoprotein is reported to be normal[29].

Computerized tomography shows a multiloculated hypertranslucent mass (Figure 1.12). Hypovascularity is indicated angiographically (Figure 1.13), contrasting with the marked hypervascular picture seen in hepatoblastoma.

With the naked eye, a large bulky mass, 10–20 cm in diameter, is clearly demarcated from the surrounding liver. The cut surface is fleshy with a mucinous tan–white or yellow appearance, and there is usually extensive haemorrhage and necrosis (Figure 1.14)[27]. The hilum of the liver is usually spared.

Microscopically, the tumour is relatively distinctive. The growth is separated from the adjacent liver by a pseudocapsule[17,27]. There is a proliferation of spindle cells loosely or densely arranged in a myxomatous matrix (Figure 1.15). Tumour cell cytoplasm is scant with ill-defined borders. Large anaplastic cells with single or multiple nuclei are found in many areas (Figure 1.16). Mitoses are frequent and are commonly atypical. Variable-sized hyaline globules occupy intracellular and extracellular locations (Figure 1.17); they are PAS positive and diastase resistant (Figure 1.18). Bile ducts, frequently cystic, together with non-neoplastic hepatocytes are commonly entrapped at the periphery of the tumour. The density of the anaplastic cells is especially marked around ducts; this relationship between tumour and epithelium is reminiscent of embryonal rhabdomyosarcoma[17]. Cytoplasmic cross-striations are absent. The absence of bile ducts in metastases suggests that they are not an integral component of the tumour[17,30].

Immunohistochemistry shows a complex antigenic profile: vimentin, desmin, muscle-specific actin, cytokeratin, α_1-antitrypsin, α_1-antichymotrypsin, lysozyme and S-100 protein[29]. Leuschner *et al.*[28] also found variable positivity for desmin and cytokeratin. Immunohistochemistry for alpha-fetoprotein has so far been negative. Electron microscopy has demonstrated fibroblastic, histiocytoid, myofibroblastic and myoblastic differentiation[29].

The microscopic differential diagnosis includes embryonal rhabdomyosarcoma, malignant fibrous histiocytoma and fibrosarcoma of the liver. Indeed, the relationship between malignant fibrous histiocytoma of the liver and undifferentiated embryonal sarcoma is still debated[29]. There are also superficial similarities to mesenchymal hamartoma of the liver[31] (compare Figures 1.15 and 1.19). The small-cell undifferentiated type of hepatoblastoma and sarcomatous areas of hepatocellular carcinoma also cause diagnostic confusion[29].

The histogenesis is uncertain but the phenotypic diversity on immunohistochemistry and electron microscopy suggests an origin from a primitive mesenchymal cell. The tumour appears to be organ-specific as primary tumours of similar appearance are not reported elsewhere. Surgical resection, together with chemotherapy, is the treatment of choice. The tumour metastasizes to the lung and bone, and may extend directly into contiguous structures. Currently, about one third of the patients survive beyond 3 years[28].

EMBRYONAL RHABDOMYOSARCOMA

This is dealt with in Chapter 12.

MESENCHYMAL HAMARTOMA

The majority of lesions occur in patients under 12 months of age and there is a predominance of boys. Patients usually present clinically with an abdominal enlargement or an abdominal mass. The tumour may attain enormous dimensions and, in Stocker's series[31], tumour weights ranged from 238–6810 g. The right lobe of the liver is more commonly affected.

The growth is readily discernible with the naked eye because of its gelatinous consistency, sharp margins and cysts containing serous or viscid fluid. Encapsulation is rare and necrosis and haemorrhage are notable for their absence. Pedunculation is not uncommon.

Four basic microscopic elements are identified[31]: a bland myxomatous stroma, irregular tortuous bile ducts, cords of normal-appearing hepatocytes and variable numbers of delicate blood vessels (Figure 1.19). The myxomatous stroma comprises scattered stellate cells in a matrix rich in mucopolysaccharide (Figure 1.20). Foci of extramedullary haemopoiesis are seen in more than 80% of tumours[31]. Bile ducts are more prominent at the periphery and frequently disclose complex branching patterns or undergo cyst formation. More commonly, however, the cysts arise in areas of stromal degeneration secondary to fluid accumulation. The lesion merges with the surrounding hepatic parenchyma, often forming satellite nodules caused by proliferation of myxoid stroma at the margin.

Undifferentiated (embryonal) sarcoma of the liver and hepatic haemangioendothelioma are considerations in the differential diagnosis. Mesenchymal hamartoma is entirely benign and surgical extirpation is curative; however,

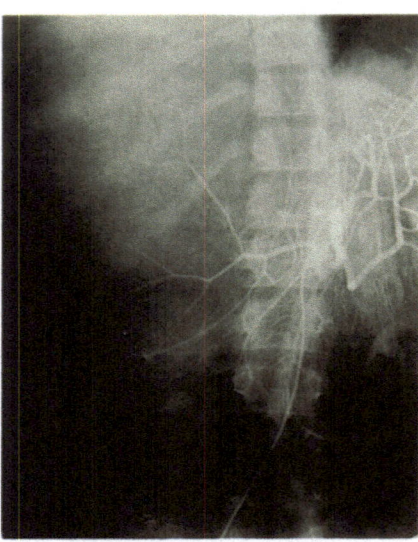

Fig. 1.13 Lack of vascularity, characteristic of undifferentiated (embryonal) sarcoma of the liver, is demonstrated angiographically in the same tumour

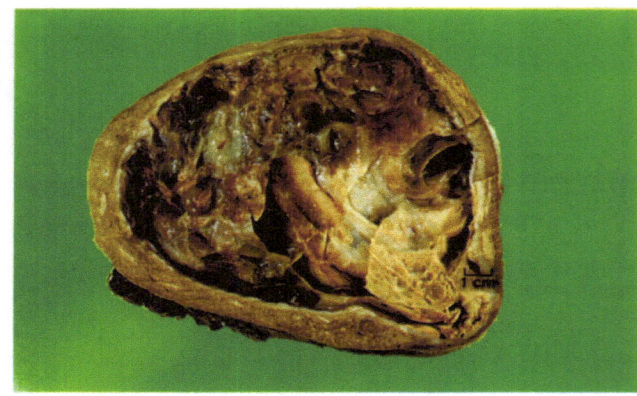

Fig. 1.14 Gross specimen of undifferentiated (embryonal) sarcoma of the right lobe of liver. The tumour is largely necrotic and haemorrhagic. It is bordered by a shell of compressed hepatic parenchyma

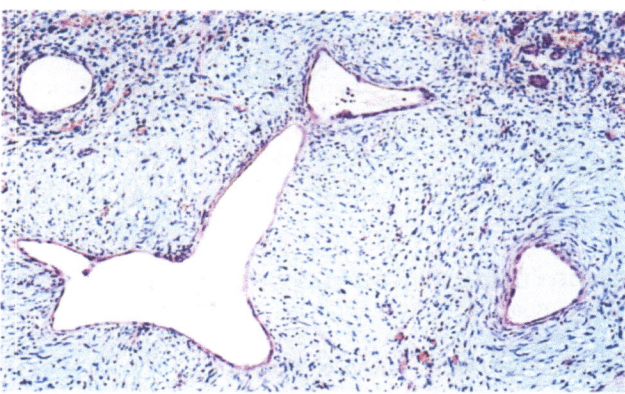

Fig. 1.15 Microscopic view of undifferentiated (embryonal) sarcoma of the liver reveals irregular bile ducts and a myxoid stroma. The picture bears a striking resemblance to mesenchymal hamartoma (compare with Figures 1.19 and 1.20). H&E × 75

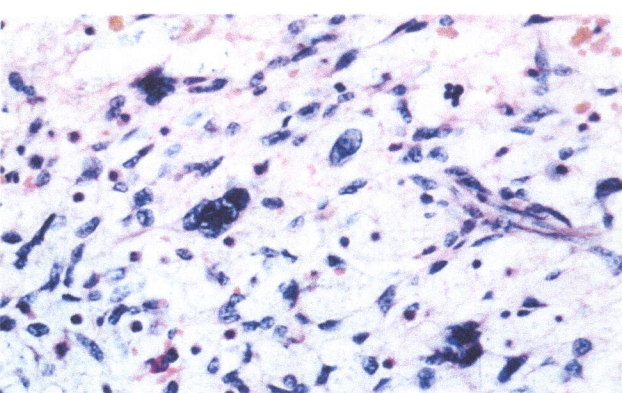

Fig. 1.16 Microscopic view of undifferentiated (embryonal) sarcoma of the liver demonstrates several large anaplastic tumour cells set in a myxoid stroma. H&E × 300

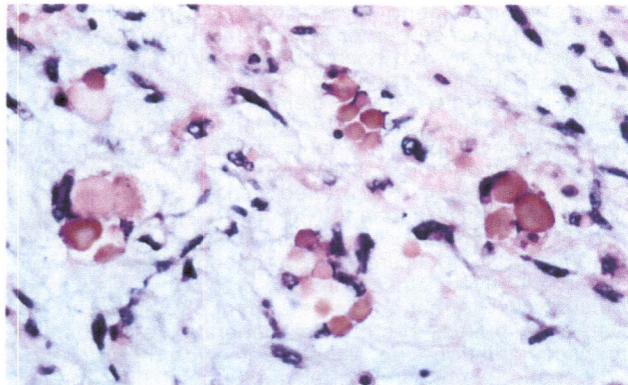

Fig. 1.17 Microscopic view of undifferentiated (embryonal) sarcoma of the liver shows eosinophilic hyaline globules which seem to occupy an intracytoplasmic and extracytoplasmic location. This is an important diagnostic feature of the tumour. H&E × 300

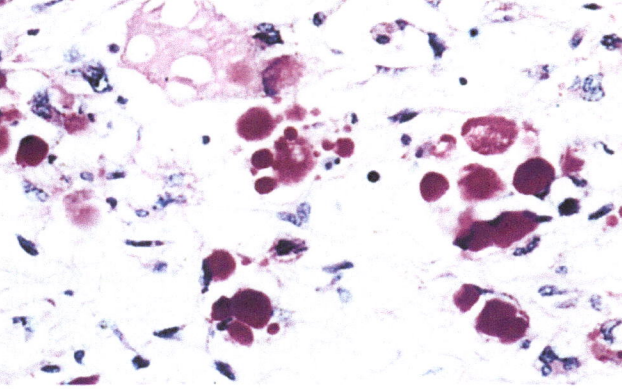

Fig. 1.18 The hyaline globules demonstrated in Figure 1.17 are associated with strong PAS positivity. PAS × 300

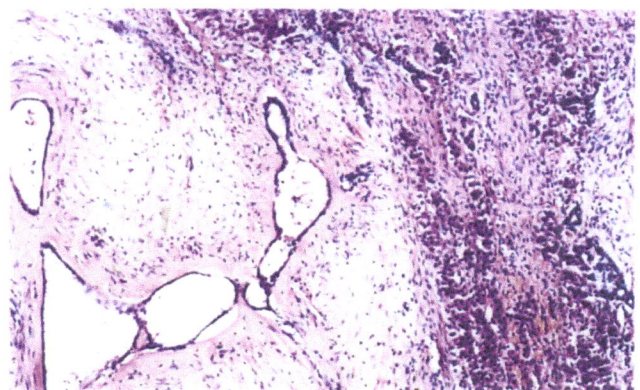

Fig. 1.19 Mesenchymal hamartoma, removed from an 18-month-old girl, shows mildly cystic gyrate ducts irregularly dispersed in mucoid stroma; the stroma contains a number of small delicate vessels. The resected specimen weighed 1680 g and measured 24 × 19 × 8 cm. H&E × 75

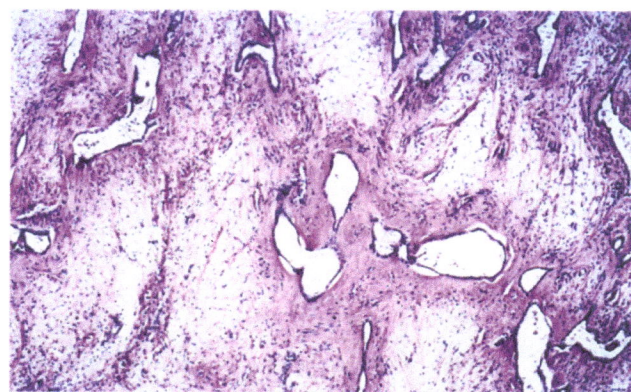

Fig. 1.20 Same specimen as in Figure 1.19. Mesenchymal hamartoma shows bile ducts surrounded by abundant mucoid stroma, reminiscent of undifferentiated (embryonal) sarcoma of the liver. H&E × 48

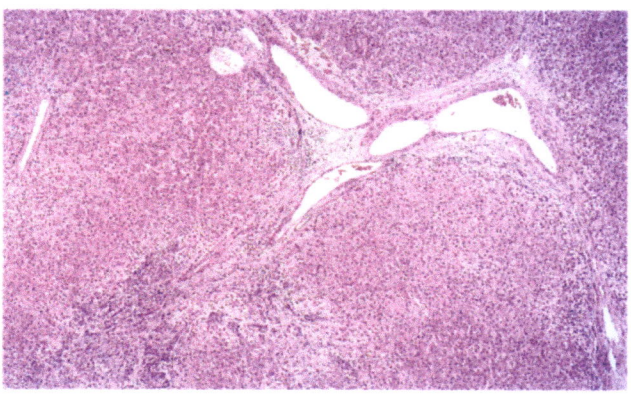

Fig. 1.21 Focal nodular hyperplasia from a 16-year-old girl is characterized microscopically by the presence of broad connective tissue septa that contain bile ducts, arteries and veins. The patient presented with a large hepatic mass that was completely resected. H&E × 48

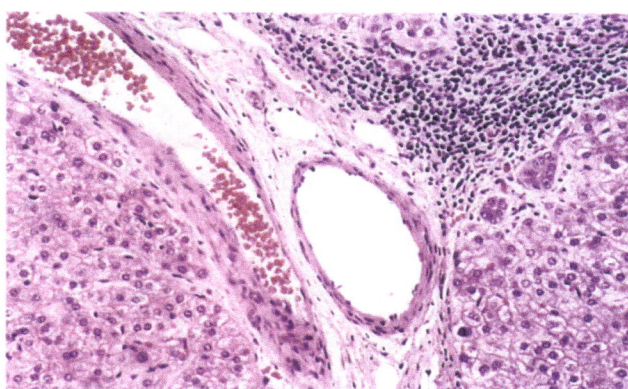

Fig. 1.22 Same tumour as seen in preceding figure. The vessels in the fibrous septum display eccentric wall thickening; a focal lymphocytic infiltrate is present. H&E × 185

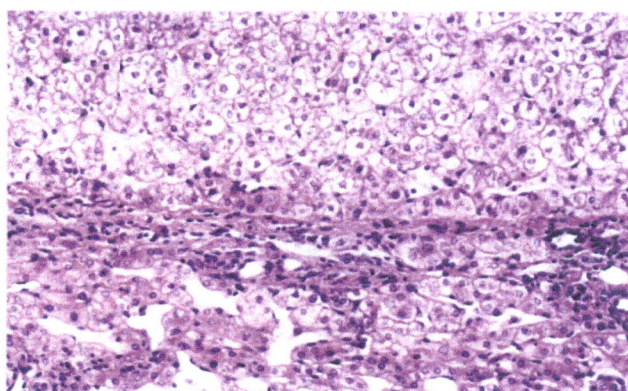

Fig. 1.23 Hepatic adenoma (upper half) from a 12-year-old girl shows benign-appearing hepatocytes that are slightly larger than normal hepatocytes (lower half). Ultrasound examination had earlier demonstrated multiple hepatic nodules, one of which was very large. The main nodule was excised. She is well and off treatment 3 years later. H&E × 185

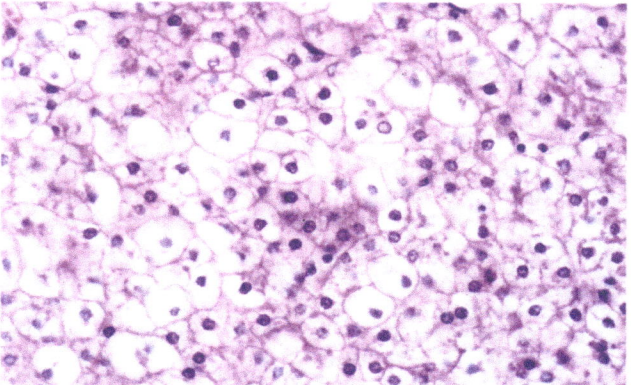

Fig. 1.24 At higher magnification, the adenoma shows large cells with unusually clear vacuolated cytoplasm. There is no significant nuclear atypia in this field. H&E × 300

fatality has been reported to follow intraoperative and postoperative complications[31].

FOCAL NODULAR HYPERPLASIA

Focal nodular hyperplasia (FNH) is a distinct histopathological entity distinguishable from liver cell adenoma[17,32]. The tumour arises rarely in children and, together with hepatic adenoma, accounts for some 2% of all childhood hepatic tumours[17]. The children reported by Stocker and Ishak[33] ranged in age from birth to 14 years. As in adults, the patients are mostly female. Liver function tests are normal. Most patients present with a non-tender mass found by parents or during routine medical examination, or they are discovered incidentally at autopsy. Angiography discloses a highly vascular lesion and the technique is useful for localizing the tumour within the liver[17].

The left lobe of the liver is more commonly involved; less often both hepatic lobes are affected[33]. The lesions are sharply demarcated, although unencapsulated, irregular in outline and of uniformly firm consistency. Their size varies from 1–15 cm in diameter and the cut surface discloses a yellow–tan to brown colour. Bile discoloration is uncommon. Larger lesions tend to bulge from the surface and may be pedunculated. The tumours are subdivided into lobules by fibrous septa which frequently converge to form a central stellate scar. Prominent vessels frequently course through the adjacent parenchyma and within larger fibrous septa. The remainder of the liver appears unremarkable apart from the effect of compression.

Microscopically[17,33], interconnecting fibrous septa divide the lesion into lobules of varying size (Figure 1.21). The lobules are composed of cords of hepatocytes slightly larger than those of adjacent normal liver. The cells frequently contain variable amounts of fat and glycogen. Mitoses are absent. The narrower fibrous septa contain small arteries, veins and bile ducts. The vessels show mild to moderate intimal thickening which is often eccentric (Figure 1.22). A relatively consistent feature is an infiltrate of neutrophils and/or lymphocytes within the septa. A biopsy diagnosis is possible but the lesion may be mistaken for cirrhosis or congenital hepatic fibrosis; in this regard a biopsy from the adjacent normal parenchyma taken at the same time should be helpful[34].

FNH must be distinguished from more common benign and malignant tumours. Resection should be attempted only if it can be carried out without risk to the patient. Long-term follow-up has shown few adverse effects. After surgical resection, recurrences are unusual. This is a non-neoplastic lesion, and instances of transition to hepatocellular carcinoma are not recorded[33].

HEPATIC ADENOMA

This is one of the least common tumours of the liver in children and may occur at any age[11]. The usual clinical presentation is an asymptomatic abdominal mass. A solitary mass in the right of the liver measuring 10 cm or less is the usual gross description[17]. The cut surface has a homogeneous pale yellow to tan colour, and encapsulation is partial or complete.

Microscopically, the tumour is composed of uniform-appearing well-differentiated hepatocytes, usually larger than normal hepatocytes (Figure 1.23), arranged in cords of two or three cells thick. The cytoplasm is usually vacuolated due to the presence of abundant glycogen or lipid, or both (Figure 1.24). Cytological atypia may be present and does not, of itself, infer malignancy. Portal structures, bile ducts and Kupffer cells are absent[34].

Most adenomas in children appear to arise sporadically[34]; less often they are associated with underlying disease. Adenomas, often multiple, may develop in pati-

ents with Type I glycogen storage disease[35], the hereditary chronic form of tyrosinaemia[21], Fanconi's anaemia[23] and galactosaemia[11]. In glycogen storage disease the number and size of adenomas tend to increase with age, but they have been known to regress with dietary therapy; rarely do they progress to hepatocellular carcinoma[11]. Anabolic steroids and maternal hormones have also been implicated in their induction[11].

Distinction from well-differentiated hepatocellular carcinoma may be impossible[11], especially when small samples of tissue are examined for histological diagnosis. In contrast with focal nodular hyperplasia, the reasons for resecting an adenoma are more compelling because of the possibility of malignant change[34].

HAEMANGIOENDOTHELIOMA

This is the second most common primary tumour of the liver in infancy. Presentation is usually within the first 6 months after birth. While the majority of cases present with asymptomatic hepatomegaly, other forms of presentation include high-output congestive cardiac failure (secondary to arteriovenous shunting within the tumour), a bleeding diathesis due to platelet consumption and rupture leading to exsanguinating haemoperitoneum[17]. In 45% of reported cases there are associated multiple cutaneous vascular tumours[36]. The hepatic lesion may be single or multiple. With the advent of modern radiological techniques the diagnosis in most cases can be made without recourse to open surgery[17].

Haemangioendothelioma (Figure 1.25) differs microscopically from cavernous haemangioma (Figure 1.26) in having smaller vascular spaces, often devoid of erythrocytes, and lined by plump endothelial cells. The vessels are separated by fibromyxomatous stroma. Extramedullary haemopoeisis may be prominent and calcification, probably a regressive feature, is often seen.

Dehner and Ishak[36] recognized two histological patterns of hepatic haemangioendothelioma. The features described above conform to their Type I lesion, which is far more common. The Type II lesion is considered to be distinct by virtue of larger vascular spaces with more irregular and complex budding and branching of its walls (Figure 1.27). Endothelium is hyperchromatic and pleomorphic. Bile ducts and small nests of hepatocytes are often interposed in the supporting stroma (Figure 1.28). Cavernous haemangiomatous foci, which seem to be a sign of maturation, occur in association with both patterns.

The importance in the recognition of the type II lesion lies in the possible confusion with angiosarcoma. Angiosarcoma is exceptionally rare in children. However, angiosarcoma arising in young children following biopsy diagnoses of haemangioendothelioma is recorded[11]. The Type II lesion is distinguished from angiosarcoma, among other features, by a paucity of mitoses, lack of a solid 'sarcomatous' component, and absence of sinusoidal or vascular invasion[17].

Type II haemangioendotheliomas, on the other hand, are reported rarely to undergo metastases[36]; but identical lesions may arise in extrahepatic sites (45% of cases) and whether these are separate lesions or represent metastases may be difficult to resolve.

OTHER PRIMARY HEPATIC NEOPLASMS

Endocrine tumours, biliary epithelial tumours, leiomyosarcomas, germ cell tumours (see Chapter 9) and lymphomas have been reported to arise rarely in the livers of children[11]. Nodular regenerative hyperplasia, a condition usually reported in adults, is rarely encountered in children[37]. Primary malignant rhabdoid tumours involving the liver have also been recorded[38].

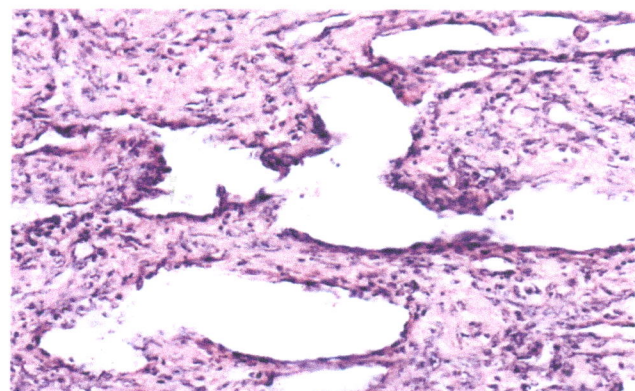

Fig. 1.25　The lesion was totally excised from a 1-month-old boy who presented with a hepatic mass. Variable-sized channels generally devoid of red blood cells, lined by plump endothelial cells, characterize Type I haemangioendothelioma. H&E × 300

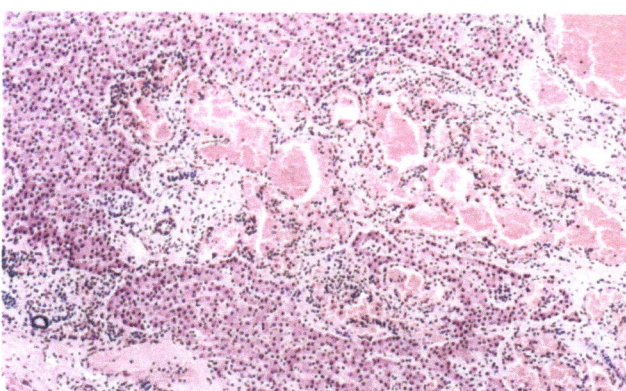

Fig. 1.26　For comparison, this shows a cavernous haemangioma which was an incidental finding at autopsy in a 21-month-old male child. The lesion is composed of variable-sized vascular spaces filled with blood and separated by fibrous stroma. H&E × 48

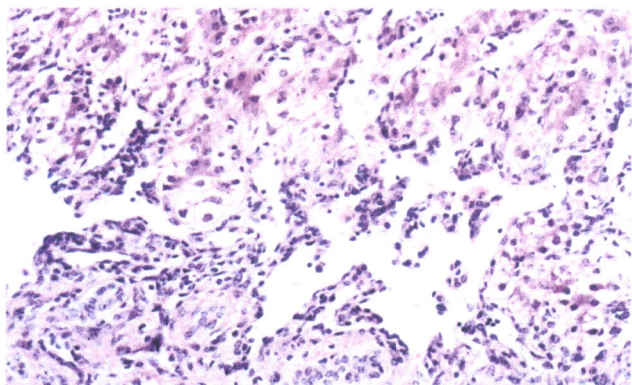

Fig. 1.27　Type II haemangioendothelioma from a 6-day-old girl who presented with a mass in the right upper quadrant of the abdomen. There are irregular vascular spaces with complex papillary infoldings and intervening hepatocytes. H&E × 185

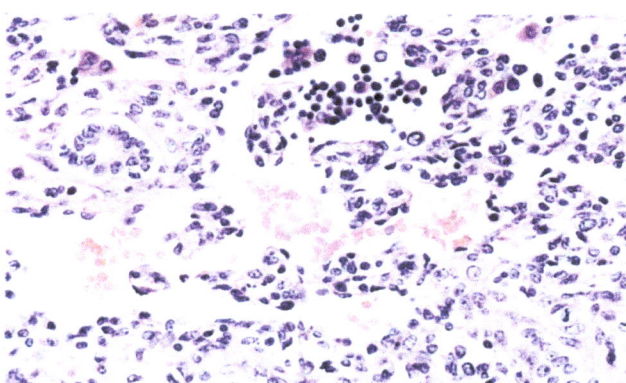

Fig. 1.28　Type II haemangioendothelioma. Same lesion as in Figure 1.27. The vascular spaces reveal a papillary configuration. A bile duct is included and haemopoietic tissue is present. H&E × 300

REFERENCES

1. Luks FI, Yazbeck S, Brandt ML, Bensoussan AL, Brochu P,- Blanchard H. Benign liver tumors in children: a 25-year experience. J Pediatr Surg. 1991;26:1326–30.
2. Exelby PR, Filler RM, Grosfeld JL. Liver tumors in children with particular reference to hepatoblastoma and hepatocellular carcinoma: American Academy of Pediatrics Surgical Section Survey – 1974. J Pediatr Surg. 1975; 3:329–37.
3. Draper GJ, Birch JM, Bithell JF, et al. Childhood cancer in Britain: incidence, survival and mortality. (Studies on medical and population subjects no. 37). London: HMSO;1982.
4. Lack EE, Neave C, Vawter GF. Hepatoblastoma. A clinical and pathological study of 54 cases. Am J Surg Pathol. 1982;6:693–705.
5. Gonzalez-Crussi F, Upton MP, Maurer HS. Hepatoblastoma. Attempt at characterization of histological subtypes. Am J Surg Pathol. 1982;6:599–612.
6. Orozco-Florian R, McBride JA, Favara BE, Steele A, Brown SJ, Steele P. Congenital hepatoblastoma and Beckwith–Wiedemann syndrome: A case study including DNA ploidy profiles of tumor and adrenal cytomegaly. Pediatr Pathol. 1991;11:131–42.
7. Fraumeni JF, Rosen PJ, Hull EW, Barth RF, Shapiro SR, O'Connor JF. Hepatoblastoma in infant sisters. Cancer. 1969;24:1086–90.
8. Napoli VM, Campbell WG. Hepatoblastoma in infant sister and brother. Cancer. 1977;39:2647–50.
9. Phillips M, Dicks-Mireaux C, Kingston J. et al. Hepatoblastoma and polyposis coli (familial adenomatous polyposis). Med Ped Oncol. 1989;17:441–7.
10. Garber JE, Li FP, Kingston JE. et al. Hepatoblastoma and familial adenomatous polyposis. J Natl Cancer Inst. 1988;80:1626–8.
11. Weinberg AG, Finegold MJ. Primary hepatic tumours of childhood. Hum Pathol. 1983;14:512–37.
12. Couran RM, Hitchcock CL, Waclawiw MA, Stocker JT, Ishak KG. Hepatoblastoma; the prognostic significance of histological type. Pediatr Pathol. 1992;12:167–83.
13. Haas J, Muczynski KA, Krailo M et al. Histopathology and prognosis in childhood hepatoblastoma and hepatocarcinoma. Cancer. 1989;64:1082–95.
14. Ishak KG, Glunz PR. Hepatoblastoma and hepatocarcinoma in infancy and childhood. Report of 47 cases. Cancer. 1967;20:396–422.
15. Dehner LP, Manivel JC. Hepatoblastoma: an analysis of the relationship between morphologic subtypes and prognosis. Am J Ped Hem Oncol. 1988;10:301–7.
16. Kasai M, Watanabe I. Histological classification of liver-cell carcinoma in infancy and childhood and its clinical evaluation. A study of 70 cases collected in Japan. Cancer. 1970;25:551–63.
17. Dehner LP. Hepatic tumors in the pediatric age group: a distinctive clinicopathologic spectrum. Perspect Pediatr Pathol. 1978;4:217–68.
18. Manivel C, Wick MR, Abenoza P, Dehner LP. Teratoid hepatoblastoma. The nosologic dilemma of solid embryonic neoplasms of childhood. Cancer. 1986;57:2168–74.
19. Fletcher JA, Kozakewich HP, Pavelka K, et al. Consistent cytogenetic aberrations in hepatoblastoma: a common pathway of genetic alterations in embryonal liver and skeletal muscle malignancies? Genes Chromosomes Cancer. 1991;3:37–43.
20. Lack EE, Neave C, Vawter GF. Hepatocellular carcinoma. Review of 32 cases in childhood and adolescence. Cancer. 1983;52:1510–15.
21. Weinberg AG, Mize CE, Worthen HG. The occurrence of hepatoma in the chronic form of hereditary tyrosinemia. J Pediatr. 1976;88:434–8.
22. Dehner LP, Snover DC, Sharp HL, Ascher N, Nakhleh R, Day DL. Hereditary tyrosinaemia type 1 (chronic form): pathologic findings in the liver. Hum Pathol. 1989;20:149–58.
23. LeBrun DP, Silver MM, Freedman MH, Phillips MJ. Fibrolamellar carcinoma of the liver in a patient with Fanconi anaemia. Hum Pathol. 1991;22:396–8.
24. Ni YH, Chang MH, Hsu HY. Hepatocellular carcinoma in childhood. Clinical manifestations and prognosis. Cancer. 1991;68:1737–41.
25. Chen WJ, Lee JC, Hung WT. Primary malignant tumor of liver in infants and children in Taiwan. J Pediatr Surg. 1988;23:457–61.
26. Berman MA, Burnham JA, Sheahan DG. Fibromellar carcinoma of the liver: an immunohistochemical study of nineteen cases and a review of the literature. Hum Pathol. 1988;19:784–94.
27. Stocker JT, Ishak KG. Undifferentiated (embryonal) sarcoma of the liver. Report of 31 cases. Cancer. 1978;42:336–48.
28. Leuschner I, Schmidt D, Harms D. Undifferentiated sarcoma of the liver in childhood. Morphology, flow cytometry, and literature review. Hum Pathol. 1990;21:68–76.
29. Aoyama C, Hachitanda Y, Sato JK, Said JW, Shimada H. Undifferentiated (embryonal) sarcoma of the liver. A tumor of uncertain histogenesis showing divergent differentiation. Am J Surg Pathol. 1991;15:615–24.
30. Keating S, Taylor GP. Undifferentiated (embryonal) sarcoma of the liver. Ultrastructural and immunohistochemical similarities with malignant fibrous histiocytoma. Hum Pathol. 1985;16:693–9.
31. Stocker JT, Ishak KG. Mesenchymal hamartoma of the liver: report of 30 cases and review of the literature. Pediatr Pathol. 1983;1:245–67.
32. Knowles DM, Wolff M. Focal nodular hyperplasia of the liver. A clinicopathologic study and review of the literature. Hum Pathol. 1976;7:533–45.
33. Stocker JT, Ishak KG. Focal nodular hyperplasia of the liver: a study of 21 pediatric cases. Cancer. 1981;48:336–45.
34. Dehner LP, Parker ME, Franciosi RA, Drake RM. Focal nodular hyperplasia and adenoma of the liver. A pediatric experience. Am J Ped Hematol/Oncol. 1979;1:85–94.
35. Poe R, Snover DC. Adenomas in glycogen storage disease type I. Two cases with unusual histologic features. Am J Surg Pathol. 1988;12:477–83.
36. Dehner LP, Ishak KG. Vascular tumours of the liver in infants and children. A study of 30 cases and review of the literature. Arch Pathol. 1971;92:101–11.
37. Mones JM, Saldana MJ. Nodular regenerative hyperplasia of the liver in a 4-month-old infant. Am J Dis Chld. 1984;138:79–81.
38. Parham DM, Peiper SC, Robicheaux G, Ribeiro RC, Douglass EC. Malignant rhabdoid tumor of the liver. Arch Pathol Lab Med. 1988;112:61–4.

Wilms' tumour and the nephroblastoma complex

2

Nephroblastoma is the most common renal neoplasm of childhood[1]. Of all childhood malignancies it has the highest probability of long-term survival with an overall cure rate of approximately 90%[2]. It is universally accepted as a malignant embryonal neoplasm arising from the primitive blastema of the kidney. In the National Wilms' Tumor Study (NWTS) in the USA, the mean age at diagnosis for sporadic unilateral cases was 45 months, with 80% of cases diagnosed in the first 5 years of life. The random risk for developing Wilms' tumour has been estimated to be 1 in 10 000 births. At diagnosis, 6% of tumours are bilateral[2]; patients with bilateral tumours tend to present at a younger age[3]. Congenital Wilms' tumours have been reported on rare occasions[4].

An abdominal mass discovered by a family member or medical practitioner is the usual mode of presentation; pain and haematuria are other symptoms. Hypertension may occur. The gross nephrectomy specimen usually includes the ipsilateral adrenal and hilar lymph nodes, together with a segment of ureter. The left kidney is affected slightly more than the right. Most tumours weigh 200–1000 g[1]. The pathologist should routinely attempt to identify the renal vein and examine its lumen for tumour. The cut surface of the tumour typically shows lobulated grey–white tissue replacing a large portion of the kidney (Figure 2.1)[1]. A clear demarcation is typically present between tumour and renal parenchyma. Focal haemorrhage and necrosis are commonly seen. The tumour may be multifocal. Structural changes of the short arm of chromosome 11 are the most common chromosome abnormality found in Wilms' tumour[50].

To ensure adequate tissue sampling, at least one tumour section should be taken for each centimetre diameter of tumour[1]. Metastatic sites usually involve regional lymph nodes (hilar and periaortic), lung and liver; bone is rarely affected[5,6]. The tumour may penetrate the renal capsule and infiltrate pericapsular tissue. Intrarenal vasculature may be invaded. The basic microscopic pattern of Wilms' tumour is a biphasic growth composed of islands of metanephric blastema separated by mesenchyme (Figure 2.2)[1]. The metanephric blastema is a compact arrangement of small oval to polygonal cells with hyperchromatic nuclei and scant cytoplasm (Figure 2.3). There may be variable epithelial differentiation, usually in the form of tubules showing degrees of lumen formation (Figure 2.4). Some of the tubules have ill-defined lumens and may resemble neural rosettes. Glomeruloid structures are infrequently encountered. When one component occupies more than 65% of the sectioned tumour, the pattern is subtyped as predominant, e.g. blastema-, epithelial-, or stromal-predominant[7]. When no single component predominates, the tumour is referred to as one of mixed pattern. The mixed pattern constitutes the largest single group (59%) according to data from the NWTS.

The stromal component covers a spectrum from immature mesenchymal to mature fibrous tissue. Other mesenchymal elements, such as fetal muscle, cartilage, adipose tissue, and occasionally bone, may occur in the stroma. Ganglion cells[8] and keratin cysts[9,10] are other histological findings.

DIFFERENTIAL DIAGNOSIS

This presents a problem only in blastema-predominant Wilms' tumour or when blastema represents the sole component. Entities to be considered in the differential diagnosis include neuroepithelial tumours (PNETs), non-Hodgkin's lymphoma (especially Burkitt's lymphoma), congenital mesoblastic nephroma, renal adenocarcinoma and teratoma[11].

A serpentine or nodular cellular arrangement can usually be found in some areas in most Wilms' tumours, and provides an important diagnostic clue. Wilms' tumour may show intracytoplasmic inclusions similar to malignant rhabdoid tumour of the kidney (MRTK)[12] (see Chapter 3). Treatment for MRTK is considerably more drastic; thus a correct diagnosis is critical.

MONOMORPHOUS EPITHELIAL WILMS' TUMOUR

This is a rare form of Wilms' tumour usually affecting patients in their first year. Grossly, the tumour is well-demarcated, lacks haemorrhage and necrosis and is generally Stage 1[13]. The neoplasm is composed of epithelium arranged in tubules that are indistinguishable from those usually seen in the triphasic tumour (Figure 2.5). The tubules are aligned back-to-back without intervening blastema or stroma[14]; flattened or columnar epithelium lines the tubules that may be microcystically dilated. This pattern of Wilms' tumour is especially associated with a favourable clinical outcome.

ANAPLASTIC WILMS' TUMOUR

Children with anaplastic Wilms' tumours have a significantly shorter survival than those with favourable histology Wilms' tumours[15]. While only about 7–8% of the NWTS-1 and -2 populations showed cellular anaplasia, they accounted for 24% of all relapses and 39% of all tumour deaths[15]. A notable exception to this poor outcome appears to be patients with cellular anaplasia in Stage 1 disease[16]. Intensified drug schedules have not significantly improved clinical outcome[2]; others have expressed an opposing view[17].

Strict criteria are laid down for the recognition of cellular anaplasia[7,11]. These include: (a) nuclear enlargement to at least three times the nuclear size of an adjacent cell of the same type; (b) marked hyperchromatism of the enlarged nuclei; (c) bizarre mitotic figures (Figure 2.6). Anaplasia may be focal (10% or less of the sectioned tumour) or diffuse (more than 10% of the sectioned tumour).

Blastemal, epithelial and stromal component may be involved, singly or in combination. The definition does not extend to skeletal muscle that may be present in the stroma[11]. Entrapped megakaryocytes, crush artifact, overlapping of cells, overstaining, foreign material or calcification may be mistaken for anaplasia[11].

Anaplasia is rare in the tumours of children aged less than 2 years and it is more commonly reported in advanced-stage disease[17]. Anaplastic tumours are unilateral in more than 90% of cases[15]. Males and females are affected with equal frequency. The lung and liver are the most common sites for first relapse[15]. Anaplastic tumours correlate with an older age (36 months or older), non-white race, and lymph node metastases at diagnosis. When cellular anaplasia is suspected by these criteria,

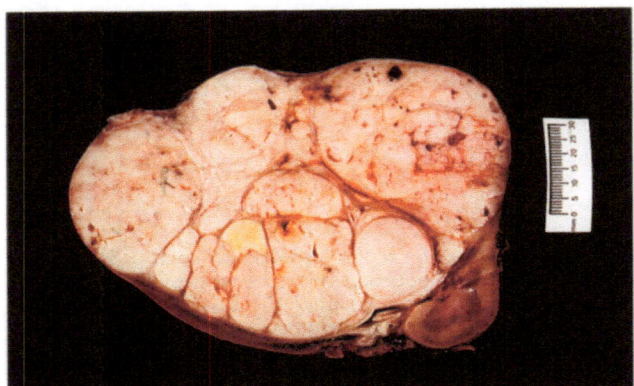

Fig. 2.1 The cut surface shows a solid lobular appearance characteristic of conventional Wilms' tumour. The patient was a 2-year-old boy who had a tumour of the right kidney

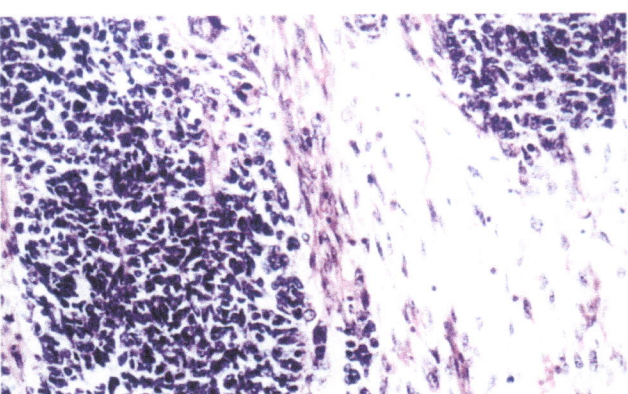

Fig. 2.2 A biphasic pattern is shown in a conventional Wilms' tumour: the tumour is composed of blastema and stroma. This was a left-sided renal tumour resected from a 3-year-old girl. H&E × 185

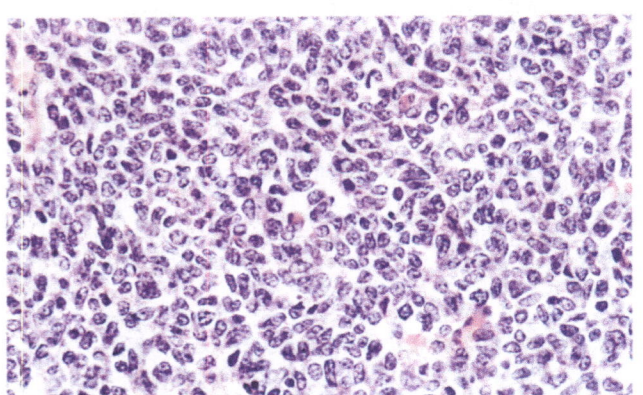

Fig. 2.3 The microscopic field displays blastema only. The tumour was a blastema-predominant Wilms' tumour removed from a 10-week-old girl. H&E × 300

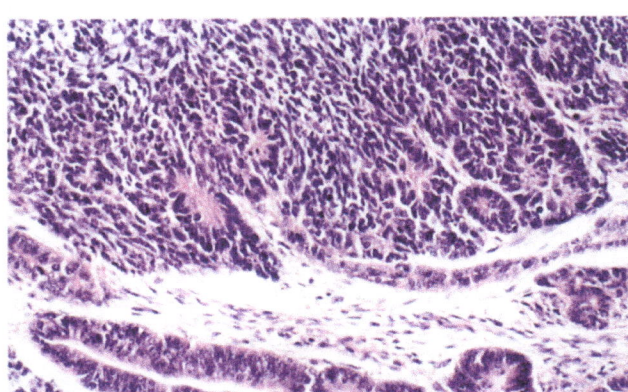

Fig. 2.4 Some of the tubules are immature and resemble neural rosettes. This may result in diagnostic confusion with neural tumours. H&E × 185

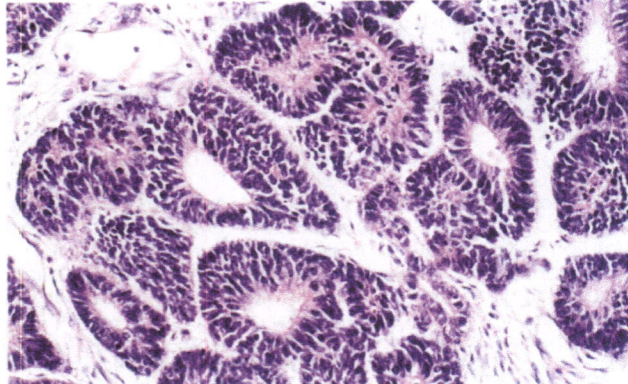

Fig. 2.5 A Wilms' tumour reveals a pattern that is largely made up of neoplastic tubules. When neoplastic tubules are the sole component, the tumour is sometimes referred to as monomorphic epithelial nephroblastoma. H&E × 185

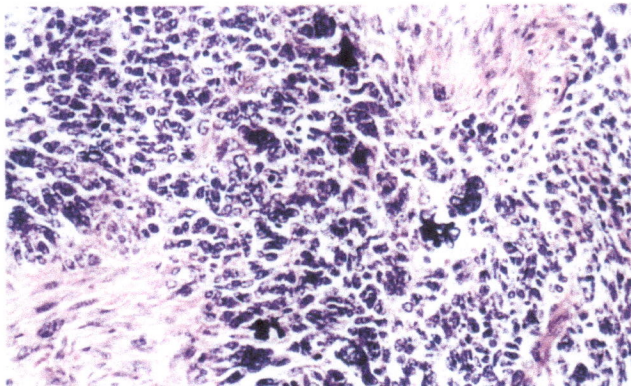

Fig. 2.6 Cellular anaplasia is seen within the blastematous component of a Wilms' tumour. H&E × 185

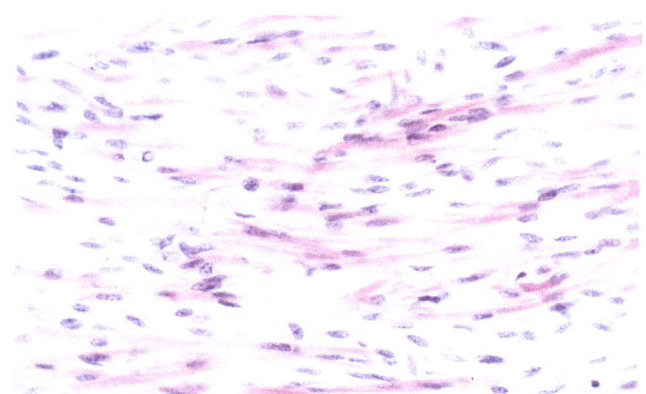

Fig. 2.7 This tumour was virtually entirely composed of fetal rhabdo-myoblasts. When this stromal component comprises more than 60% of cross-sectional area of representative sections, the tumour is referred to as fetal rhabdomyomatous Wilms' tumour. H&E × 300

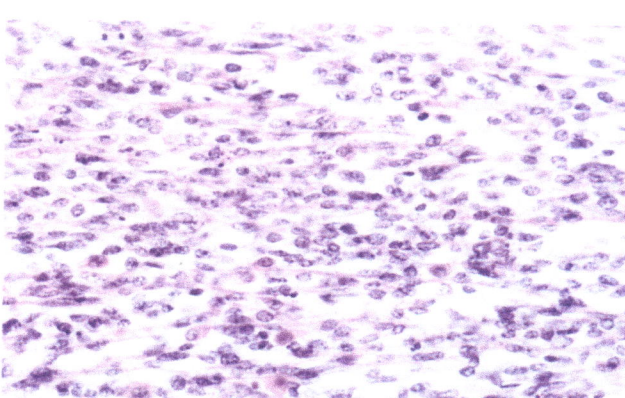

Fig. 2.8 Fetal rhabdomyomatous Wilms' tumour showing a more cellular area comprising an admixture of blastema and fetal rhabdomyo-blasts. Same tumour as shown in Figure 2.7. H&E × 300

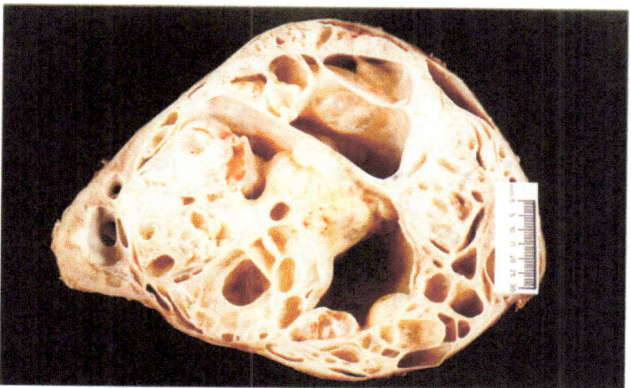

Fig. 2.9 The cut surface shows a cystic tumour largely replacing the kidney, characteristic of cystic partially differentiated nephroblastoma (CPDN). The patient was an 11-month-old girl with a tumour of the right kidney. The excised specimen weighed 1004 g

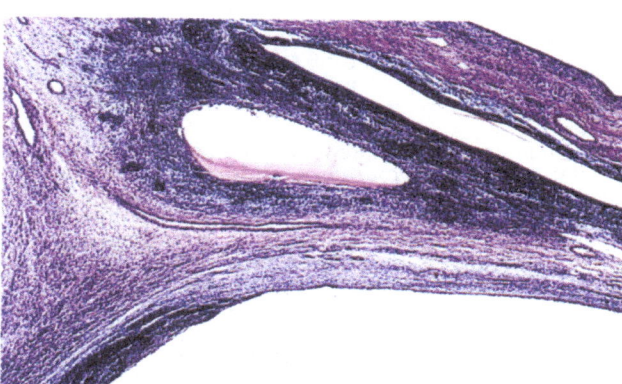

Fig. 2.10 The wall of a cyst of CPDN is seen to contain a large amount of blastematous tissue. H&E × 30

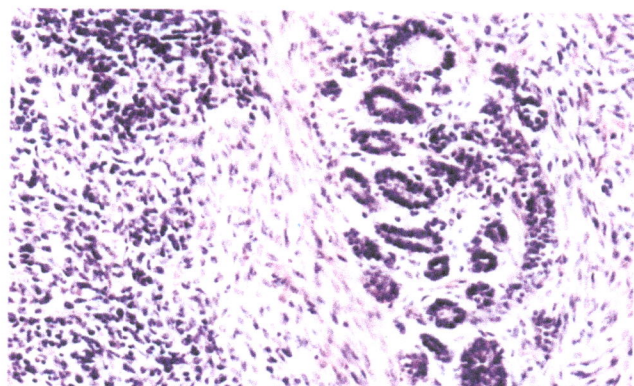

Fig. 2.11 Higher magnification of the cyst wall in a CPDN shows stroma, immature tubules and blastema. H&E × 185

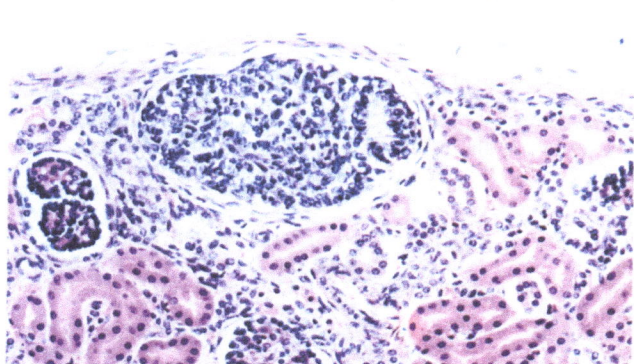

Fig. 2.12 A nascent or dormant nephrogenic rest composed of a microscopic-sized nodule of blastemal cells occupying a subcapsular location (an incidental finding in an 11-week-old boy whose death was attributed to SIDS). H&E × 185

Bonadio et al.[15] advise studying two or three times more sections than that ordinarily recommended for Wilms' tumour. These authors were also concerned that cellular anaplasia may follow preoperative chemotherapy; Beckwith[11], on the other hand, claimed that anaplasia is rare following chemotherapy.

The extent of anaplasia (i.e. whether focal or diffuse) does not appear to be relevant[16]. Anaplasia present in the primary tumour is almost invariably also seen in metastases[11]. The converse is not necessarily true, but poor tissue sampling may be an explanation.

DNA INDEX

Increased DNA content of tumour cells (aneuploidy) in Wilms' tumour determined by flow cytometry and/or image analysis is strongly coupled with cellular anaplasia. On the other hand, aneuploidy may be present in tumours that would otherwise be categorized as favourable histology[18,19]. Numerous complex chromosome translocations have been demonstrated in tumours with focal and diffuse anaplasia[18].

FETAL RHABDOMYOMATOUS WILMS' TUMOUR

This unusual variant of Wilms' tumour is virtually limited to children under 2 years of age. Thirty per cent of the tumours are bilateral[20]. They tend to be large and polypoid tumour may be seen projecting into the pelvicalyceal system.

The microscopic picture is dominated by the presence of fetal-type skeletal muscle, arranged in bundles against a background of fibroblasts and collagen (Figure 2.7)[20]. Foci of undifferentiated blastema are often intermixed (Figure 2.8). For the diagnosis to be acceptable the picture should occupy 60% or more of the surface area of representative sections[20]. With some exceptions the clinical outcome is very favourable; bilateral involvement would obviously adversely affect prognosis.

Fetal rhabdomyomatous Wilms' tumour should be distinguished from 'pure' rhabdomyosarcoma of the kidney[21]. This latter entity seems to be exceedingly rare, as there were only three such cases collected by the NWTS Pathology Centre between 1969 and 1990[12]. Metanephric blastema is absent in renal rhabdomyosarcoma and the muscle constituent is described as unequivocally malignant.

CYSTIC PARTIALLY DIFFERENTIATED NEPHROBLASTOMA (CYSTIC NEPHROMA; BENIGN CYSTIC NEPHROBLASTOMA; RENAL MULTILOCULAR CYST)

There is little question that cystic partially differentiated nephroblastoma (CPDN) is a neoplastic condition histogenetically related to Wilms' tumour, and probably represents a well-differentiated counterpart[22]. Its incidence is low compared with conventional Wilms' tumour. Gallo and Penchansky[22] found four examples among 165 renal tumours in children that included 143 Wilms' tumour. The tumour usually affects infants less than 2 years of age[23,24]. The clinical course is benign. As in Wilms' tumour, an abdominal mass is the usual mode of clinical presentation.

Grossly, a well-circumscribed multicystic structure replaces part of the kidney (Figure 2.9). The diameter of the lesions varies from 4.5–21 cm, and weights of 58–1440 g are recorded[24]. The cysts vary in size and usually contain pale yellow or clear fluid; they do not communicate with each other, nor do they communicate with the renal pelvis. Microscopically, the cysts are lined by cuboidal, flattened or hobnail epithelium, but a specific lining epithelium may be absent. The lining is often interrupted by minute excrescences protruding into the cyst lumina. The intervening septa contain variable amounts of immature renal blastema (Figure 2.10) showing degrees of epithelial differentiation (Figure 2.11). The latter may include primitive tubules and glomeruli, often focally distributed. Rhabdomyocytes are frequently present[22,24]. The tumour is often surrounded by a zone of compressed renal parenchyma that clearly demarcates the tumour from the rest of the kidney. Recently, attention has been drawn to a papillonodular variant of CPDN which has a similar benign course to that of the conventional type[25].

The cysts of CPDN are probably an expression of tubular differentiation of metanephric blastema in which the tubules have undergone cystic dilatation[23]; alternatively, they may be derived from the dysplastic tubules commonly found in the intralobar type of nephroblastomatosis[26] (see below). Precursor lesions of Wilms' tumour have not so far been described in association with CPDN. Metastases are not known to occur, but recurrence in one case has been reported[24]. Total nephrectomy followed by regular follow-up is the treatment of choice[23]. CPDN may coexist with frank Wilms' tumour[24].

The differential diagnosis lies mainly in separating CPDN from cystic nephroma (benign multilocular cyst)[24]. The absence of immature renal elements in the septal stroma of the latter condition is the principal distinguishing feature. The septa of cystic nephroma are generally thin and composed of mature fibrous tissue that may contain mature tubular structures. It stands to reason that in order to separate CPDN from cystic nephroma adequate tissue should be sampled for microscopy. Histogenetic separation of these two entities has been questioned[24]. Other conditions that should be considered in the differential diagnosis are cystic congenital mesoblastic nephroma, cystic forms of bone metastasizing renal tumour of childhood, and cystic change in conventional nephroblastoma[2].

NEPHROGENIC RESTS AND NEPHROBLASTOMATOSIS

Terminological confusion has for a long time overshadowed this category of renal lesions; for the purposes of this description the nomenclature used is that proposed by Beckwith, Kiviat and Bonadio[27] (Table 2.1). Accordingly, a nephrogenic rest (previously referred to as nodular renal blastema) is a focus of persistent nephrogenic cells that can be induced to form a Wilms' tumour (Figure 2.12). These lesions are found in nearly 1% of routine perinatal autopsies and in 25–40% of kidneys with Wilms' tumour[2].

Table 2.1 Nephroblastomatosis nomenclature

Nephrogenic rests (perilobar or intralobar)
  —dormant
  —maturing
  —hyperplastic
  —neoplastic:
         adenomatous
         nephroblastomatous
Diffuse nephrogenic rests or nephroblastomatosis
  —perilobar
  —intralobar
  —combined

Nephrogenic rests may be categorized as perilobar or intralobar depending on their distribution in the renal lobule[2]. Nephrogenic rests are also separated according to their outcome; hence, they may be viewed as dormant (nascent), maturing (sclerosing, obsolescent) (Figure 2.13), hyperplastic or neoplastic[27].

Neoplastic rests arise as expanding nodules within a pre-existent rest that usually becomes compressed at the periphery (Figures 2.14 and 2.15). Neoplastic rests, depending on their cytological features, are either adenomatous or nephroblastomatous. Many mitoses and closely packed cells characterize the nephroblastomatous rest (Figure 2.16). Adenomatous nephrogenic rests, by comparison, have less 'aggressive' cytological features (Figure 2.17); the cells are less mitotically active and are less closely packed.

This subdivision of nephrogenic rests applies equally to perilobar and intralobar lesions. Intralobar nephrogenic rests are located anywhere within the renal cortex or medulla. Because they are frequently compressed by tumour, these rests are more difficult to identify. Most rests are predominantly stromal and contain small clusters of blastemal cells; mature fat is often present. The boundary between the lesion and renal parenchyma is typically blurred; renal tubules are often encompassed by the nephrogenic rest.

When the nephrogenic rests (or their derivatives) are diffuse or multifocal the condition is referred to as nephroblastomatosis[27]. Nephroblastomatoses are also separated according to their relation to lobar topography[27], i.e. perilobar nephroblastomatosis or intralobar nephroblastomatosis (Figures 2.18 and 2.19). The term 'combined nephroblastomatosis' is used when perilobar and intralobar types coexist.

Exceptionally, the entire renal parenchyma is uniformly involved, and, for such cases, universal or panlobar nephroblastomatosis is the recommended designation. Wilms' tumour may arise in association with perilobar or intralobar nephrogenic rests. Most tumours arising in association with the latter show prominent stromal development, often including skeletal muscle. Against this background, structures resembling collecting ducts and ampullae are frequently present (Figure 2.20).

Intralobar nephroblastomatosis is thought to be related to an event early in embryogenesis; perilobar nephroblastomatosis, on the other hand, is linked to an event in later embryogenesis[2]. Both lesions predispose to bilateral disease, more so in relation to intralobar nephroblastomatosis[2].

Nodular renal blastema (nephrogenic rests) has been reported in association with congenital obstructive nephropathy, with or without accompanying dysplasia, but it is unclear whether these lesions predispose to the development of Wilms' tumour[28]. Nephrogenic rests are also strongly related to congenital anomalies of the kidney[29], often associated with trisomy 18.

CONGENITAL MESOBLASTIC NEPHROMA (FETAL MESENCHYMAL HAMARTOMA; FIBROUS HAMARTOMA; LEIOMYOMATOUS HAMARTOMA)

This entity was included in the overall category of Wilms' tumour until its distinctive clinical and microscopic features were recognized[30]. It presents typically at birth or during the first week[31]; it is less often discovered later in infancy. The rarity of the tumour is evidenced by the reported identification of 29 mesoblastic nephromas among 889 Wilms' tumours[31]. Despite accounting for only some 3% of all childhood renal tumours, it constitutes the most common solid renal tumour at birth. An asymptomatic abdominal mass, discovered incidentally, is the usual clinical presentation. The pregnancy may be complicated by prematurity or polyhydramnios. Males and females are affected with equal frequency and the right kidney is involved more often than the left. Hypercal-

caemia is recorded in some cases[32]. The precise nature and histogenesis of the tumour remain unsettled.

The involved kidney is usually found to be enormously enlarged and the renal capsule is stretched tightly over the tumour; resected specimens weigh 35–450 g[33]. The growth has a firm rubbery consistency and the cut surface is typically trabeculated, and has been likened to a uterine fibroid (Figure 2.21). The tumour is not itself encapsulated. Not infrequently it replaces up to 90% of the renal parenchyma, distorting the remaining renal structures. Softening, haemorrhage and necrosis are unusual features. Occasional cysts may be grossly discernible and in some cases may be the dominant feature[34].

The microscopic picture has been compared with that of infantile fibromatosis[35], showing tightly interdigitating bundles of fibroblasts and myofibroblasts (Figure 2.22). Mitotic activity is variable. An infiltrative growth pattern is a distinctive feature and finger-like projections of the lesion penetrate the normal renal parenchyma (Figure 2.23). Normal glomeruli and tubules are often entrapped along the tumour/kidney interface[36] and may appear dysplastic[33]. The renal capsule may be breached and the growth may extend into the perirenal tissue; this is especially likely to occur at the renal hilum. Prominent lymphatics, foci of haemopoiesis, rhabdomyocytic differentiation and islands of cartilage, are other recognized elements and a myxoid pattern is sometimes prominent[33].

Local recurrence is rare after surgical resection. As the single most important factor determining recurrence is the presence of a positive surgical margin, it is imperative that the surgeon secures a wide margin of excision.

Microscopically, congenital mesoblastic nephroma may superficially resemble clear-cell sarcoma of the kidney[31]. As the prognoses associated with the two entities are so vastly different, an erroneous diagnosis would be disastrous.

A less common but potentially aggressive form of congenital mesoblastic nephroma is referred to as the cellular (or atypical) variant[31,37,38]. This subtype seems to make up about a third of all cases[2]. On naked eye inspection, cellular congenital mesoblastic nephroma is less reminiscent of a uterine fibroid, and haemorrhage and necrosis are generally more common. Patients tend to present later in infancy and the tumours are generally larger[31]. The histology is characterized by a greater degree of cellularity (Figure 2.24) and enhanced mitotic activity. Conventional congenital mesoblastic nephroma may show areas of increased cellularity indistinguishable from the cellular variant, suggesting overlap between the two patterns.

Local recurrence and even metastases have been reported in association with the cellular variant[2]. According to the latter author, tumours that should be viewed with concern are those with incomplete resection (including intraoperative rupture), and when the patient's age exceeds 3 months.

TERATOID WILMS' TUMOUR

This is a recently recognized entity that by virtue of a significant presence of nephroblastomatous tissue is quite distinct from renal teratoma[39]. It is also separate from Wilms' tumour due to the inclusion of a significant proportion of heterologous structures, more so than is usually found in Wilms' tumour. Bilaterality, frequent involvement of the renal pelvis and a close relationship with nephroblastomatosis, are other attributes. Its occurrence in three out of 290 patients with Wilms' tumour at the St Jude Children's Research Hospital (Tennessee) attests to its rarity[40].

CLINICAL SYNDROMES ASSOCIATED WITH WILMS' TUMOUR

The most notable of these associations is the WAGR syndrome (Wilms' tumour, aniridia, genitourinary anomal-

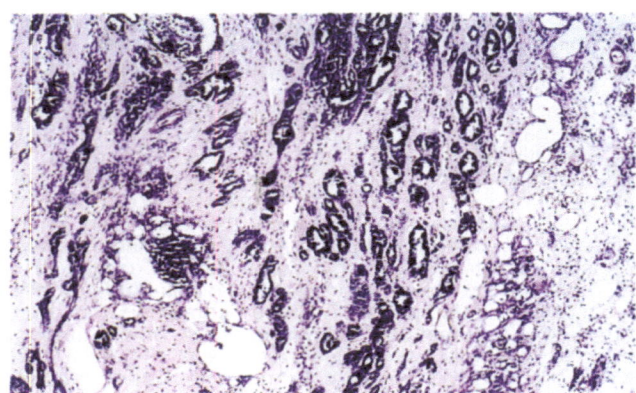

Fig. 2.13 This microphotograph shows a maturing or sclerosing rest; it consists of epithelial tubules set in a background of stromal hyalinization with few, if any, blastemal cells. H&E × 75

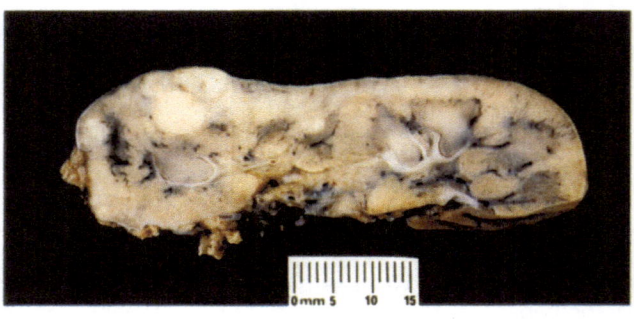

Fig. 2.14 A hyperplastic rest is grossly visible beneath the renal capsule of the cut surface of the kidney

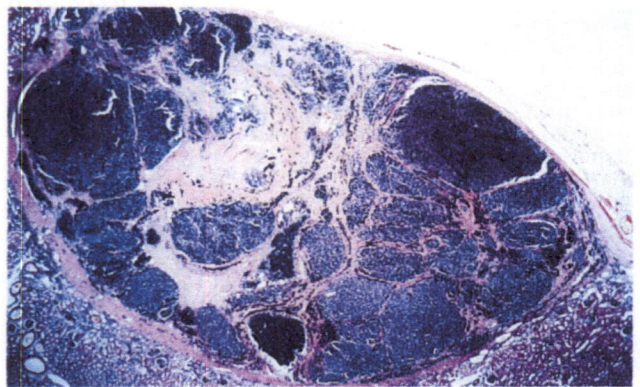

Fig. 2.15 Microscopic view of hyperplastic rest shown in the preceding figure is seen to be composed of nodules of blastema located within a sclerosing lesion. H&E × 13

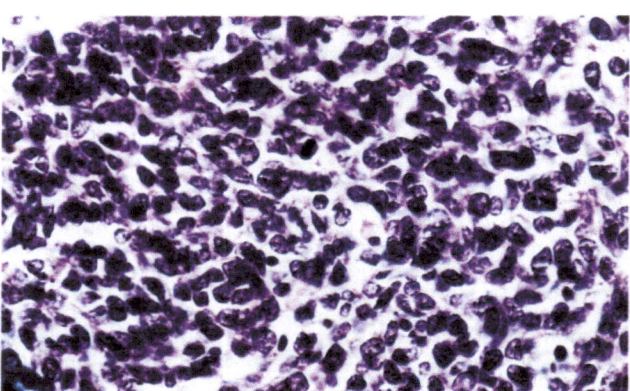

Fig. 2.16 Neoplastic rest showing nephroblastomatous cytological features, with closely apposed cells containing dark nuclei and scant cytoplasm; mitoses are evident. H&E × 480

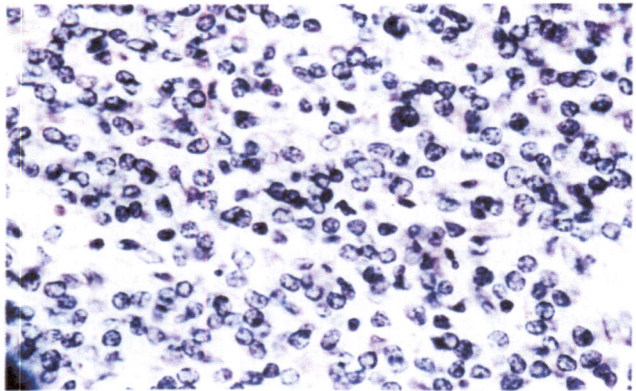

Fig. 2.17 Neoplastic rest showing less aggressive cytological features, consistent with an adenomatous rest; the tumour cells are more widely spaced, the nuclei are pale and there is more cytoplasm. H&E × 480

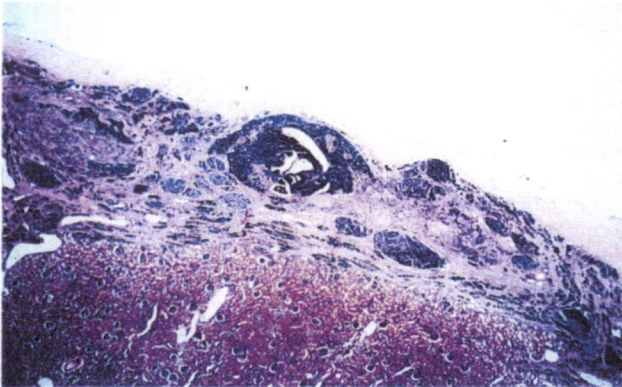

Fig. 2.18 A diffuse superficial zone of nephrogenic rests is demonstrated beneath the renal capsule; this pattern is referred to as perilobar nephroblastomatosis. H&E × 13

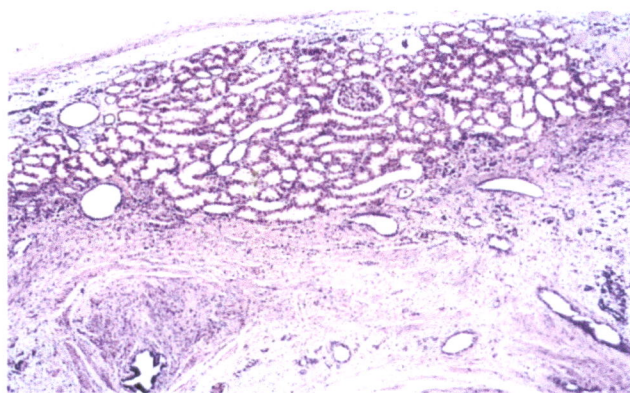

Fig. 2.19 Intralobar nephroblastomatosis showing an overlying zone of normal superficial cortex. The patient, a 2-year-old boy, with bilateral loin masses, presented in renal failure. There was no associated Wilms' tumour. H&E × 48

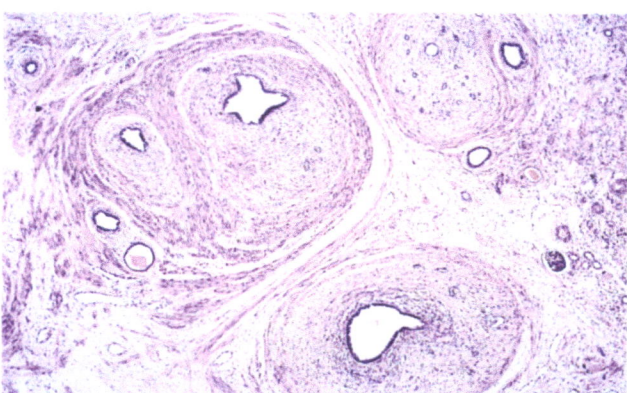

Fig. 2.20 Embryonal-appearing tubules, resembling conventional renal dysplasia, sometimes cuffed with blastema, are a common feature of intralobular nephroblastomatosis. Entrapped renal tubules and glomeruli are seen on the right. H&E × 48

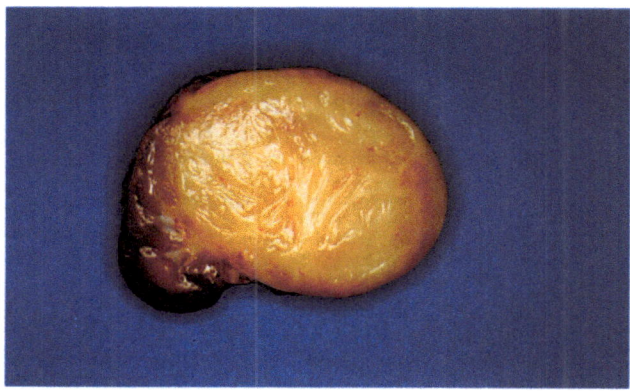

Fig. 2.21 Macroscopic view of cut surface of a congenital mesoblastic nephroma partially replacing the renal substance. A solid trabecular appearance, reminiscent of a uterine fibroid, is characteristic of the tumour

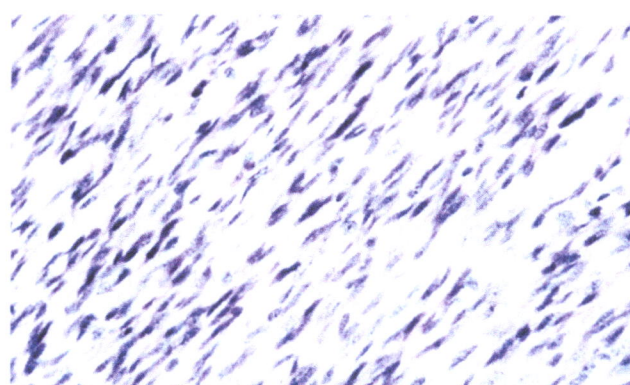

Fig. 2.22 Microscopically, the tumour is composed of spindle cells with a degree of cellularity generally associated with the conventional form of congenital mesoblastic nephroma. H&E × 300

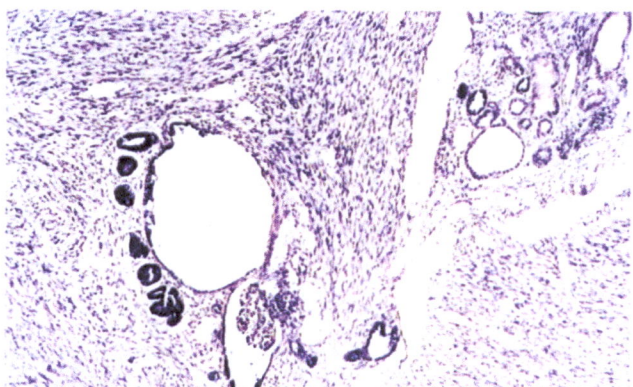

Fig. 2.23 Margin of a conventional congenital mesoblastic nephroma demonstrates the infiltrative character of the growth, seen here to encircle renal tubules and glomeruli. H&E × 75

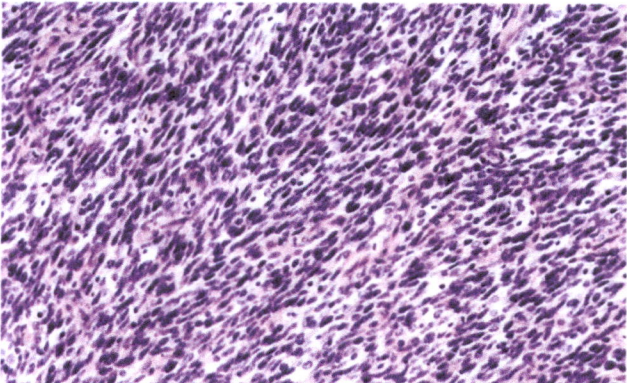

Fig. 2.24 Compared with the two preceding figures, the degree of cellularity is considerably greater in this example of congenital mesoblastic nephroma; it represents the so-called cellular (or atypical) variant of the tumour. H&E × 185

ies, mental retardation)[27] (Table 2.2). A distinctive interstitial deletion of the p13 region of chromosome 11 is usually found. Approximately one third of patients with aniridia and 11p13 deletion go on to develop Wilms' tumour.

Table 2.2 Clinical syndromes associated with Wilms' tumour

WAGR syndrome
Drash syndrome
Hemihypertrophy
Beckwith–Wiedemann syndrome
Perlman syndrome
Familial Wilms' tumour

The Drash syndrome refers to a combination of Wilms' tumour, pseudohermaphroditism and abnormal renal function[41]. Affected children are born with ambiguous genitalia and all patients reveal a 46XY karyotype. The gonads are commonly dysgenetic and there is a strong propensity to develop gonadoblastoma. The most common underlying glomerular lesion is diffuse mesangiosclerosis[41]. Increasingly, incomplete forms of Drash syndrome are reported.

Hemihypertrophy, Beckwith–Wiedemann syndrome and Perlman syndrome are associated with sporadic Wilms' tumour[42]. These conditions also commonly show perilobar nephroblastomatosis. Familial Wilms' tumour, a rarely reported entity, affects about 1% of Wilms' tumours.

Although perilobar nephrogenic rests are frequently encountered in trisomy 18, it is unusual for Wilms' tumour to affect such patients[42]. An association between Wilms' tumour and von Recklinghausen's neurofibromatosis has been suggested[43]. An analysis of 547 patients with Wilms' tumour showed 24 (4.4%) with genitourinary anomalies, including defects of the kidney, hypospadias, cryptorchidism and duplications of the collecting system[44]. However, as the prevalence of genitourinary anomalies in the general population is unknown, a definite association with Wilms' tumour cannot be established with certainty.

EXTRARENAL WILMS' TUMOUR

Wilms' tumour rarely arises at extrarenal sites[45–47]. Exclusion of a primary renal tumour is implicit in the diagnosis. The most common sites are the retroperitoneum and inguinal region. The embryogenesis is controversial but those found in the juxtarenal location may originate in a supernumerary kidney[47].

Wilms' tumour arising in teratomas should be classified separately[47]. They have been reported most commonly in the sacrococcygeal region[47–49]. The teratomatous tissue may be difficult to identify microscopically, due to dominant growth of the renal element or incomplete sampling of the tumour.

REFERENCES

1. Kidd JM. Wilms' tumour: gross characteristics, extent of disease at time of initial diagnosis, and some factors affecting prognosis. In: Pochedly C, Baum ES, editors. Wilms' tumor, clinical and biological manifestations. New York, Amsterdam, Oxford: Elsevier; 1984: 251–64.
2. Beckwith JB. Wilms' tumor and other renal tumors of childhood: an update. J Urol. 1986;36:320–4.
3. Breslow N, Beckwith JB, Ciol M, Sharples K. Age distribution of Wilms' tumor: report from the National Wilms' Tumor Study. Can Res. 1988;48:1653–7.
4. Hrabovsky EE, Othersen HB, deLorimier A, Kelalis P, Beckwith JB, Takashima J. Wilms' tumor in the neonate: a report from the National Wilms' Tumor Study. J Pediatr Surg. 1986;21:385–7.
5. Marsden HB, Lawler W, Kumar PM. Bone metastasizing renal tumour of childhood. Morphological and clinical features, and differences from Wilms' tumour. Cancer. 1978;42:1922–8.
6. Marsden HB, Lennox EL, Lawler W, Kinnier-Wilson LM. Bone metastases in childhood renal tumours. Br J Cancer. 1980;41:875–9.
7. Beckwith JB, Palmer NF. Histopathology and prognosis of Wilms' tumor. Results from the First National Wilms' Tumor Study. Cancer. 1978;41:1937–48.
8. Magee F, Mah RG, Taylor GP, Dimmick JE. Neural differentiation in Wilms' tumor. Hum Pathol. 1987;18:33–7.
9. Vakil VV, Sirsat MV, Dalal SJ. Nephroblastoma (Wilms' tumour) with keratinizing cysts. Ind J Pathol Bacteriol. 1965;8:149–54.
10. Dabke KV, Vishnoi KR, Agarwal S. Nephroblastoma with keratinizing cysts (a case report). Ind J Cancer. 1974;11:50–3.
11. Beckwith JB. Wilms' tumor and other renal tumors of childhood: a selective review from the National Wilms' Tumor Study Pathology Center. Hum Pathol. 1983;14:481–92.
12. Weeks DA, Beckwith JB, Mierau GW, Zuppan CW. Renal neoplasms mimicking rhabdoid tumor of the kidney. A report from the National Wilms' Tumor Study Pathology Center. Am J Surg Pathol. 1991; 15:1042–54.
13. Ugarte N, Gonzalez-Crussi F, Hsueh W. Wilms' tumor: its morphology in patients under one year of age. Cancer. 1981;48:346–53.
14. Chatten J. Epithelial differentiation in Wilms' tumor: a clinicopathological appraisal. Perspect Pediatr Pathol. 1976;3:225–51.
15. Bonadio JF, Storer B, Norkool P, Farewell VT, Beckwith JB, D'Angio GJ. Anaplastic Wilms' tumour: clinical and pathologic studies. J Clin Oncol. 1985;3:513–20.
16. Zuppan CW, Beckwith JB, Luckey DW. Anaplasia in unilateral Wilms' tumor: a report from the National Wilms' Tumor Study Pathology Center. Hum Pathol. 1988;19:1199–209.
17. Corey SJ, Andersen JW, Vawter GF, Lack EE, Sallan SE. Improved survival for children with anaplastic Wilms' tumors. Cancer. 1991;68:970–4.
18. Douglass EC, Look AT, Webber B et al. Hyperdiploidy and chromosomal rearrangements defined the anaplastic variant of Wilms' tumor. J Clin Oncol. 1986;4:975–81.
19. Kumar S, Marsden HB, Cowan RA, Barnes JM. Prognostic relevance of DNA content in childhood renal tumors. Br J Cancer. 1989;59:291–5.
20. Wigger HJ. Fetal rhabdomyomatous nephroblastoma – a variant of Wilms' tumor. Hum Pathol. 1976;7:613–23.
21. Penchansky L, Gallo G. Rhabdomyosarcoma of the kidney in children. Cancer. 1979;44:285–92.
22. Gallo G, Penchansky L. Cystic nephroma. Cancer. 1977;39:1322–7.
23. Joshi VV, Banerjee AK, Yadav K, Pathak IC. Cystic partially differentiated nephroblastoma. A clinicopathologic entity in the spectrum of infantile renal neoplasia. Cancer. 1977;40:789–95.
24. Joshi VV, Beckwith JB. Multilocular cyst of the kidney (cystic nephroma) and cystic partially differentiated nephroblastoma. Terminology and criteria for diagnosis. Cancer. 1989;64:466–79.
25. Joshi VV, Beckwith JB. Pathologic delineation of the papillonodular type of cystic partially differentiated nephroblastoma. A review of 11 cases. Cancer. 1990;66:1568–77.
26. Walford N. Panlobar nephroblastomatosis: a distinctive form of renal dysplasia associated with Wilms' tumour. Histopathology. 1990;17:37–44.
27. Beckwith JB, Kiviat NB, Bonadio JF. Nephrogenic rests, nephroblastomatosis, and the pathogenesis of Wilms' tumor. Pediatr Pathol. 1990;10:1–36.
28. Craver R, Dimmick J, Johnson H, Nigro M. Congenital obstructive uropathy and nodular renal blastema. J Urol. 1986;136:305–7.
29. Bove KE, Koffler H, McAdams AJ. Nodular renal blastema. Definition and possible significance. Cancer. 1969;24:323–32.
30. Bolande RP, Brough AJ, Izant RJ. Congenital mesoblastic nephroma of infancy. Pediatrics. 1967;40:272–8.
31. Sandstedt B, Delemarre JFM, Krul EJ, Tournade MF. Mesoblastic nephromas: a study of 29 tumours from the SIOP nephroblastoma file. Histopathology. 1985;9:741–50.
32. Jayabose S, Iqbal K, Newman L et al. Hypercalcaemia in childhood renal tumors. Cancer. 1988;61:788–91.
33. Bolande RP. Congenital mesoblastic nephroma of infancy. Perspect Pediatr Pathol. 1973;1:227–50.
34. Ganick DJ, Gilbert EF, Beckwith JB, Kiviat N. Congenital cystic mesoblastic nephroma. Hum Pathol. 1981;12:1039–43.
35. Beckwith JB. Wilms' tumor and other renal tumors of childhood. In: Finegold M, editor. Pathology of neoplasia in children and adolescents. Philadelphia: WB Saunders; 1986:313–26.
36. Beckwith JB, Weeks DA. Congenital mesoblastic nephroma. When should we worry? Arch Pathol Lab Med. 1986;110:98–9.
37. Gormley TS, Skoog SJ, Jones RV, Maybee D. Cellular congenital mesoblastic nephroma: what are the options. J Urol. 1989;142: 479–83.

38. Beckwith JB. Mesenchymal renal neoplasms of infancy revisited. J Pediatr Surg. 1974;9:803–5.
39. Variend S, Spicer RD, MacKinnon AE. Teratoid Wilms' tumour. Cancer. 1984;53:1936–42.
40. Fernandes ET, Parham DM, Ribeiro RC, Douglass EC, Kumar APM, Wilimas J. Teratoid Wilms' tumour: the St Jude experience. J Pediatr Surg. 1988;23:1131–4.
41. Manivel JC, Sibley RK, Dehner LP. Complete and incomplete Drash syndrome: a clinicopathologic study of five cases of a dysontogenetic-neoplastic complex. Hum Pathol. 1987;18:80–9.
42. Bove K. Nephroblastomatosis. An overview. Arch Pathol Lab Med. 1989;113:723–4.
43. Stay EJ, Vawter G. The relationship between nephroblastoma and neurofibomatosis (von Recklinghausen's disease). Cancer. 1977;39:2550–5.
44. Pendergrass TW. Congenital anomalies in children with Wilms' tumor. A new survey. Cancer. 1976;37:403–9.
45. Akhtar M, Kott E, Brooks B. Extrarenal Wilms' tumor. Report of a case and review of the literature. Cancer. 1977;40:3087–91.
46. Lai HS, Hung WT, How SW. Extrarenal Wilms' tumor – a case report. J Pediatr Surg. 1988;23:454–6.
47. Andrews PE, Kelalis PP, Haase GM. Extrarenal Wilms' tumor: results of the National Wilms' Tumor Study. J Pediatr Surg. 1992;27:1181–84.
48. Gonzales-Crussi F. Case 6. Retroperitoneal tumor. Pediatr. Pathol. 1985;4:181–5.
49. Tebbi K, Ragab AH, Ternberg JL, Vietti TJ. An extrarenal Wilms' tumor arising from a sacrococcygeal teratoma. Clin Pediatr. 1974;13: 1019–21.
50. Slater RM, Mannens MMAM. Cytogenetics and molecular genetics of Wilms' tumor of childhood. Cancer Genet Cytogenet. 1992;61:111–21.

Variable patterns of behaviour in relation to 'Wilms' tumour' had been recognized for many years[1]. The identification of several new entities then led to gradual attrition of the tumour category. Congenital mesoblastic nephroma was the first such entity to be identified. Others followed, including a small subgroup with a distinct microscopy that had been recognized earlier for its propensity to metastasize to bone[1]. Subsequently, the first National Wilms' Tumor Study (NWTS) reported three sarcomatous patterns associated with a poor outcome[2]. These patterns were referred to as rhabdomyosarcomatoid, clear-cell pattern and the hyalinizing pattern. The term 'rhabdomyosarcomatoid' was based on the light microscopic features that suggested muscle differentiation; ultrastructural studies, however, subsequently failed to confirm muscle differentiation and the tumours were renamed rhabdoid tumours[3]. Tumours with a similar microscopic pattern were later described in extrarenal locations[4]; their precise relationship to the renal tumours has yet to be clarified[5].

The NWTS confirmed the marked propensity of the tumours with a clear-cell pattern to metastasize to bone. About the same time, similar tumours had been reported by Marsden et al. in the United Kingdom[6,7] as 'bone metastasizing renal tumour of childhood' (BMRTC).

Compared with conventional Wilms' tumours, these sarcomatous patterns tend to involve younger patients and are collectively referred to as 'unfavourable histology' renal tumours because of their poor response to therapy. Current opinion holds that they are histogenetically distinct and should be considered separate from Wilms' tumours.

BONE METASTASIZING RENAL TUMOUR OF CHILDHOOD (BMRTC; CLEAR-CELL SARCOMA OF THE KIDNEY)

This rare tumour of the kidney has a distinctive histology[1,2,6,7]. Its association with aggressive behaviour and an unfavourable outcome is well recognized, as is a marked propensity to metastasize to bone. An abdominal mass with haematuria is the usual clinical presentation[8]. BMRTC comprises about 2–4% of all renal neoplasms of childhood[6,8,9]. Males are moderately more often affected than females[8]. Bilateral tumours and extrarenal tumours with a similar microscopic appearance have not been documented[8].

Of the cases entered in the NWTS-I and NWTS-II, osseous metastases were encountered in 42% of cases; Marsden et al.'s series[7] revealed a figure of 60%. This contrasts with Wilms' tumour which is hardly ever associated with osseous metastases[6,7]. Osseous metastases in BMRTC may be single or multiple and the skull is most commonly affected[7,8]. The lung, liver and lymph nodes are other common metastatic sites. With increasing survival following more intensive therapy, brain metastases are increasingly recognized[10]. Flow cytometry on a limited number of tumours has so far consistently revealed a diploid DNA pattern[11].

Pathological features

The gross features of BMRTC lack specificity. The cut surface of the illustrated tumour is tan, smooth and partially lobulated (Figure 3.1). Haemorrhage is uncommon[8]. Many authors emphasize the tendency for the tumours to localize centrally, with many of the neoplasms apparently arising in the medulla of the kidney[2,12]. There is usually clear demarcation between tumour and adjacent normal kidney, but cysts are common at the tumour–kidney interface. The tumours tend to be very large and tumour weights in excess of 1000 g have been recorded[8].

Microscopically, the classic pattern shows sheets of small monomorphic cells with round to oval uniform nuclei, indistinct nucleoli and sparse mitoses (Figure 3.2)[9,13]. The cytoplasm shows ill-defined boundaries, is moderate in amount and vacuolated. Clear-cell sarcoma of the kidney, the alternative terminology, takes its name from the latter feature. Tumour cell cytoplasm stains negatively with PAS[8] (contrasting with other clear-cell tumours, such as renal cell carcinoma). A network of small blood vessels, usually the size of capillaries, arranged in parallel rows, characteristically divides the tumour into cords and columns of more or less equal breadth (Figure 3.3)[2,9]. Beckwith and Larson[13] refer to these cells as 'cord cells'.

These parallel arrays are usually connected at several points by prominent side branches to form arcades, and this is a distinctive and important diagnostic feature. However, the vascular component may be inconspicuous or may be accentuated by a collar of perivascular spindle cells (Figure 3.4). These cells were referred to as 'septal cells' by Beckwith and Larson[13]. According to these authors, transition between the 'cord cells' and the 'septal cells' may be observed. The vascular pattern is sharply outlined by a reticulin stain (Figure 3.5).

The bland nuclei and sparse mitoses of the tumour cells impart a deceptively banal appearance. Some specimens show areas in which the cells are eosinophilic and non-vacuolated, defying the designation 'clear-cell sarcoma of the kidney'. To date, immunohistochemical studies have not been helpful in diagnosis, or in elucidating the cell of origin.

There is no evidence that the tumour undergoes tubular differentiation; when tubules are present they are usually found peripherally and are likely to represent pre-existent entrapped nephrons. These tubules have a well-defined basement membrane and are lined by basophilic cuboidal epithelium, thought to result from metaplasia. The entrapped tubules frequently undergo dilatation (Figure 3.6) and may form grossly discernible cysts; alternatively, cysts may form within a myxoid stroma[9,12]. The tumour typically displays an infiltrative border, contrasting with the 'pushing' border typical of a Wilms' tumour[9].

Histological variations

The foregoing description corresponds to the 'classic pattern' of BMRTC. Changes of an epithelioid or stromal nature produce a picture which deviates from the basic classic pattern[9,13]. These variants may resemble a number of other neoplastic entities and may cause diagnostic confusion. Evidence of the classic pattern will usually be revealed on diligent searching of multiple sections.

Aggregation of the tumour cells into cords or ribbons may mimic an epithelial pattern. This has been referred to as the 'epithelioid trabecular pattern' of BMRTC and

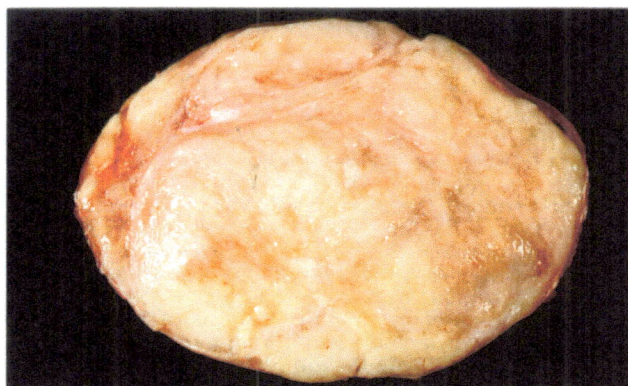

Fig. 3.1 The cut surface of the BMRTC is tan, smooth and partly lobulated. The nephrectomy specimen weighed 920 g and was removed from a boy aged 22 months

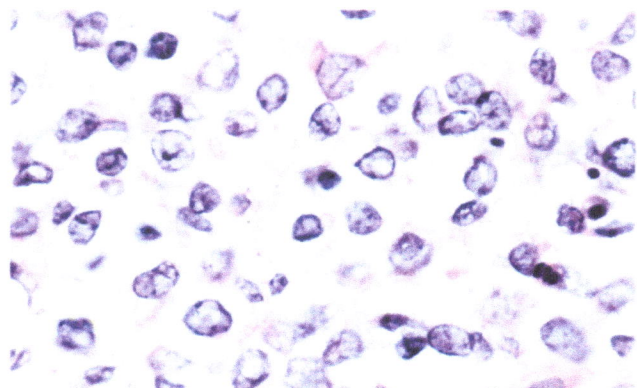

Fig. 3.2 BMRTC shows a bland appearance of the tumour cells. The cytoplasm stains poorly and cell boundaries are ill-defined. Nuclei are round to oval with moderate variation in size; nuclear chromatin is evenly granular. Mitotic figures are scarce. H&E × 750

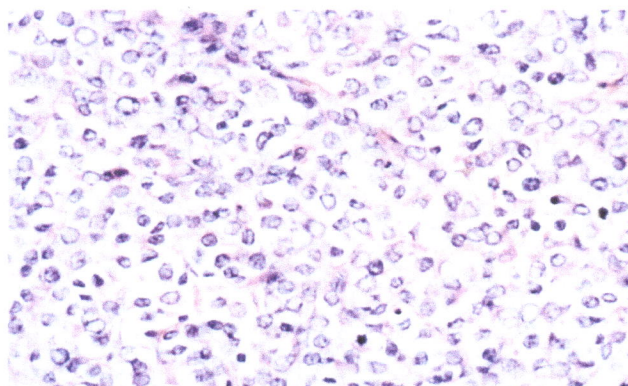

Fig. 3.3 A low-power view shows an occasional delicate blood vessel coursing through a sheet of tumour cells. Such blood vessels, often arranged in parallel rows, are an important diagnostic feature of the tumour. H&E × 300

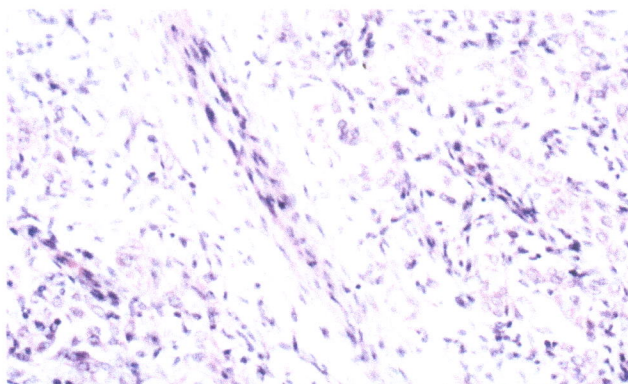

Fig. 3.4 BMRTC shows a blood vessel in the centre of the field surrounded by spindle cells and finer more delicate vessels are seen on either side. This is probably an early phase of the fibrotic pattern shown in Figure 3.8. H&E × 185

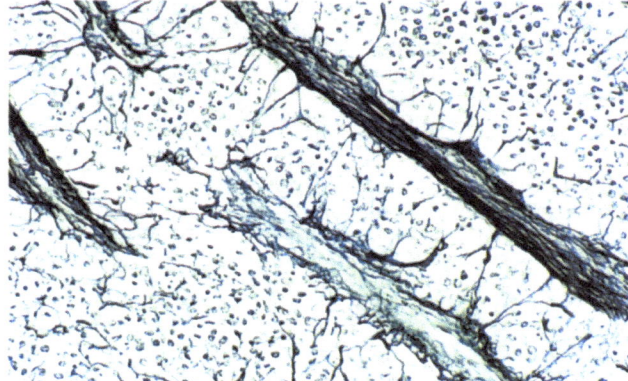

Fig. 3.5 Reticulin stain accentuates the distinctive vascular pattern of BMRTC. In addition to reticulin fibres outlining the vessels, strands of reticulin are also seen to enter the tumour parenchyma at right angles to the vessels. Gomori reticulin × 185

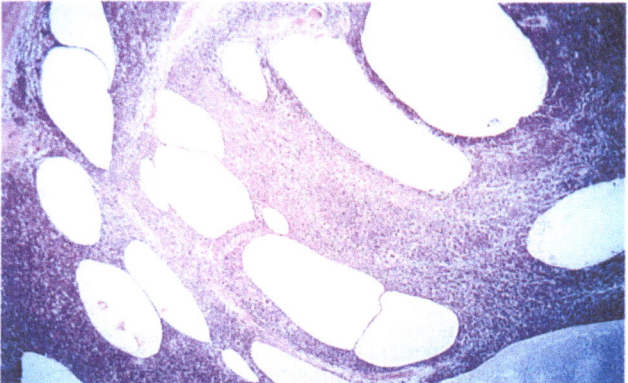

Fig. 3.6 BMRTC of the kidney shows several prominent cysts almost certainly due to dilatation of entrapped collecting tubules. H&E × 13

the importance of its recognition is that it may be mistaken for Wilms' tumour. Stromal changes are related to one or more mechanisms, including sclerosis of the 'cord cells', proliferation of the 'septal cells' or secretion of mucosubstances by the tumour[13]. When the cord cells are replaced by collagen, the vascular arcades are preserved or exaggerated. Proliferation of the septal cells initially results in exaggeration of the classic pattern, that later becomes compressed and obliterated (Figure 3.8). (The gross appearance of this specimen is shown in Figure 3.7.) Secretion of mucosubstances produces a myxoid or cystic appearance which often disrupts and masks the classic pattern, but the change is usually only focal[13]. Other patterns have been reported, including 'angiomatous' and 'neurolemmomatous'[9].

Marked stromal hyalinization may impart an osteoid appearance, a feature originally responsible for designating these tumours 'osteosarcomatoid'. The stromal cells of the fibrohyalinized pattern may be spindled and resemble congenital mesoblastic nephroma, a tumour with a profoundly different prognosis (see Chapter 2).

Differential diagnosis of BMRTC

When proliferation of septal cells is extensive the tumour may be difficult to distinguish from congenital mesoblastic nephroma[13]. The neoplasm may also be confused with cystic partially differentiated nephroblastoma, or, when the cysts are sufficiently prominent, the cystic variant of congenital mesoblastic nephroma[14]. Pre-existing vessels in the tumour may undergo dilatation and form an angiectatic pattern[9].

Distinction between BMRTC and Wilms' tumour

It is imperative to distinguish BMRTC from Wilms' tumour as the two tumours are widely different in prognosis and demand different therapeutic modalities. Beckwith and Larson[13] have outlined pointers to facilitate this differentiation:

(a) A monomorphous pattern favours BMRTC, contrasting with the 'aggregated pattern' of Wilms' tumour.

(b) Wilms' tumour tends to have a 'pushing' border forming a dense pseudocapsule and rounded contours compared with BMRTC, which tends to have 'smoothly irregular' borders with rounded tumour masses isolating individual renal elements. The renal elements are not compressed or pushed aside as in Wilms' tumour.

(c) In BMRTC, the nuclear chromatin is finely dispersed; this contrasts with the coarser chromatin pattern of Wilms' tumour, but exceptions do occur.

(d) The presence of skeletal muscle or foci of definite Wilms' tumour effectively excludes BMRTC.

(e) Bilateral tumours in association with BMRTC, so far, have not been described and nephrogenic rests (nodular renal blastema) (see Chapter 2) are rarely seen with BMRTC.

Ultrastructure of BMRTC

Electron microscopy reveals large vesicular nuclei that are occasionally indented[8,12]. Chromatin is finely granular and evenly dispersed. Nucleoli are inconspicuous. The cytoplasm contains small numbers of mitochondria, rough endoplasmic reticulum and intermediate filaments. Glycogen is absent. True desmosomes are not seen. The optically clear cytoplasm appears to equate with slender cytoplasmic processes (filopodia) extending into 'pools' of pale extracellular matrix.

MALIGNANT RHABDOID TUMOUR OF THE KIDNEY (MRTK)

This is a highly aggressive neoplasm and one of the most lethal of early infancy[15,16]. The largest collection of cases is held by the National Wilms' Tumor Study (NWTS) Center in the United State[16] which reports death rates of about 90%, despite the implementation of modern treatment schedules[14]. Of 111 cases recently reviewed from this source, the tumour was found to predominate in infancy and childhood with a median age of 11 months. MRTK comprised 1.8% of all renal tumours entered in the NWTS. Five patients were under 1 month of age. Males outnumber females (1.5:1). Hypercalcaemia may be the presenting feature[16,17]. The histogenesis of MRTK is still obscure; theories include origin from muscle, neuroectoderm, the histiocyte, epithelium, mesenchyme and mixed mesenchyme/epithelium[16]. Serious consequences of overtreatment are likely to follow an erroneous diagnosis of MRTK.

The tumour was originally designated 'rhabdomyosarcomatoid pattern of Wilms' tumour'[2]. It is encountered less frequently than BMRTC. In common with BMRTC, MRTK has been reported to show a diploid DNA pattern on flow cytometry[11].

Pathology of MRTK

MRTK forms bulky masses largely replacing the kidney[16] (Figure 3.9). Bilateral renal tumours have not been reported. Advanced-stage disease is frequently found at initial presentation and metastases usually involve multiple sites[15]. The medial aspect of the kidney is commonly involved and the pelvic structures consequently are often distorted[16]. The cut surface is usually grey or tan, and haemorrhage and necrosis are observed commonly. The tumour–kidney interface is usually ill-defined. Metastatic disease usually involves multiple sites[15]; the lung is the most commonly involved, followed by liver, brain and bone.

Microscopy reveals a monomorphous tumour composed of sheets, cords or nests of large round or polygonal cells with large eccentric vesicular nuclei and prominent ('owl's eye') nucleoli; the nucleoli are usually single and centrally placed (Figure 3.10)[16]. Mitoses are numerous, but multipolar and bizarre forms are encountered rarely and nuclear pleomorphism is of only moderate degree. Cytoplasm is abundant and eosinophilic. Intracytoplasmic globular hyaline inclusions are a striking feature and an important diagnostic aid (Figure 3.11)[16]. Sclerosing infiltration of the renal medulla is characteristic.

PAS staining shows the inclusions to be negative or only faintly positive[5]. The inclusions vary in number from one area of the tumour to another, and also between different tumours. Their number in the primary tumour and corresponding metastases may be markedly discrepant. Extensive searching may be necessary to find inclusions.

On the other hand, cytoplasmic inclusions may not be detected and reliance should then be placed on other cytological features, notably large nucleoli and abundant cytoplasm[16]. The inclusions in the absence of other cytological features lack specificity since they are found in a number of other (non-rhabdoid) neoplasms; these include favourable histology Wilms' tumour, renal cell carcinoma, transitional cell and collecting duct carcinoma, renal oncocytoma, rhabdomyosarcomas and neuroepithelial tumour[18]. Of these, the most common 'pseudorhabdoid' category is favourable histology Wilms' tumour. Many of these entities may be excluded by virtue of their usual involvement of older patients. Macronucleoli found in some cellular congenital mesoblastic nephroma and renal lymphoma are also a potential source of diagnostic confusion[18].

Immunohistochemically, the tumour cells express vimentin generally corresponding to the location of the intracytoplasmic inclusions (Figure 3.12). The cells are also often positive for epithelial markers (cytokeratin and EMA), and immunoreactivity for muscle-associated antigens (myoglobin and desmin) has been reported[5].

The tumour edge is typically infiltrative and often encompasses pre-existing renal tubules, unlike the edge of most Wilms' tumours which is compressed and accompanied by a pseudocapsule. In common with BMRTC and congenital mesoblastic nephroma, the entrapped renal tubules may undergo a form of embryonal metaplastic epithelial change. Dilatation of the entrapped tubules may produce a multicystic appearance. In some areas the tumour cells of MRTK are spindled and, consequently, congenital mesoblastic nephroma may be mimicked[9].

Histological variation in MRTK

The foregoing description corresponds to the 'classic' microscopic pattern of MRTK. A number of histological variables have been described[16]. These include a sclerosing pattern, epithelioid pattern, spindled pattern, lymphomatoid pattern, and vascular pattern. While most tumours display one or more of these patterns, diligent searching will usually uncover features of the 'classic' pattern. These various groups were outlined in detail by Weeks et al.[16]; they were not significant independent prognostic variables. This wide range of histological patterns raises problems in differential diagnosis, especially so when limited material is presented for diagnosis.

Ultrastructure of MRTK

Ultrastructurally, the most notable feature of the tumour is the presence within the cytoplasm of parallel filaments arranged in concentric large whorled masses (Figure 3.13), often indenting the nucleus[3,5,15,19]. The filaments are of intermediate size (8–10 nm). Lipid droplets, mitochondria or fragments of ergastoplasm are occasionally incorporated within the concentric filamentous array. Nucleolar prominence is confirmed and rudimentary cell junctions and dilated rough endoplasmic reticulum are common. Alternating thick and thin filaments or Z-band material diagnostic of contractile cells are not seen.

MRTK vs. Wilms' tumour

In contrast to Wilms' tumour, MRTK has no known association with dysmorphic syndromes[16]. The tumour usually affects infants and younger children. MRTK is invariably associated with biological aggressiveness and resistance to current forms of therapy. The tumours are also always unilateral and there is no association with nephrogenic rests, or with other histological accompaniments of Wilms' tumour, such as skeletal muscle, adipose tissue or cartilage[16].

MRTK as part of the multiple primary tumour syndrome

An interesting aspect of MRTK is the association with neuroepithelial tumours of the brain, most of which morphologically resemble medulloblastomas[20]. Of the NWTS cases of MRTK, 13.5% are documented as having associated brain tumours[16]. These tumours are usually located in or near the midline, either in the posterior fossa or just above. The brain tumours may precede, coincide with or follow the diagnosis of the renal neoplasm. The primary brain neoplasm should not be mistaken for MRTK metastatic to the brain; as well as being histologically different, the latter also usually occupies the cerebrum[16].

EXTRARENAL RHABDOID TUMOUR

Primary tumours of similar microscopic appearance involving extrarenal sites are discussed in Chapter 13. The sites involved include the thymus, subcutaneous tissue, liver and vulva. The relationship between MRTK and extrarenal rhabdoid tumours is currently enigmatic[21].

REFERENCES

1. Morgan E, Kidd JM. Undifferentiated sarcoma of the kidney. A tumour of childhood with histopathologic and clinical characteristics distinct from Wilms' tumor. Cancer. 1978;42:1916–21.
2. Beckwith JB, Palmer NF. Histopathology and prognosis of Wilms' tumor. Results from the First National Wilms' Tumor Study. Cancer. 1978;41:1937–48.
3. Haas JE, Palmer NF, Weinberg AG et al. Ultrastructure of malignant rhabdoid tumor of the kidney. Hum Pathol. 1981;12:646–57.
4. Gonzalez-Crussi F, Goldschmidt RA, Hsueh W et al. Infantile sarcoma with intracytoplasmic filamentous inclusions. Cancer. 1982;49:2365–75.
5. Tsokos M, Kouraklis G, Chandra RS, Bhagavan BS, Triche TJ. Malignant rhabdoid tumour of the kidney. Arch Pathol Lab Med. 1989;113:115–20.
6. Marsden HB, Lawler W, Kumar PM. Bone metastasizing renal tumor of childhood. Morphological and clinical features, differences from Wilms' tumor. Cancer. 1978;42:1922–8.
7. Marsden HB, Lawler W. Bone-metastasizing renal tumour of childhood. Br J Cancer. 1978;38:437–41.
8. Sotelo-Avila C, Gonzalez-Crussi F, Sadowinski S, Gooch WM, Pena R. Clear cell sarcoma of the kidney: a clinicopathologic study of 21 patients with long-term follow-up evaluation. Hum Pathol. 1986;16:1219–30.
9. Beckwith JB. Wilms' tumor and other renal tumors of childhood: a selective review from the National Wilms' Tumor Study Pathology Center. Hum Pathol. 1983;14:481–92.
10. D'Angio GJ, Breslow N, Beckwith JB et al. Treatment of Wilms' tumor. Results of the Third National Wilms' Tumor Study. Cancer. 1989;64:349–60.
11. Kumar S, Marsden HB, Cowan RA, Barnes JM. Prognostic relevance of DNA content in childhood renal tumours. Br J Cancer. 1989;59:291–5.
12. Haas JE, Bonadio JF, Beckwith B. Clear cell sarcoma of the kidney with emphasis on ultrastructural studies. Cancer. 1984;54:2978–87.
13. Beckwith JB, Larson E. Case 7. Clear cell sarcoma of kidney. Pediatr Pathol. 1989;9:211–18.
14. Beckwith JB. Wilms' tumor and other renal tumors of childhood: an update. J Urol. 1986;136:320–4.
15. Palmer NF, Sutow W. Clinical aspects of the rhabdoid tumor of the kidney: a report of the National Wilms' Tumor Study Group. Med Pediatr Oncol. 1983;11:242–5.
16. Weeks DA, Beckwith JB, Mierau GW, Luckey DW. Rhabdoid tumor of the kidney. A report of 111 cases from the National Wilms' Tumor Study Pathology Center. Am J Surg Pathol. 1989;13:439–58.
17. Jayabose S, Iqbal K, Newman L et al. Hypercalcemia in childhood renal tumors. Cancer. 1988;61:788–91.
18. Weeks DA, Beckwith JB, Mierau GW, Zuppan CW. Renal neoplasms mimicking rhabdoid tumour of the kidney. A report from the National Wilms' Tumor Study Pathology Center. Am J Surg Pathol. 1991;15:1042–54.
19. Fung CHF, Gonzalez-Crussi F, Yonan TN, Martinez N. 'Rhabdoid' Wilms' tumour. Arch Pathol Lab Med. 1981;105:521–3.
20. Bonnin JM, Rubinstein LJ, Palmer NF, Beckwith JB. The association of embryonal tumors originating in the kidney and in the brain. A report of seven cases. Cancer. 1984;54:2137–46.
21. Weeks DA, Beckwith JB, Mierau GW. Rhabdoid tumor. An entity or a phenotype? Arch Pathol Lab Med. 1989;113:113–14.

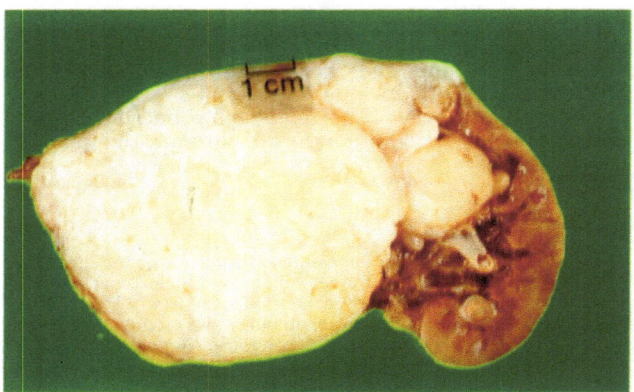

Fig. 3.7 Gross appearance of BMRTC involving the left kidney of an 18-month-old girl. Extensive areas of white fibrous tissue are seen replacing the tumour. Nephrectomy followed a 3-month course of chemotherapy

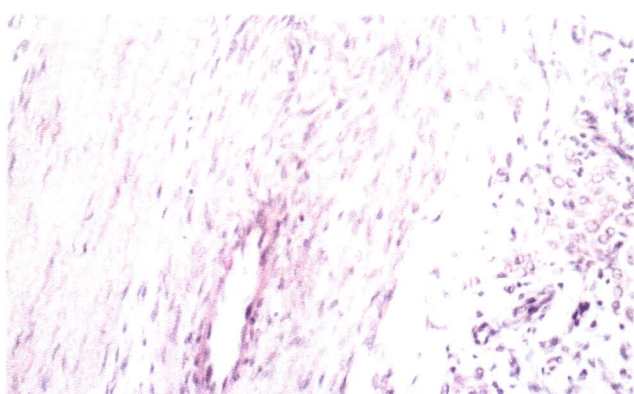

Fig. 3.8 Microscopic view from the same specimen demonstrated in the preceding figure shows an isolated vessel surrounded by dense fibrous tissue in the centre of the field; the 'classic pattern' of the tumour is just seen on the right. H&E × 185

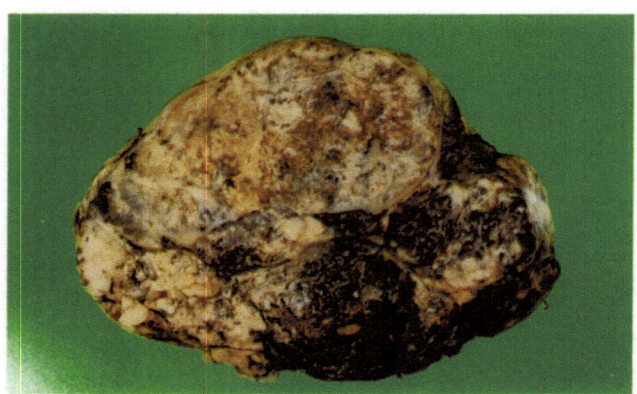

Fig. 3.9 Malignant rhabdoid tumour involving the left kidney of a 3-year-old boy. The cut surface is extensively necrotic and haemorrhagic. The excised specimen weighed 1089 g and measured 16 × 12.5 × 10 cm

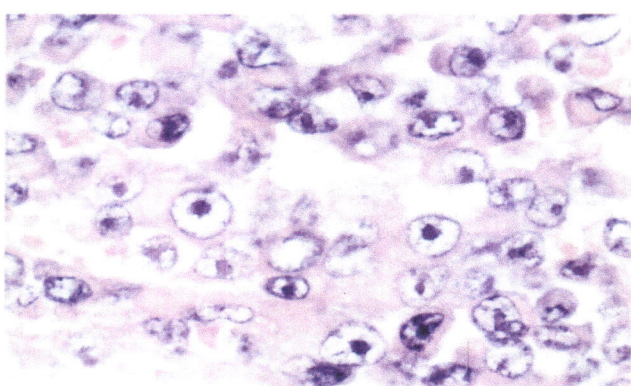

Fig. 3.10 Microscopic view of malignant rhabdoid tumour of the kidney shows a diffuse growth pattern with medium-sized cells in which the nuclei contain large single prominent nucleoli ('macronucleoli'). Cytoplasm is copious and eosinophilic. H&E × 750

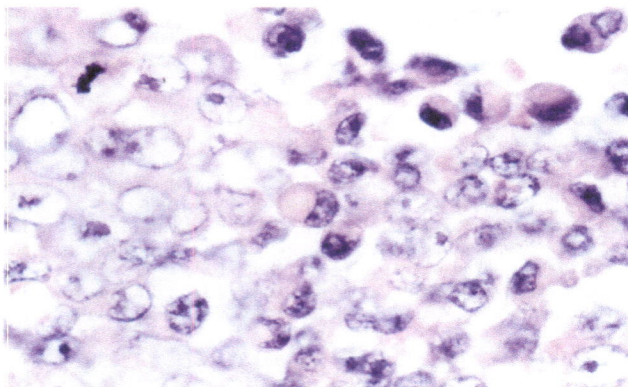

Fig. 3.11 High-magnification view of malignant rhabdoid tumour of the kidney shows several cells with conspicuous intracytoplasmic hyaline globular inclusions. H&E × 750

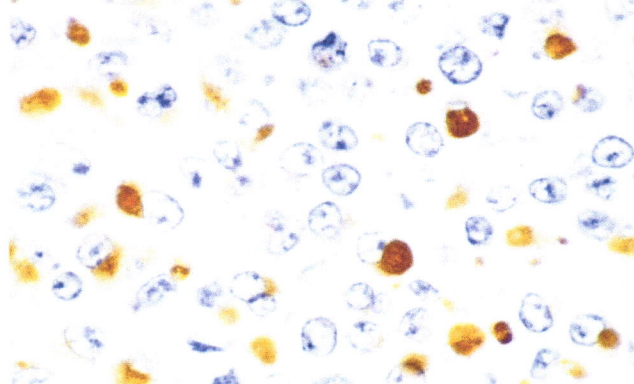

Fig. 3.12 Immunohistochemistry for vimentin demonstrates punctate positivity that corresponds to the cytoplasmic inclusion seen in standard sections. × 750

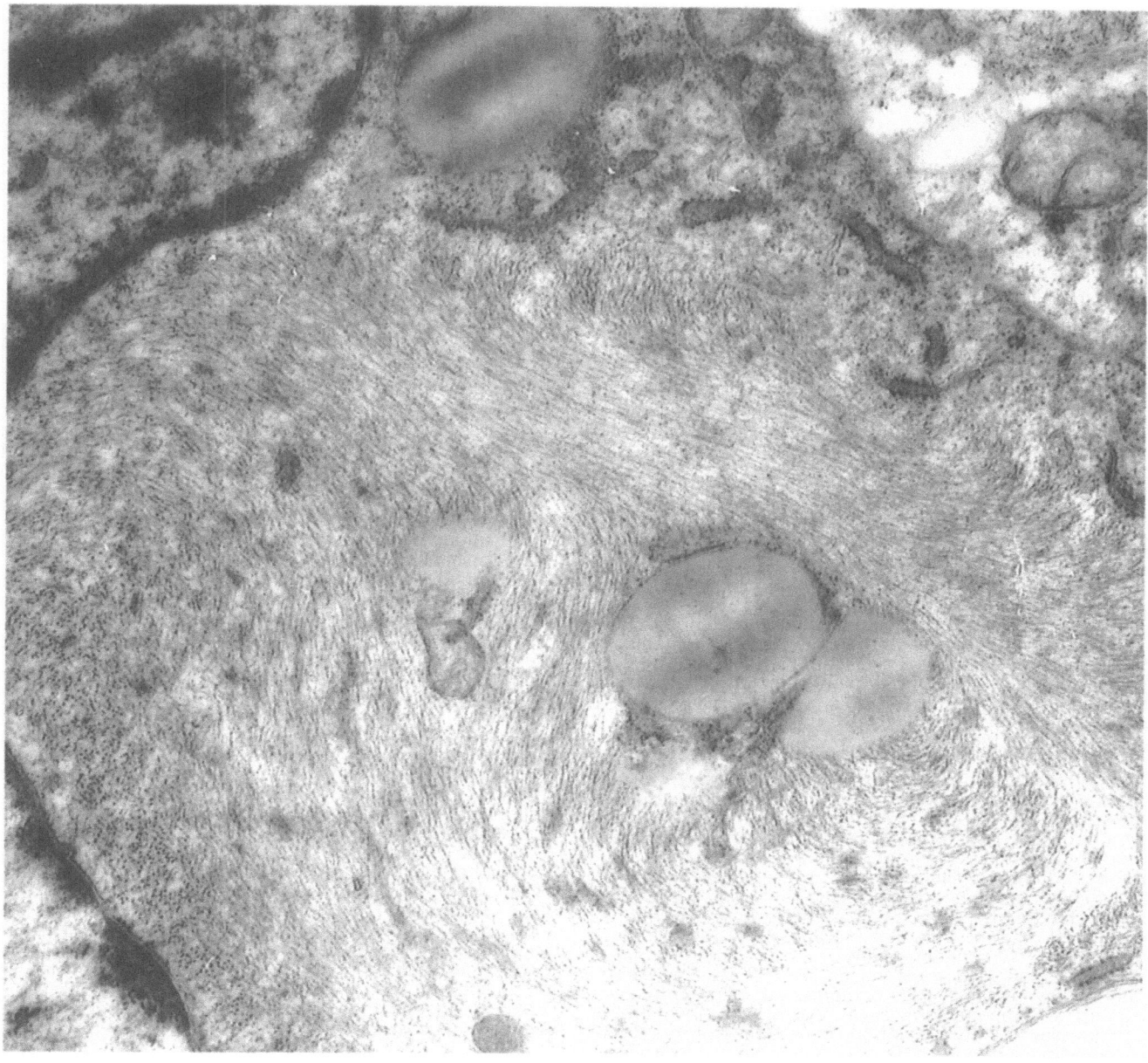

Fig. 3.13 Ultrastructural view of a tumour cell from malignant rhabdoid tumour of kidney reveals an intracytoplasmic whorl of intermediate filaments indenting the nucleus. × 43 000

Malignant lymphoma

4

NON-HODGKIN'S LYMPHOMA

In childhood, non-Hodgkin's lymphoma (NHL) accounts for approximately 60% of lymphomas[1], and for about 10% of all paediatric cancers[2]. These are neoplasms of the immune system in which the malignant cells recapitulate their normal counterparts, morphologically and functionally. The majority of tumours fall within three major subcategories; lymphoblastic lymphoma, Burkitt's lymphoma and large cell ('histiocytic') lymphoma[1,3]. Lymphoblastic and Burkitt's lymphoma account for 80–85% of cases.

Childhood NHL differ from their adult counterparts insofar as they are predominantly extranodal, rarely follicular and often leukaemic[1,3]. They are usually high-grade malignancies, exhibiting rapid cellular proliferation. Paraproteins are rarely secreted and there is a high clinical response rate to treatment. A strong correlation exists between certain histological types and anatomical location, contrasting with the situation usually found in adults.

The vast majority of NHL in children are committed to B- and T-cell lineage[4], and the majority of patients have no apparent underlying disease[2]. Current therapy for NHL is based on careful pathological categorization and accurate clinical staging.

LYMPHOBLASTIC LYMPHOMA

Lymphoblastic lymphoma involves all age groups but is most prevalent in children and adolescents. It accounts for some 35–40% of all childhood NHL[1,3]. In the past, lymphoblastic lymphoma was referred to variously as 'poorly differentiated lymphocytic lymphoma of childhood', 'Sternberg sarcoma', 'lymphosarcoma of childhood' and 'convoluted lymphocytic lymphoma'. Boys are affected more often than girls and the peak age incidence is about 11 years. A mediastinal mass, with or without upper body lymphadenopathy, is a common finding (Figure 4.1)[1,3], and a pleural effusion is often present. The mediastinal mass may compress adjacent structures leading to superior vena cava syndrome or respiratory embarrassment[2]. Spread to bone marrow and progression to leukaemia is seen in at least 50% of patients. Extensive disease at diagnosis is found in most patients with lymphoblastic lymphoma.

A diffuse monomorphous pattern of small cells with round to oval or convoluted nuclei and scant barely discernible cytoplasm is the usual microscopic picture (Figure 4.2)[5]. Chromatin is finely dispersed and there are usually two or more (usually indistinct) nucleoli. Nuclear convolutions are characteristic and are found in more than 80% of tumours (Figure 4.3)[6], but they may be sparse[7,8]. Mitotic figures generally are numerous (about four per high-power field) and a 'starry sky' pattern is related to the presence of macrophages containing phagocytosed cellular debris. This feature is less prominent compared with Burkitt's lymphoma.

Cytoplasmic vacuolation, as seen in Burkitt's lymphoma, is not a feature. Tumour cell cytoplasm displays minimal methyl green pyronine staining. Diffuse diastase-sensitive PAS-positive cytoplasmic staining for glycogen is sometimes present. A paranuclear dot-like acid phosphatase positivity is usually revealed in enzyme histo-chemical preparations.

Immunochemical markers show that the majority of lymphoblastic lymphomas are of T-cell lineage[9]; a smaller number are of B-cell lineage or do not express any such markers (non-B and non-T). Compared with adult cases, paediatric cases show a greater tendency towards a T-cell phenotype[9]. Non-B, non-T lymphoblastic lymphomas often present as skin tumours commonly involving the head and neck region. Intracytoplasmic en-bloc PAS (diastase-sensitive) positivity, similar to that seen in Ewing's sarcoma and rhabdomyosarcoma, may be encountered in non-B, non-T lymphoblastic lymphomas (Figure 4.4).

Forty per cent of T-cell lymphoblastic lymphomas express the common acute lymphoblastic lymphoma surface antigen (CALLA). In tissue sections and bone marrow aspirate preparations, the lymphoblasts of ALL and lymphoblastic lymphoma are indistinguishable[10]. This lack of distinction is also encountered ultrastructurally. These observations have led some investigators to suggest that the two conditions are simply different manifestations of the same disease.

On the other hand, clinical differences do exist between lymphoblastic lymphoma and acute lymphoblastic leukaemia. For example, the majority of patients with lymphoblastic lymphoma have a mediastinal mass and the bone marrow and peripheral blood are usually spared or minimally involved. By contrast, patients with ALL present with massive bone marrow involvement and often blood invasion. The antigenic profile of T-cell lymphoblastic lymphoma and T-cell ALL are similar, but T-cell ALL shows a tendency towards a more immature phenotype[9].

Nuclear convolutions in lymphoblastic lymphoma do not appear to correlate with clinical outcome, nor do they correlate with any pattern of immunostaining[6]. Griffith et al.[6] reported a large-cell variant in 11% of 106 cases of lymphoblastic lymphoma. In the large-cell variant, the lymphoblasts were either larger in size, and/or displayed one or two relatively prominent nucleoli. This variant tended to involve the abdomen. However, the disease-free survival was no different from that of conventional lymphoblastic lymphoma.

BURKITT'S LYMPHOMA

Burkitt's lymphoma (small non-cleaved cell malignant lymphoma), a monoclonal tumour of early B lymphocytes, accounts for about one-third of cases of NHL in childhood[1]. With a cell doubling time of 24 hours, it is the fastest-growing of all human tumours. Burkitt's lymphoma is endemic in para-equatorial Africa and New Guinea, but may occur sporadically throughout the world. This latter form is referred to as sporadic, non-African, non-endemic or American Burkitt's lymphoma.

Endemic and sporadic Burkitt's lymphoma are histologically and immunologically indistinguishable[11] but there are significant clinical differences[12] (Table 4.1). The endemic form affects younger patients and is more frequently associated with Epstein–Barr virus[1,3]. Jaw and gonadal involvement is more common in African Burkitt's lymphoma[12]. The sporadic cases show a higher incidence of pleuropulmonary, gastrointestinal, lymph nodal and bone marrow involvement. An intra-abdominal mass is the usual mode of presentation and the tumour often takes origin from Peyer's patches of the ileocaecal region or mesenteric lymph nodes. Intestinal obstruction or intussusception are recognized complications[3].

Table 4.1 Differences between sporadic and endemic Burkitt's lymphoma

	Sporadic	Endemic
Age	5–10 year age peak	Age incidence more evenly distributed over first 2 decades
Male : female ratio	3 : 1	2 : 1
Anatomical site	Predominantly abdominal	High incidence of jaw tumours
Disease stage at presentation	Limited	Advanced
EBV-DNA+	About 20% of tumours	> 90% of tumours

EBV = Epstein–Barr virus

A diffuse pattern of uniform small non-cleaved cells typifies the histological picture (Figure 4.5)[13]. The cells are larger than normal lymphocytes (but smaller than those of large-cell lymphoma). The nuclei are round to oval, centrally positioned, and display a coarse chromatin pattern with one to several basophilic nucleoli. Nuclear convolutions are absent. The tumour cells reveal a narrow rim of basophilic or amphophilic cytoplasm in which, on close inspection, a coarse vacuolation is most readily appreciated in imprint preparations (Figure 4.6). Mitotic activity is vigorous, and a 'starry sky' pattern is imparted by the many non-neoplastic macrophages containing phagocytosed material (Figure 4.7). This feature of the tumour is non-specific and may be found in the other types of non-Hodgkin's lymphoma; it is especially conspicuous in Burkitt's lymphoma, but is not present in all cases.

Characteristically, the cell cytoplasm is strongly pyroninophilic (Figure 4.8), and neutral fat is commonly demonstrated in the cytoplasmic vacuoles (Figure 4.9). PAS staining is consistently negative.

Burkitt's lymphoma expresses the cytoplasmic and surface immunoglobulin characteristics of a B-cell neoplasm[14]. Other features that support a B-cell origin include morphological similarity with the small non-cleaved germinal centre cell and a tendency for the growth to localize in the germinal centres of focally or partially involved lymph nodes (Figure 4.10). The common acute lymphoblastic lymphoma surface antigen (CALLA) is also frequently present[3]. A 8–14q translocation is commonly observed in the tumour cells[3] and serves as a useful diagnostic marker.

Undifferentiated lymphoma, which predominates in adults, exhibits a similar anatomical distribution, cell morphology and immunological profile to that of Burkitt's lymphoma. However, current opinion questions the value of distinguishing between Burkitt's lymphoma and undifferentiated lymphoma[15].

A leukaemic variant of Burkitt's lymphoma (B-ALL), the smallest group of ALL, constitutes 0.8–2.3% of all leukaemias in children. Extramedullary tumour masses are often coexistent, especially involving the gastrointestinal tract. The cytology of the leukaemic cells is indistinguishable from that seen in Burkitt's lymphoma and, as in Burkitt's lymphoma, cells conform to L3 morphology of the FAB classification of acute lymphoblastic leukaemias in childhood[16]; cytogenetically, they also manifest a 8–14q translocation[16].

Prognosis in Burkitt's lymphoma is compromised by advanced clinical stage, age less than 12 years, and bone marrow involvement[1]. In both endemic and sporadic

forms, using intense combination chemotherapy, a complete response rate can be expected in more than 90% of cases; a relapse rate of 45% is reported and an overall 2-year survival of 54% is obtainable[1].

LARGE-CELL LYMPHOMA

This group of NHL is morphologically and immunologically heterogeneous[1,3], and, of the different types of lymphoma found in children, it is the least well characterized. The different designations that have been applied to this category of lymphoma include 'reticulum cell sarcoma' and 'histiocytic lymphoma'. Large-cell lymphomas make up some 15% of all lymphomas in childhood[3].

Compared with lymphoblastic lymphoma and Burkitt's lymphoma, large-cell lymphoma has a more random anatomical distribution. About 40% of cases affect extranodal sites, including the gastrointestinal tract, bone, skin, nasopharynx, tonsil, lung, mediastinum, gonads and soft tissue[3]. The extranodal tumours tend to be bulky and circumscribed. At diagnosis, osseous and hepatic involvement are unusual and tumour is often limited to one side of the diaphragm.

Microscopically, the size of the nuclei is an important feature in the diagnosis of large-cell lymphoma[3]. The nuclei are larger and cytoplasm is less than seen in reactive histiocytes (Figure 4.11). The mitotic index may be high and a 'starry-sky' pattern and focal necrosis may be encountered[3].

Large-cell lymphoma includes a proportion of tumours with a distinctive antigenic phenotype: Ki-1 (CD30) +ve (Figure 4.12), HLA-DR +ve and EMA +ve[17,18]; a number are negative for leukocyte common antigen (CD45). The tumours are referred to as anaplastic (Ki-1) large-cell lymphomas (or simply Ki-1 lymphoma) and seem to correspond to the largest category of large-cell NHL in the National Cancer Institute Working Formulation – the immunoblastic, polymorphous subtype[19]. The majority express T-cell markers, occasionally a B-cell lineage. Children and adolescents are often affected[17,18,20,21]. In one series of 41 patients with Ki-1 lymphomas, six (15%) were under the age of 17 years[22]. In this age group, Ki-1 lymphoma is the most common peripheral T-cell lymphoma. Peripheral lymphadenopathy and skin lesions are the most common form of clinical presentation[23], often accompanied by systemic symptoms, such as fever, weight loss and nausea. Tumour limited to the skin has a potential for spontaneous regression[20]. The translocation (t(2;5)(p23;q35)) appears to be specific for Ki-1 lymphoma[24].

Microscopically[17,22,23], the tumour shows a cohesive growth pattern of large cells with prominent pleomorphic nuclei, abundant basophilic cytoplasm, and a high mitotic rate. The lymph node is often only partially involved and follicles may be spared. There is a predilection for paracortical involvement and intrasinusoidal dissemination. Multinucleate giant cells are common, as are fibrosis, plasma cell infiltrates and wreath-like cells, the latter sometimes resembling Reed–Sternberg cells (Figure 4.13)[17,23]. Erythrophagocytosis by tumour cells may be seen (Figure 4.14)[18,21], mimicking a histiocytic malignancy. In a case reported by Dehner[20], overt anaplasia was lacking and the microscopic picture was 'histiocytic'.

Regressive atypical histiocytosis of skin reported by Flynn et al.[25] (see Chapter 8) is almost certainly an example of anaplastic (Ki-1) lymphoma[23]. In the past, many Ki-1 lymphomas were probably misdiagnosed as malignant histiocytosis or metastatic carcinoma[17]. Some cases may be difficult to distinguish from Hodgkin's disease[17]. Histiocytic sarcoma, granulocytic sarcoma, Ewing's sarcoma, alveolar rhabdomyosarcoma, malignant

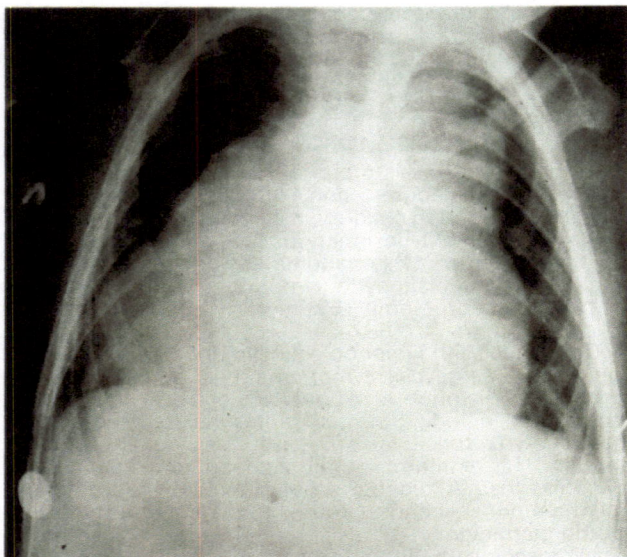

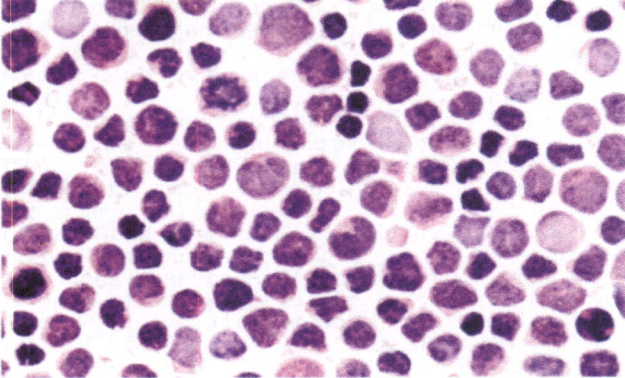

Fig. 4.2 Microscopically, lymphoblastic lymphoma shows a diffuse monomorphous small cell pattern with round-to-ovoid nuclei and a rim of barely discernible cytoplasm. Chromatin is finely dispersed and two or more indistinct nucleoli are present. H&E × 750

Fig. 4.1 Chest X-ray reveals a large anterior mediastinal mass in a young child with lymphoblastic lymphoma

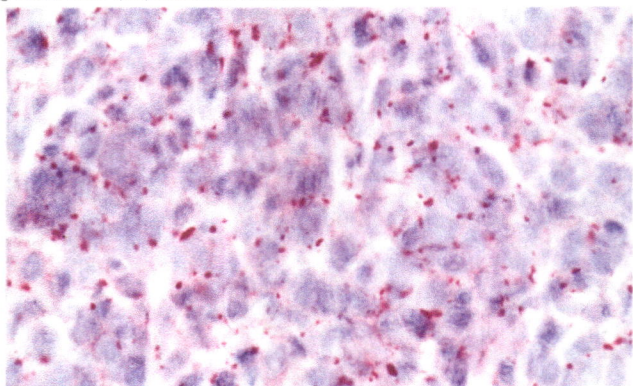

Fig. 4.3 Cytological preparation from lymphoblastic lymphoma reveals tumour cells with scant cytoplasm and frequent nuclear convolutions. H&E × 750

Fig. 4.4 Cutaneous lymphoma of lymphoblastic type from the forehead of a child. Immunohistochemistry showed a non-B,non-T phenotype. Intracytoplasmic *en bloc* PAS positivity is shown in frozen section. The picture should not be confused with other small-cell tumours known to be associated with intracytoplasmic *en bloc* positivity (e.g. Ewing's sarcoma and rhabdomyosarcoma). PAS × 750

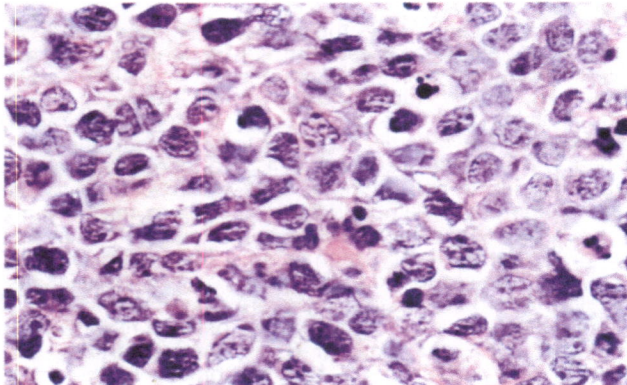

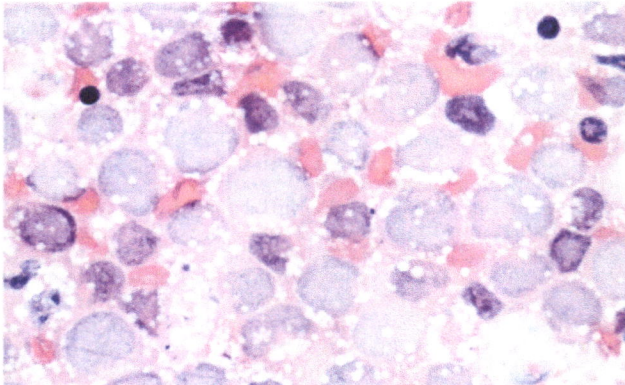

Fig. 4.5 The tumour cells of Burkitt's lymphoma are uniform in size with a round-to-ovoid centrally positioned nucleus and a thin rim of basophilic cytoplasm. Nuclear convolutions are absent and two or more nucleoli are generally present. H&E × 750

Fig. 4.6 Imprint preparation of Burkitt's lymphoma reveals small but prominent vacuoles in the cytoplasm of the tumour cells. H&E × 750

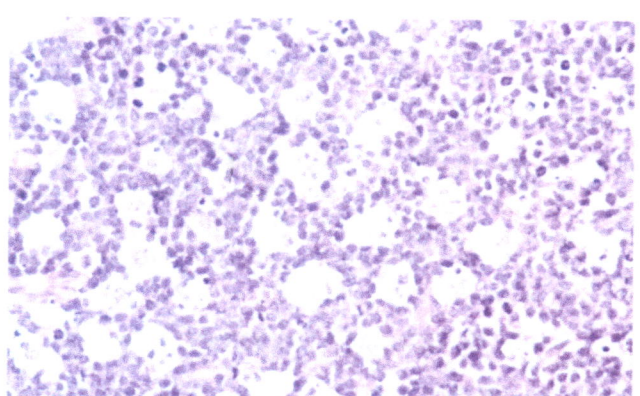

Fig. 4.7 The biopsied tissue shows Burkitt's lymphoma in which there are scattered macrophages with ingested cellular debris, imparting a 'starry-sky' pattern. The patient was a 13-year-old boy who was found to have a large anterior mediastinal mass (an atypical location for Burkitt's lymphoma). H&E × 300

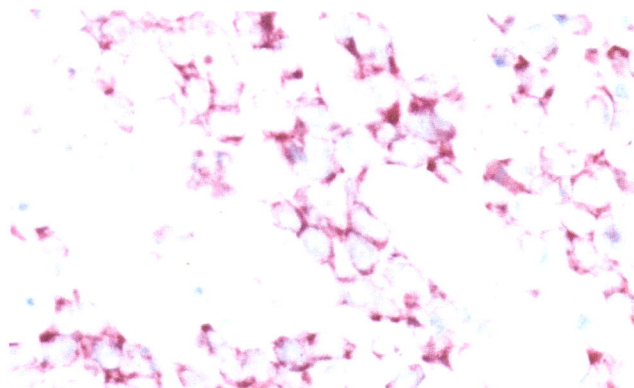

Fig. 4.8 Strong cytoplasmic pyroninophilia is demonstrated in the tumour cells from a Burkitt's lymphoma. Methyl green-pyronin × 750

Fig. 4.9 Cytological preparation of Burkitt's lymphoma stained with Oil-red O shows neutral fat within the numerous cytoplasmic vacuoles. ORO × 750

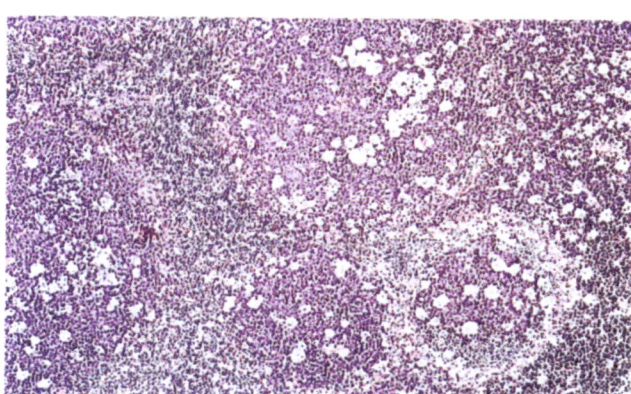

Fig. 4.10 A relatively low-magnification view of intra-abdominal Burkitt's lymphoma to show partial involvement of lymphoid follicles. H&E × 75

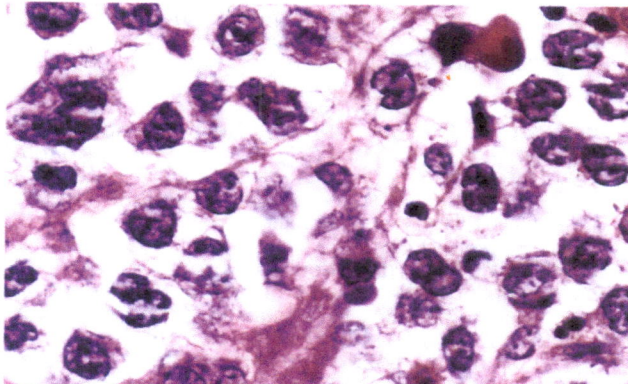

Fig. 4.11 The microscopic field is of large-cell lymphoma. The large size of the nuclei is an important diagnostic feature. The nuclei are also vesicular with prominent nucleoli; the cytoplasm is relatively scant. The patient was a 3-year-old boy who presented with a large mass in the right iliac fossa which was diagnosed as anaplastic (Ki-1) lymphoma. H&E × 750

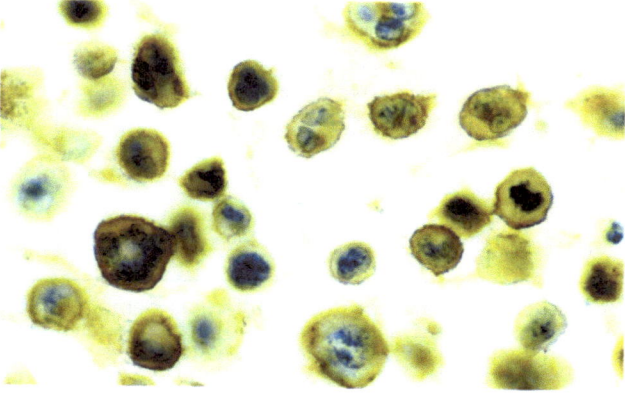

Fig. 4.12 Prominent membranous positivity for Ki-1 antigen is observed in the tumour cells of anaplastic large-cell lymphoma. × 750

histiocytosis, (dys)germinoma and undifferentiated carcinoma are other tumours that enter the differential diagnosis.

HISTIOCYTIC LYMPHOMA

A small number of large-cell lymphomas express markers that conform to a histiocytic lineage[3]. Such markers include lysozyme (muramidase) and α_1-antichymotrypsin, as well as enzyme histochemistry for acid phosphatase. Tumours expressing this profile should be regarded as truly histiocytic. In contrast with malignant histiocytosis, the tumour is localized[26], although progression to malignant histiocytosis may occur.

HODGKIN'S DISEASE

This is primarily a disease of young adults but an appreciable number of cases involve children and adolescents[27]. Children make up about 10% of all cases of Hodgkin's disease, although the incidence among children is considerably greater in underdeveloped countries[28,29]. Hodgkin's disease rarely arises in children less than 2 years old. The youngest patient in Poppema and Lennert's series[27] was 22 months. A cure rate of some 80% may be expected with current therapeutic regimens. Childhood Hodgkin's disease affects significantly more boys than girls[30,31]. The aetiology of the disease remains enigmatic.

Painless lymph node enlargement, generally affecting the cervical region, is the usual mode of clinical presentation[30]. Extranodal involvement is rare. Concomitant involvement of the mediastinal lymph nodes, identified by imaging techniques, is found in almost half of the patients. However, primary mediastinal lymph node involvement is unusual. Involvement of bone, liver and lung is usually part of widespread disease. The Ann Arbor system is currently widely used for staging purposes[32] (Table 4.2). The stages are further divided into A and B categories, in which A indicates the absence of symptoms and B indicates the presence of symptoms, such as weight loss, unexplained fever or night sweats. Systemic features occur in about 40% of patients. The extent of the disease at first presentation is the most important determinant of clinical outcome. With the marked improvement in treatment, histological grading has taken on less prognostic significance[3]. A change in histological subtype during the course of the disease is reported to occur in 2–10% of cases[33].

Table 4.2 Ann Arbor staging system for Hodgkin's disease

Stage I:	Involvement of a single lymph node region (I) or of a single extralymphatic organ or site (Ie).
Stage II:	Involvement of one or two lymph node regions on the same side of the diaphragm or localized involvement of extralymphatic organ or site and one or more lymph node regions on the same side of diaphragm.
Stage III:	Involvement of lymph node regions on both sides of diaphragm, which may also be accompanied by localized involvement of an extralymphatic organ or site, or of the spleen, or both.
Stage IV:	Diffuse or disseminated involvement of one or more extralymphatic organs or tissues, with or without associated lymph node involvement.

Diagnosis depends on the histological demonstration of Reed–Sternberg cells. These are large binucleate or multinucleate cells with moderately abundant cytoplasm and a characteristic halo around a large eosinophilic or amphophilic nucleolus (Figure 4.15). The cytoplasm is strongly pyroninophilic. Mononuclear variants of the Reed–Sternberg cell, also referred to as Hodgkin's cells, are also usually present. Reed–Sternberg-like cells are diagnostically non-specific and may be seen in other conditions, e.g. infectious mononucleosis, metastatic carcinoma[3] and some forms of large-cell lymphoma[17]. Hodgkin's disease should therefore be diagnosed against the background cellularity as well as adhering strictly to criteria in identifying the Reed–Sternberg cell. The precise nature of the Reed–Sternberg cell is unknown. Different morphological types of Reed–Sternberg cell are associated with the different subtypes of Hodgkin's disease. 'Mummified' Reed–Sternberg cells are cells that have undergone degeneration (Figure 4.16); their nuclei are pyknotic and the cytoplasm hyalinized and deeply eosinophilic.

IMMUNOHISTOCHEMISTRY OF HODGKIN'S DISEASE

The Reed–Sternberg cell of Hodgkin's disease and the Hodgkin's cell (mononuclear variant) manifest strong immunoreactivity for Ki-1 (CD30). Reed–Sternberg cells also express intracytoplasmic IgG kappa and lambda chains[3] as well as Leu-M1 (CD 15), an antibody that reacts primarily with cells of granulocytic lineage[33]. None of these antibodies, however, mark specifically for Hodgkin's disease. Variability in staining pattern is reported and immunohistochemical results should not be accepted uncritically[33]. About 80% of the small lymphocytes in Hodgkin's disease are T cells. The antigenic profile of the L&H variant of the Reed–Sternberg cell is discussed below.

CLASSIFICATION OF HODGKIN'S DISEASE

The histological system most widely accepted is that originally proposed by Lukes and Butler[34], later modified at the Rye symposium[35].

Nodular sclerosing Hodgkin's disease

This is the most common subtype of Hodgkin's disease found in childhood in Europe and North America where it accounts for some 50–75% of all cases[33]. The mediastinum is commonly involved. Naked eye study may reveal coarse nodularity on the cut surface of the lymph node (Figure 4.17). The microscopic diagnosis depends on demonstrating a banded type of sclerosis that completely or partially divides the lymphoid tissue into nodules[33]. This pattern may be enhanced with a stain for reticulin (Figure 4.18). The nodules are composed of a mixture of varying combination of neoplastic and reactive cells. The neoplastic component is represented by lacunar cells and classic Reed–Sternberg cells (Figure 4.15); lymphocytes, plasma cells, histiocytes and eosinophils comprise the reactive component. Classic Reed–Sternberg cells are often sparse; pleomorphic Reed–Sternberg cells are more readily detected (Figure 4.19).

The lacunar cell, a variant of the Reed–Sternberg cell, is characterized by abundant pale-staining cytoplasm that frequently retracts in formalin-fixed paraffin-embedded tissues, leaving a clear space or 'lacuna' around the cell (Figure 4.20). The lacunar cells may occur singly, in clusters or sheets (Figure 4.21)[33].

The sclerosis takes precedence over other criteria and a single band of collagen is sufficient for the diagnosis. Fibrosis often commences in the capsule and later extends into the nodal parenchyma. The degree of fibrosis correlates with the duration of disease and may be so extensive that lacunar cells and Reed–Sternberg cells are difficult to identify. The reactive component of nodular sclerosis varies considerably from being lymphocyte predominant, through mixed cellularity to lymphocyte depletion.

Two patterns of nodular sclerosing Hodgkin's disease are recognized. The Type 1 pattern shows nodules that exhibit lymphocyte predominance or mixed cellularity. An extensive search may be necessary to detect classic Reed–Sternberg cells. In the Type 2 pattern, more than half of the nodules show lymphocyte depletion or a mixed cellularity pattern. The majority of the Reed–Sternberg cells are of the lacunar type but pleomorphic Reed–Sternberg cells are also frequently found. There is conspicuous infiltration by polymorphs and plasma cells, and necrosis, which is often present, may simulate necrotizing lymphadenitis or cat-scratch disease[3].

Lymphocyte predominance Hodgkin's disease

Histologically, lymphocytic and histiocytic (L&H) predominance subtype of Hodgkin's disease shows effacement of the normal nodal architecture. There is a background of normal-looking mature lymphocytes admixed with a variable population of reactive histiocytes and the L&H variant of the Reed–Sternberg cell. The latter cells, also referred to as 'popcorn' cells, are an important factor in the diagnosis; they have a large complex polypoid nucleus with a fine chromatin pattern and small indistinct nucleoli (Figure 4.22). The L&H cell has a distinctive immunological profile: CD 45 +ve, CD 30 +ve, EMA +ve, J chain +ve; Leu-M1 (CD 15) −ve[33]. Classic Reed–Sternberg cells are required to establish the diagnosis, however, but are generally difficult to find. A few normal follicles may be seen at the edge of the tissue.

Nodular and diffuse variants of lymphocyte predominance Hodgkin's disease are recognized[3,33]. A nodular pattern occurs in about one third of cases. In this pattern, the nodules are larger, more irregular than normal follicles, and generally ill-defined, but may be enhanced by reticulin staining. They are separated by less cellular areas containing scattered blood vessels. Epithelioid histiocytes, which may occur singly or form microgranulomata, and the L&H cells, impart a mottled appearance to the nodules. L&H cells are numerous in this variant whereas plasma cells and eosinophils are generally sparse.

In the diffuse pattern the nodal architecture is effaced by an infiltration of lymphocytes. The L&H variant of Reed–Sternberg cells and classic Reed–Sternberg cells are usually difficult to find.

Hodgkin's disease mixed cellularity

The microscopic picture of this subtype covers a wide spectrum between lymphocyte predominance and lymphocyte depletion Hodgkin's disease[3]. Classic Reed–Sternberg cells and Hodgkin's cells are easy to find and, while other variants of Reed–Sternberg cells may also be seen, they are in the minority. The reactive component comprises lymphocytes, histiocytes, plasma cells, neutrophils and eosinophils that are often present in considerable numbers (Figure 4.23). A connective tissue reaction lacks the banded pattern found in the nodular sclerosis subtype.

Identification of mixed cellularity is subject to error as the microscopic picture is likely to overlap other subtypes[33]; these include the lymphocyte predominance subtype with undue prominence of classic Reed–Sternberg cells, nodular sclerosis in the cellular phase with lacunar cells but lacking banded sclerosis, or lymphocyte depletion with an undue prominence of pleomorphic Reed–Sternberg cells.

Lymphocyte depletion Hodgkin's disease

This uncommon subtype of Hodgkin's disease is seen mainly in late adult life[33]. It is the least common subtype found in children. Reticular and diffuse fibrosis are recognized subcategories. Extranodal sites are often involved and, microscopically, mononuclear cells, Reed–Sternberg cells and disorderly fibrosis are characteristic features, in addition to a depletion of lymphocytes. Atypical pleomorphic Reed–Sternberg cells are seen frequently. When fibrosis is severe, Reed–Sternberg cells may be difficult to find. Many of the cases previously diagnosed as lymphocyte depletion Hodgkin's disease, in fact, may have been examples of T-cell lymphoma or nodular sclerosis Hodgkin's disease[3].

GRANULOCYTIC SARCOMA (CHLOROMA)

This is a rare tumour composed of granulocytic precursors[36]; it involves a wide age range, but children are often affected. 'Chloroma' is an alternative designation, based on the greenish colour of the tumour produced by myeloperoxidase in the tumour cells. The colour fades on exposure to air.

Leukaemia, usually myeloid in type, is frequently associated, or may even follow the appearance of the tumour[37,38]. The usual anatomical sites are bone, soft tissue, lymph node and skin[36]. The orbit is most commonly affected and is seen in 2–8% of all patients with acute myelogenous leukaemia.

A range of histological appearances is determined by the degree of cellular differentiation of the tumour[36]. Poorly differentiated tumours (Figure 4.24) resemble non-Hodgkin's lymphoma. Abundant granulocytes, including eosinophils, are present in the better-differentiated tumours. The presence of eosinophils is an important clue to diagnosis in the less differentiated tumours, and histochemistry for chloroacetate esterase (CAE) and lysozyme may be helpful[36].

REFERENCES

1. Callihan TR, Berard CW. Childhood non-Hodgkin's lymphomas in current histological perspective. Perspect Pediatr Pathol. 1982;7:259–77.
2. Kjeldsberg CR, Wilson JF, Berard CW. Non-Hodgkin's lymphoma in children. Hum Pathol. 1983;14:612–27.
3. Bernard A, Murphy SB, Melvin S et al. Non-T, non-B lymphomas are rare in childhood and associated with cutaneous tumor. Blood. 1982;59:549–54.
4. Smith SD, Rubin CM, Horvath A, Nachman J. Non-Hodgkin's lymphoma in children. Semin Oncol. 1990;17:113–19.
5. Wright DH, Isaacson PG. Biopsy pathology of the lymphoreticular system. London: Chapman and Hall, 1983; 230.
6. Griffith RC, Kelly DR, Nathwani BN et al. A morphological study of childhood lymphoma of the lymphoblastic type. The Pediatric Oncology Group Experience. Cancer. 1987;59:1126–31.
7. Nathwani BN, Diamond LW, Winberg CD et al. Lymphoblastic lymphoma: a clinicopathologic study of 95 patients. Cancer. 1981;48:2347–57.
8. Long JC, McCaffrey RP, Aisenberg AC, Marks SM, Kung PC. Terminal deoxynucleotidyl transferase positive lymphoblastic lymphoma. Cancer. 1979;44:2127–39.
9. Weiss LM, Bindl JM, Picozzi VJ, Link MP, Warnke RA. Lymphoblastic lymphoma: an immunophenotype study of 26 cases with comparison to T cell acute lymphocytic leukemia. Blood. 1986;67:474–8.
10. Pinkel D, Johnson W, Aur RJA. Non-Hodgkin's lymphoma in children. Br J Cancer. 1975;31(Suppl.2):298–323.
11. Wright DH, Isaacson PG. Biopsy pathology of the lymphoreticular system. London: Chapman & Hall; 1983:190.
12. Magrath IT. African Burkitt's lymphoma. History, biology, clinical features, and treatment. Am J Pediatr Hematol/Oncol. 1991;13:222–46.
13. Crist WM, Kelly DR, Ragab AH et al. Predictive ability of Lukes-Collins classification for immunologic phenotypes of childhood non-Hodgkin's lymphoma: an institutional series and literature review. Cancer. 1981;48:2070–5.
14. Mann RB, Jaffe ES, Braylan RC et al. Non-endemic Burkitt's lymphoma: a B-cell tumor related to germinal centers. N Engl J Med. 1976;295:685–91.

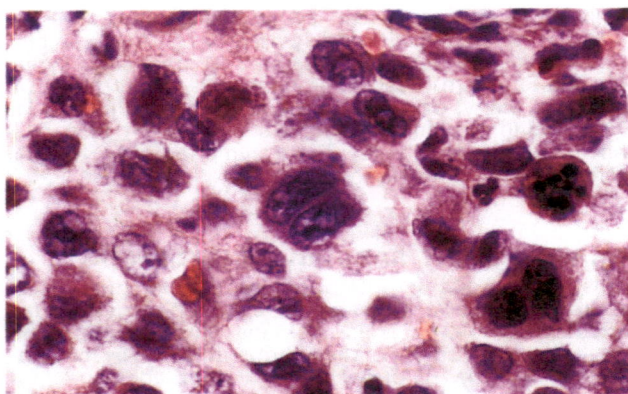

Fig. 4.13 Anaplastic (Ki-1) lymphoma. Same tumour as that shown in Figure 4.12. The binucleate cell in the centre of the field is reminiscent of a Reed–Sternberg cell. H&E × 750

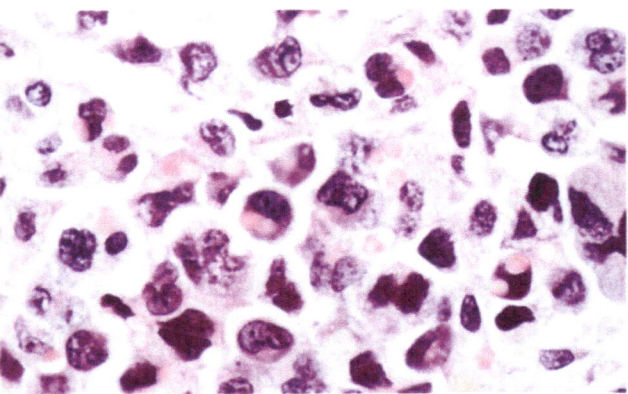

Fig. 4.14 Microscopic view of anaplastic (Ki-1) lymphoma demonstrates several of the tumour cells undergoing erythrophagocytosis; this appearance may lead to an erroneous diagnosis of malignant histiocytosis. H&E × 750

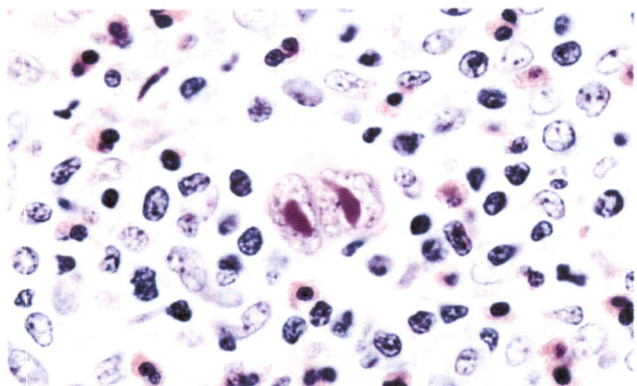

Fig. 4.15 A classic binucleated Reed–Sternberg cell from a lymph node in a 10-year-old boy with mixed-cellularity Hodgkin's disease. The patient presented with an enlarged node in the right axilla. H&E × 750

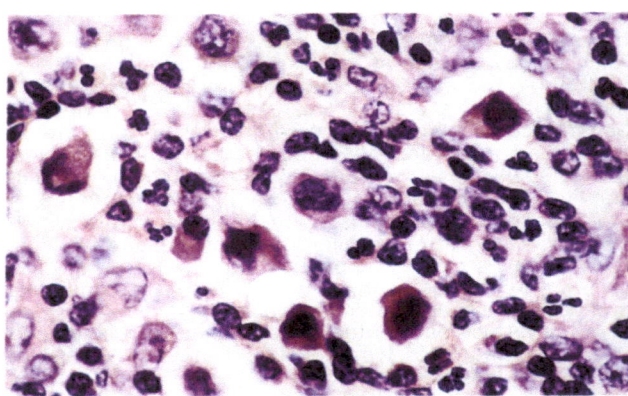

Fig. 4.16 Degenerate Reed–Sternberg cells with pyknotic nuclei and condensed deeply eosinophilic cytoplasm have diminished diagnostic potential and are referred to as 'mummified' cells. H&E × 750

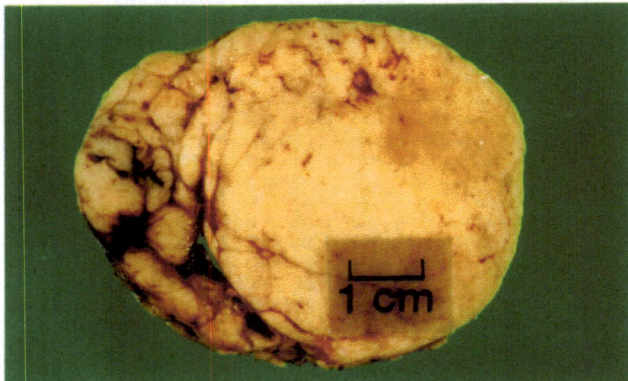

Fig. 4.17 The nodularity is conspicuous on the cut surface of this enlarged lymph node from the right axilla of a 6-year-old girl with nodular sclerosing Hodgkin's disease

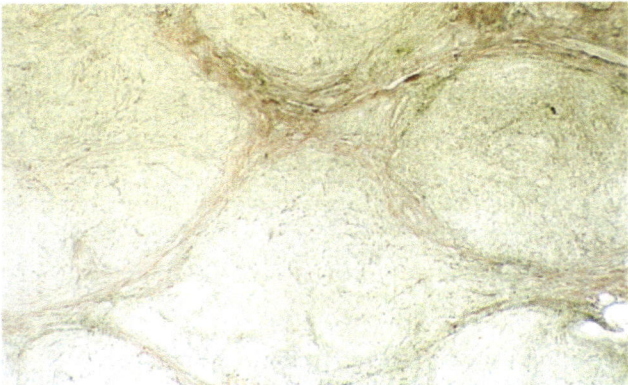

Fig. 4.18 The nodularity of nodular sclerosing Hodgkin's disease is accentuated by a stain for reticulin. The patient was a 10-year-old boy who presented with left cervical lymphadenopathy. Gomori reticulin × 30

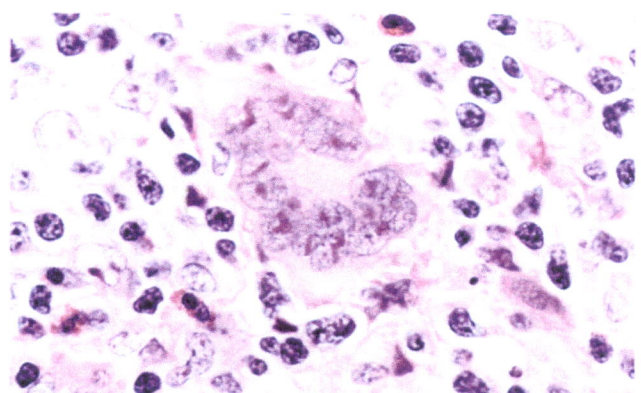

Fig. 4.19 The microscopic field reveals a large multinucleate cell with a peripheral distribution of nuclei representing the so-called 'penny on a platter' appearance. This multinuclear (or pleomorphic) variant of the Reed–Sternberg cell is a feature of nodular sclerosing Hodgkin's disease. H&E × 750

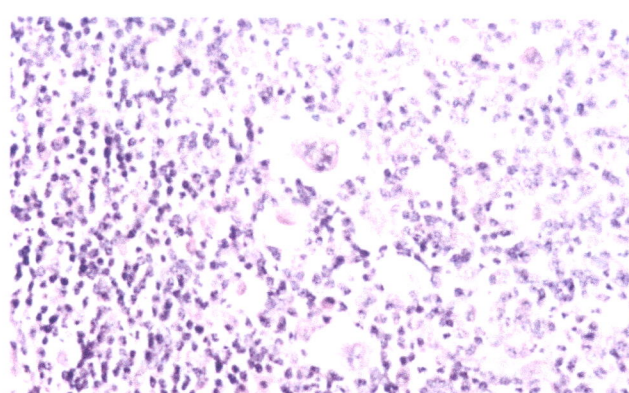

Fig. 4.20 This shows a cluster of lacunar-type Reed–Sternberg cells in a lymph node from a child with nodular sclerosing Hodgkin's disease. H&E × 300

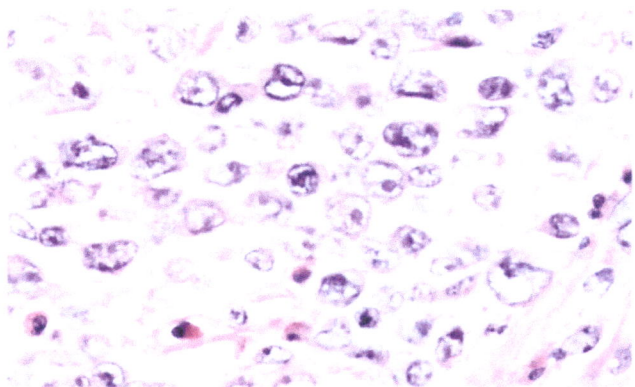

Fig. 4.21 This demonstrates a sheet of lacunar cells in a lymph node from a child with nodular sclerosing Hodgkin's lymphoma. This microscopic appearance, if widespread, may cause diagnostic confusion. H&E × 750

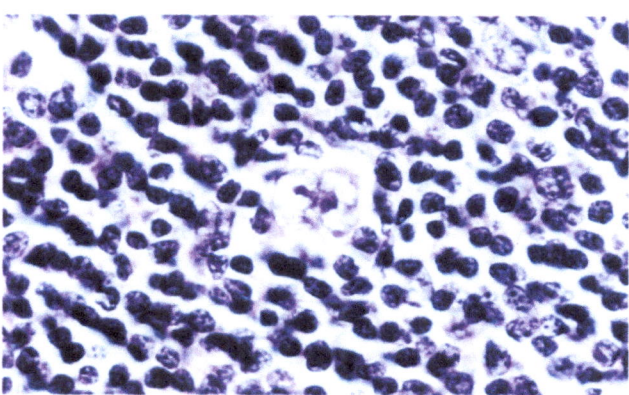

Fig. 4.22 The polylobated cell in the centre of the field is the L&H variant of the Reed–Sternberg cell and is characteristic of lymphocyte-predominant Hodgkin's disease. The enlarged cervical lymph node was resected from a 4-year-old boy. H&E × 750

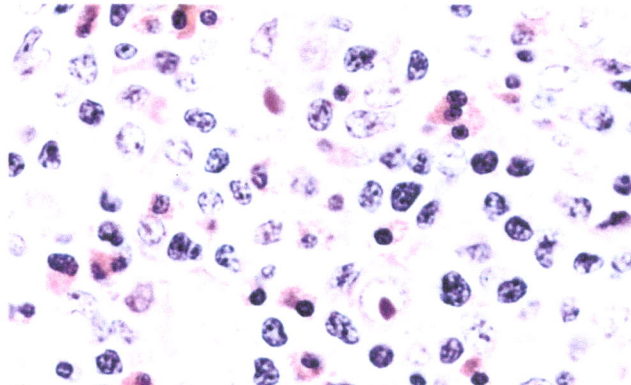

Fig. 4.23 Microscopic view of mixed-cellularity Hodgkin's disease showing mononuclear Reed–Sternberg cells set against a background of lymphocytes and many eosinophils. H&E × 750

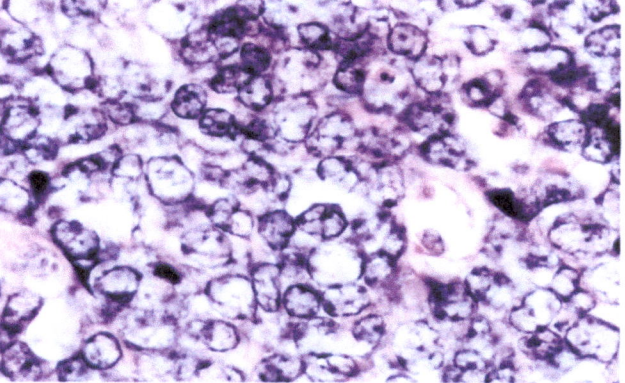

Fig. 4.24 Microscopic view of granulocytic sarcoma shows tumour cells without distinctive histological features. The patient was a 3-year-old boy who had a large retro-orbital tumour on the right side causing marked proptosis. The blood count was at first normal, but subsequently changed to one of acute myelogenous leukaemia. H&E × 750

15. Kelly DR, Nathwani BN, Griffith RC et al. A morphological study of childhood lymphoma of the undifferentiated type. The Pediatric Oncology Group Experience. Cancer. 1987;59:1132–7.
16. Gresik MV, Fernbach DJ. Leukemia in childhood. In: Finegold M, editor. Pathology of neoplasia in children and adolescents. Philadelphia: W B Saunders; 1986:46–86.
17. Schnitzer B, Roth MS, Hyder DM, Ginsburg D. Ki-1 lymphomas in children. Cancer. 1988;61:1213–21.
18. Oka K, Mori N, Kojima M, Iijima T, Hanada T, Tsuchida M. Childhood Ki-1 lymphoma. A report of two cases. Arch Pathol Lab Med. 1989;113:998–1002.
19. Hutchinson RE, Fairclough DL, Holt H, Pui CH, Sandlund JT, Berard CW. Clinical significance of histology and immunophenotype in childhood diffuse large cell lymphoma. Am J Clin Pathol. 1991;95:787–93.
20. Dehner LP. Case 5. Ki-1 lymphoma. Pediatr Pathol. 1991;11:183–90.
21. Kadin ME, Sako D, Berliner N et al. Childhood Ki-1 lymphoma presenting with skin lesions and peripheral lymphadenopathy. Blood. 1986;68:1042–9.
22. Chott A, Kaserer K, Augustin I et al. Ki-1-positive large cell lymphoma. A clinicopathologic study of 41 cases. Am J Surg Pathol. 1990;14:439–48.
23. Agnarsson BA, Kadin ME. Ki-1 positive large cell lymphoma. A morphologic and immunologic study of 19 cases. Am J Surg Pathol. 1988;12:264–74.
24. Bitter MA, Franklin WA, Larson RA et al. Morphology in Ki-1 (CD30)-positive non-Hodgkin's lymphoma is correlated with clinical features and the presence of a unique chromosomal abnormality, t(2;5)(p23;q35). Am J Surg Pathol. 1990;14:305–16.
25. Flynn KJ, Dehner LP, Gajl-Peczalska KJ, Dahl MV, Ramsay N, Wang N. Regressing atypical histiocytosis: a cutaneous proliferation of atypical neoplastic histiocytes with unexpected indolent biological behaviour. Cancer. 1982;49:959–70.
26. Wright DH, Isaacson PG. Biopsy pathology of the lymphoreticular system. London: Chapman & Hall; 1983:246.
27. Poppema S, Lennert K. Hodgkin's disease in childhood. Histopathologic classification in relation to age and sex. Cancer. 1980; 45:1443–7.
28. Solidoro A, Guzman C, Chang A. Relative increased incidence of childhood Hogkin's disease in Peru. Cancer Res. 1966;26:1204–8.
29. Olweny CLM, Katongole-Mbidde E, Kirre C, Lwanga SK, Magrath I, Ziegler J. Childhood Hodgkin's disease in Uganda: a 10 year experience. Cancer. 1978;42:787–92.
30. White L, McCourt BA, Isaacs H, Siegel SE, Stowe SM, Higgins GR. Patterns of Hodgkin's disease at diagnosis in young children. Am J Pediatr Hematol/Oncol. 1983;5:251–7.
31. Kung FH. Hodgkin's disease in children 4 years of age or younger. Cancer. 1991;67:1428–30.
32. Murphy SB. Classification staging and end-results of treatment of childhood non-Hodgkin's lymphomas: dissimilarities from lymphomas in adults. Semin Oncol. 1980;7:332–9.
33. Lee FD. Hodgkin's disease revisited. In: Anthony PP, McSween RNM, editors. Recent advances in histopathology. Edinburgh: Churchill Livingstone; 1989:79–96.
34. Lukes RJ, Butler JJ. The pathology and nomenclature of Hodgkin's disease. Cancer Res. 1966;26:1063–81.
35. Lukes RJ, Craver LF, Hall TC et al. Report of the nomenclature committee. Cancer Res. 1966;26:1311.
36. Neiman RS, Barcos M, Berard C et al. Granulocytic sarcoma: a clinicopathologic study of 61 biopsied cases. Cancer. 1981; 48:1426–37.
37. Brooks HW, Evans AE, Glass RM, Pang EM. Chloromas of the head and neck in childhood. Arch Otolaryngol. 1974;100:306–8.
38. Rajantie J, Tarkkanen A, Rapola J, Merenmies L, Perkkio M, Siimes MA. Orbital granulocytic sarcoma as a presenting sign in acute myelogenous leukemia. Ophthalmologica, Basel. 1984;189:158–61.

Neuroblastoma complex

5

Neuroblastoma is the archetypal and most common variant of peripheral primitive neuroectodermal tumour[1]. The third commonest solid malignant tumour of infancy and childhood, it is surpassed only by neoplasms of the lymphoid tissue and cerebral tumours[2,3]. It constitutes some 8–10% of all cancers seen in patients up to the age of 15 years. Ninety per cent of neuroblastomas occur in patients less than 10 years old[4]. The usual age at presentation is between birth and 5 years and boys are slightly more often affected than girls.

The tumour arises from the neuroblast, the precursor cell of autonomic neurons. Most probably derive from adrenergic neuroblasts, although some tumours may take origin from cholinergic neuroblasts[5]. Intra-abdominal tumours are the most common, arising in the adrenal medulla or paraspinal sympathetic ganglia. Extra-abdominal locations, in order of decreasing frequency, are the posterior mediastinum[6] and cervical region[7]. Large adrenal tumours may be difficult to distinguish from those arising from the paraspinal sympathetic chain. Paraspinal tumours may insinuate through the intervertebral foramina and cause spinal cord compression[8]. Such dumb-bell tumours may originate directly from the posterior root ganglia[9]. A staging system by Brodeur et al.[10] is outlined in Table 5.1. At diagnosis, the majority of patients have Stage IV disease[5]. Calcification within the tumour is often demonstrated radiologically.

Table 5.1 Staging system for neuroblastoma

Stage I:	Localized tumour confined to the area of origin; complete gross excision, with or without microscopic residual disease; identifiable ipsilateral and contralateral nodes negative microscopically
Stage IIA:	Unilateral tumour with incomplete gross excision; identifiable ipsilateral and contralateral lymph nodes negative microscopically
Stage IIB:	Unilateral tumour with complete or incomplete gross excision; with positive ipsilateral regional nodes; identifiable contralateral nodes negative microscopically
Stage III:	Tumour infiltrating across the midline with or without regional lymph node involvement; or unilateral tumour with contralateral regional lymph node involvement; or midline tumour with bilateral regional node involvement
Stage IV:	Dissemination of tumour to distant lymph nodes, bone, bone marrow, liver and/or other organs (except as defined for stage IVS). Any infant with greater than 10% tumour cells in bone marrow is stage IV and not IVS
Stage IVS:	Localized primary tumour as defined for Stage I or II with dissemination limited to liver, skin, and/or bone marrow. Bone marrow infiltration must be less than 10%

The midline is the lateral border of the vertebral column on the side opposite the origin of the primary tumour

A spectrum of histology reflects progressive histogenesis from undifferentiated neuroblastoma, through 'differentiating neuroblastoma' and ganglioneuroblastoma, to ganglioneuroma. Undifferentiated neuroblastoma shows a structureless array of small round-to-oval cells frequently compartmentalized by strands of vascular fibrous connective tissue (Figure 5.1). Nuclei show a coarse chromatin pattern with variable mitotic activity.

Homer–Wright rosettes and patches of pink fibrillary material indicate early neural differentiation ('differentiating neuroblastoma') (Figure 5.2A,B). Early neuronal

development is accompanied by cellular enlargement, nuclear vesiculation, and the emergence of prominent nucleoli. Necrosis and calcification are common. There may be intracytoplasmic positivity but the *en-bloc* or punctate positivity commonly seen in rhabdomyosarcoma and Ewing's tumour is not described.

Cytological preparations may show clumping of small groups of tumour cells with tapering cytoplasmic extensions directed radially, or linking adjacent individual tumour cells (Figure 5.3).

GANGLIONEUROBLASTOMA

Neuroblastoma that displays varying degrees of neuronal differentiation is referred to as ganglioneuroblastoma. There is no consensus as to the degree of neuronal differentiation that separates neuroblastoma from ganglioneuroblastoma[11]. Two patterns of ganglioneuroblastoma are recognized:

(a) A composite pattern consisting of one or two discrete nodules of pure neuroblastoma in a setting of a ganglioneuroma (Figure 5.4), and
(b) A diffuse pattern composed of a mixture of undifferentiated and differentiated neuroblasts (immature ganglion cells (Figure 5.5).

The importance in making this distinction lies in the better outlook for patients with the diffuse pattern. The composite pattern is much less frequent and in Adam and Hocholzer's series[6] comprised 10% of mediastinal ganglioneuroblastomas.

Shimada et al.[12] separated composite ganglioneuroblastoma into 'intermixed' and 'nodular' types. The former is associated with microscopic foci of neuroblastoma while the latter is associated with one or more grossly visible nodules of neuroblastoma. The nodular type of composite ganglioneuroblastoma is linked with a less favourable outcome.

Neuroblastoma is usually metastatic to lymph nodes, bone marrow and liver, and while isolated pulmonary metastases do occur, they are usually part of more widespread dissemination, and indicate a poor prognosis[13].

INVOLVEMENT OF THE BONE MARROW

Bone marrow is examined in cases of neuroblastoma to assess the extent or stage of disease, and to evaluate response to therapy. Involvement of bone marrow is usually focal and without radiological changes. Samples may be obtained by aspiration or trephine biopsy but, in practice, a combination of these methods is generally employed[14]. Trephine biopsies supersede specimens obtained by aspiration in terms of their rate of detection of neuroblastoma. Immunohistochemistry may be valuable in the detection of metastases, especially when only a few neoplastic cells are involved[15].

Three patterns of marrow involvement are recognized[14]. The most common is the 'myelofibrotic' pattern, characterized by distorted cords of tumour cells compressed by a desmoplastic reaction. The 'focal' or 'multifocal' pattern shows discrete rounded islands of small cells which are seen to be distinct from the surrounding normal

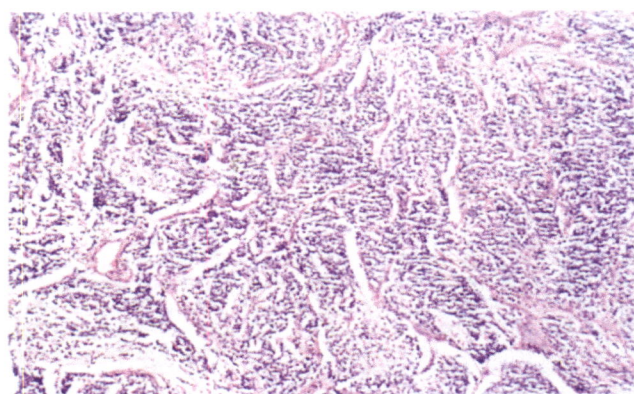

Fig. 5.1 Low-magnification view of poorly differentiated neuroblastoma shows sheets of small cells frequently compartmentalized by a delicate fibrovascular network. H&E × 75

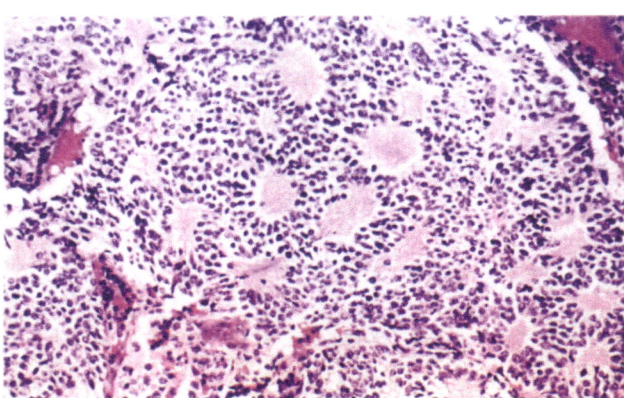

Fig. 5.2A Microscopy of 'differentiating neuroblastoma' shows prominent neural rosettes and patches of intercellular pink fibrillary material. The patient was a 4½-month-old boy who presented with a palpable left-sided abdominal mass that, on X-ray, was speckled with calcification. H&E × 185

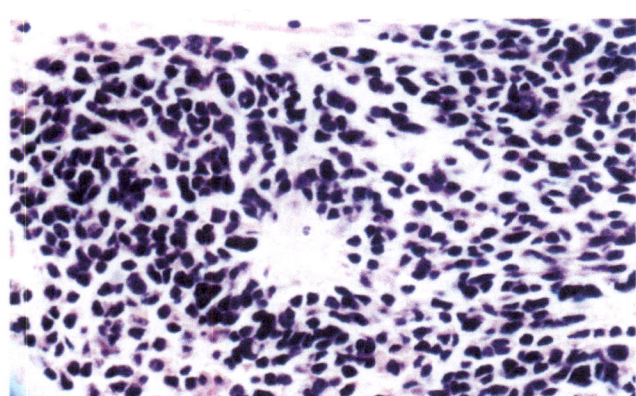

Fig. 5.2B A higher-magnification view of a Homer–Wright rosette showing a central tangle of pink neurofibrillary material surrounded by neuroblasts. Same tumour as in preceding figure. H&E × 480

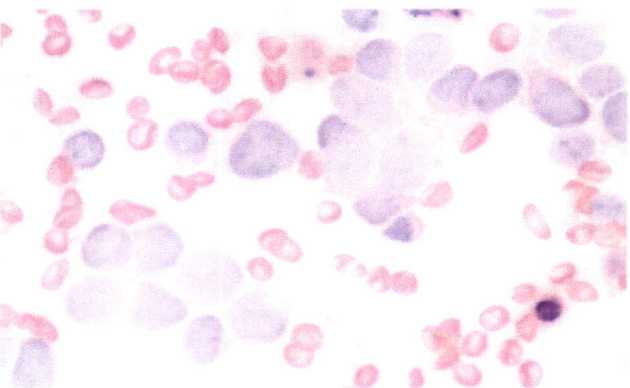

Fig. 5.3 Cytological preparation from poorly differentiated neuroblastoma shows tumour cells with generally scant cytoplasm and eccentric nuclei. Cytoplasmic extensions of the tumour cells are frequent, apparently forming a rudimentary rosette. H&E × 750

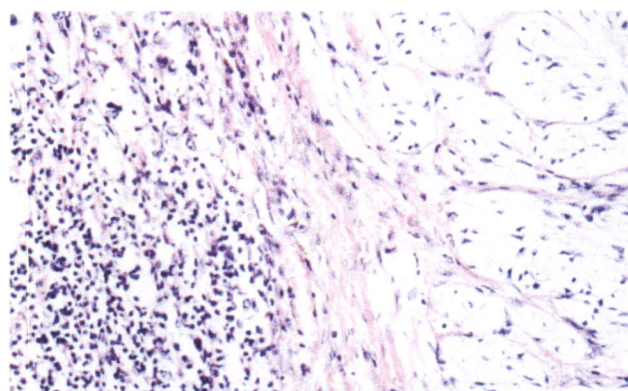

Fig. 5.4 Composite ganglioneuroblastoma shows part of a nodule of poorly differentiated neuroblastoma on the left, and ganglioneuromatous tissue on the right. H&E × 185

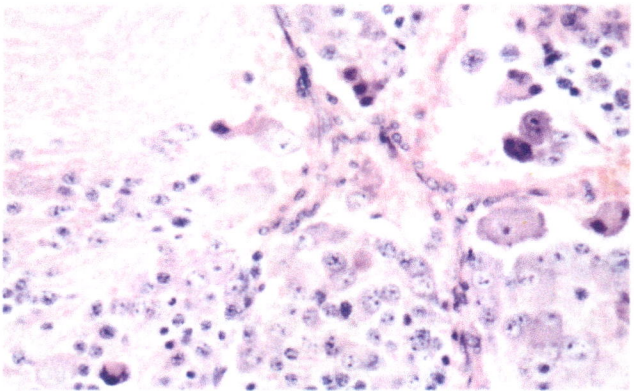

Fig. 5.5 Diffuse ganglioneuroblastoma comprises cells that represent a gradation from immature neuroblasts to relatively well-developed neurones. The tumour was removed from the posterior mediastinum of a 2-year-old girl; it weighed 131 g and measured 8.5 × 5.5 × 4.5 cm. H&E × 300

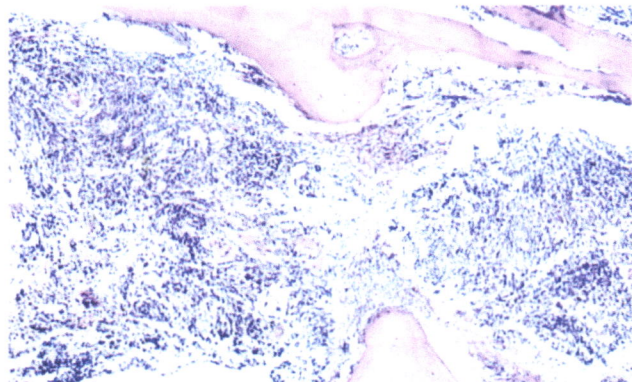

Fig. 5.6 Bone marrow shows sheets of metastatic neuroblastoma merging with haemopoietic tissue constituting the so-called 'interstitial' pattern of marrow involvement. H&E × 75

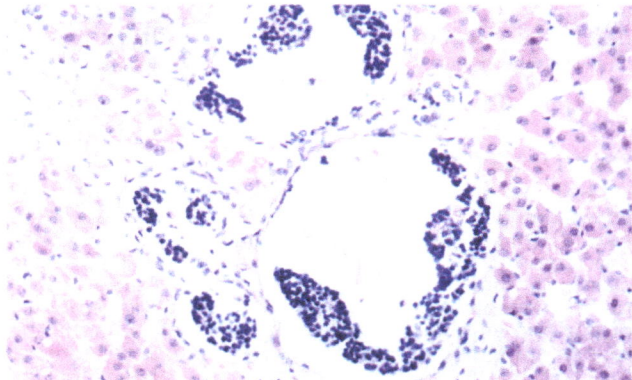

Fig. 5.7 Clusters of neuroblasts are a normal finding in the central region of the immature adrenal medulla. The adrenal gland is from a 21-week gestation morphologically normal female fetus. H&E × 185

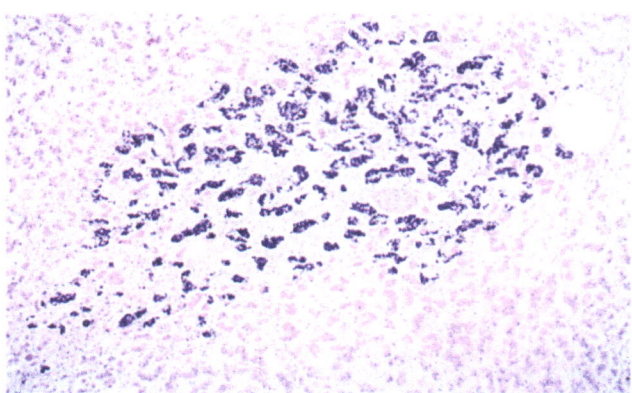

Fig. 5.8 Neuroblasts in the central medullary region of the adrenal rarely persist to term. This was an incidental finding in an infant who died 30 min after birth with a complex heart malformation. H&E × 48

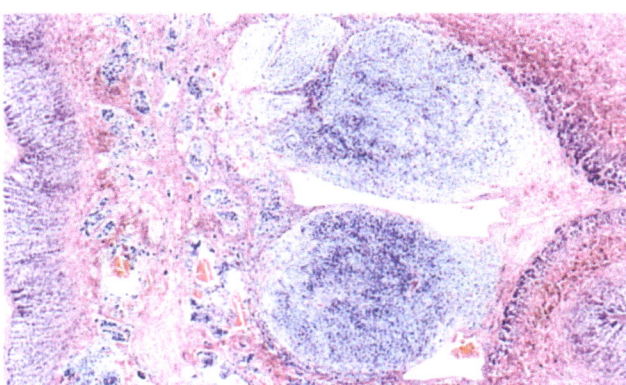

Fig. 5.9A Neuroblastoma *in-situ* is represented by several expanding nodules of neuroblastomatous tissue in the centre of the adrenal. (An incidental finding in a 20-week-old female infant who had small kidneys) H&E × 30

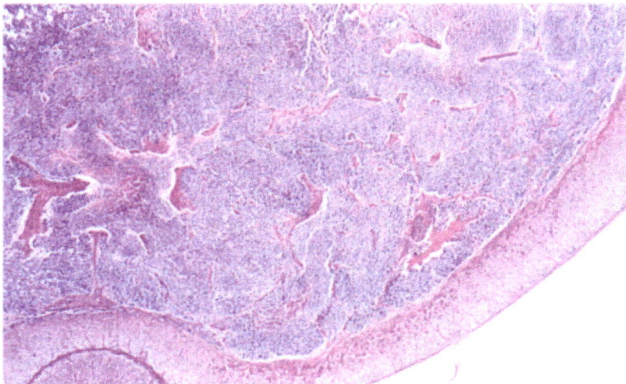

Fig. 5.9B Microscopy shows part of a relatively large neuroblastoma *in-situ* expanding the adrenal cortex. The microscopy is indistinguishable from conventional neuroblastoma (an incidental finding in a 5-week-old male cot death). H&E × 19

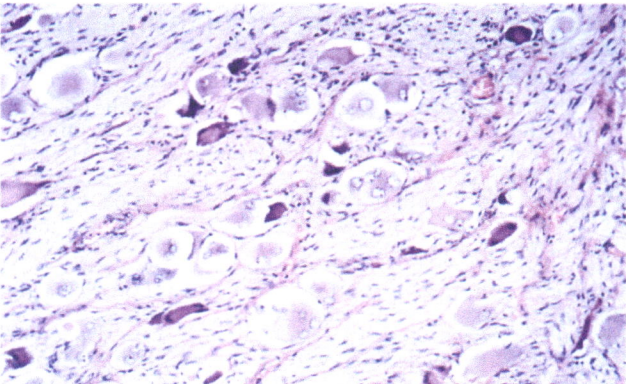

Fig. 5.10 Ganglioneuroma shows a group of relatively mature ganglion cells present within a neurocollagenous stroma. Occasional cells reveal multinuclearity and no obvious satellite cells are seen; these latter features should not detract from the microscopic diagnosis. H&E × 120

haemopoietic tissue. There is minimal increase in reticulin deposition. The 'interstitial' pattern shows sheets of small round cells which merge with the surrounding haemopoietic tissue (Figure 5.6) and are unassociated with reticulin.

IN-SITU NEUROBLASTOMA

Clusters of neuroblasts are found normally in the preterm adrenal medulla[16] (Figure 5.7) and rarely persist beyond term (Figure 5.8). Expansile nodules may develop in this region and, cytologically, are indistinguishable from classic neuroblastoma[17,18] (Figure 5.9A,B). They are rarely found incidentally at autopsy in infants less than 3 months of age and are referred to as neuroblastoma-in-situ. The lesions are regarded as preneoplastic and correspond to the first hit in Knudson's two-hit hypothesis for the genesis of neoplasia[19]. The incidence has been calculated to be some 40 times greater than clinically overt neuroblastoma, suggesting that many such nodules involute with increasing age through cytodifferentiation or necrosis[17].

GANGLIONEUROMA

Ganglioneuromas are benign, generally circumscribed, often encapsulated tumours[20]. The patients are older than those with neuroblastoma, with mean age at diagnosis of 10 years. There is usually no prior history of neuroblastoma. Catecholamines or their products are only rarely secreted. The neoplasms have an anatomical distribution similar to that of neuroblastoma and they may attain an enormous size[20]. The cut surface is usually firm yellow—grey and lobulated.

Microscopically, relatively mature neurons are seen either singly or clustered in a matrix which is fibrillary, neuromatous or neurocollagenous (Figure 5.10). The ganglion cells may or may not be surrounded by satellite cells. There may be some degree of multinuclearity but mitoses are uniformly absent. Foci of cystic degeneration (Figure 5.11), haemorrhage or calcification are encountered occasionally.

Multiple sections should be studied in order to exclude the presence of residual neuroblasts. Focal lymphocytic infiltration is fairly frequent (Figure 5.12) and may be mistaken for neuroblasts; the problem may be resolved by means of immunochemistry for leukocyte common antigen. However, the presence of a few scattered neuroblasts should not detract from a favourable prognosis.

ANCILLARY METHODS IN THE DIAGNOSIS OF NEUROBLASTOMA
Biochemical aspects

Neuroblastoma and its congeners are frequently biologically active and are capable of secreting catecholamines and their metabolites[21]. Vanilylmandelic acid (VMA) or homovanillic acid (HVA), or both, are secreted by a large majority of patients[22], and are usually measured as biochemical markers in the urine to assist diagnosis and monitor therapy. Hypertension in patients with neuroblastoma may be related to the secretion of these compounds[23], although an alternative explanation is compression of the renal pedicle by a retroperitoneal tumour[9,23]. Some tumours, especially those with advanced differentiation, are also capable of producing and secreting VIP, with intractable diarrhoea as the main symptom[24].

Immunohistochemistry

A number of neural markers has been developed to facilitate the diagnosis of undifferentiated neuroblastoma and its segregation from tumours of similar microscopic appearance. Useful antibodies include those directed at neuron-specific enolase, synaptophysin, chromogranin, protein-gene product 9.5, Leu 7 and HSAN 1.2[25,26]. These immunomarkers vary in their specificity and sensitivity and, as no single antibody is totally adequate for the diagnosis of neuroblastoma, an immunoprofile using several different antibodies is recommended[25]. Anti-S-100 protein antibody also marks cells of the supporting stroma of undifferentiated neuroblastoma and may indicate early tumour differentiation[27].

Ultrastructure

Ultrastructurally, the tumour cell nuclei are large with dispersed chromatin and occasionally prominent nucleoli[28,29]. The cytoplasm is scant and contains abundant free ribosomes, rough endoplasmic reticulum, some mitochondria, microfilaments and occasional Golgi complexes.

Catecholamine granules (neurosecretory or electron-dense granules) measuring 50–200 nm in diameter, and a compact meshwork of interdigitating neurites (Figure 5.13) are the principal features that distinguish neuroblastoma[26–29].

Neurotubules (about 25 nm in diameter) are usually found in the cytoplasmic processes. The intertwining cytoplasmic processes correspond to the eosinophilic fibrillar material seen in routine sections of 'differentiating neuroblastoma', and Schwann cells may be observed[30]. The secretory granules, while present in the cell body, are more frequently found in the cytoplasmic extensions (Figure 5.14)[28]; they should be distinguished from lysosomes. Clear vesicles about the size of catecholamine granules may be present and probably correspond to acetylcholine activity[28,29]. Increasing tumour differentiation is associated with a greater number of catecholamine granules and neurite extensions[29,30]. The neurite extensions contain longitudinally orientated neurofilaments and neurotubules[29,30]. The number and length of the neuritic processes also increase with increasing tumour differentiation, and they are particularly pronounced in ganglioneuroma[29].

Junctional complexes are often present between plasma membranes of adjacent tumour cells, or their processes[11]. Synaptic structures have been reported, but true desmosomes are rare.

Tissue culture morphology

The property of tumour cells to form neurite processes and cell clumping in tissue culture has been exploited as a diagnostic method[32]. Glyoxylic acid-induced fluorescence of tumour cells is reported in over 80% of cases and has been exploited as a diagnostic aid[32].

PROGNOSTIC DETERMINANTS OF NEUROBLASTOMA

Neuroblastoma is known for its unpredictable clinical behaviour[33] with, at one end of the spectrum, a tendency for the tumour to mature spontaneously (or even regress) and, at the other end, tumour behaviour that relentlessly progresses to a fatal outcome. The biological mechanisms responsible for this variable behaviour are unclear. A number of parameters are considered useful in predicting outcome and may be important in selecting optimal therapy. These prognostic variables are discussed below.

Clinical

The age of the patient, stage of disease and anatomical location are regarded widely as important clinical determinants of prognosis[34]. Patients under 1 year of age with neuroblastoma tend to have less extensive disease and a correspondingly better clinical outcome[22].

Adrenal neuroblastoma is generally associated with a poor outcome, possibly related to the high incidence of poorly differentiated growth at this site[9], contrasting with the better prognosis among patients with supradiaphragmatic neoplasms.

The outlook for 'metastatic' growth in the first year after birth is not necessarily as gloomy as might be expected, as the disease often undergoes spontaneous resolution. This is partly attributed to the inclusion of individuals with Stage IVS disease[35], which is defined by the presence of 'metastases' in the liver, skin and bone marrow, but without osseous involvement. In Stage IVS disease, the adrenal is the primary tumour site in the majority of cases[36].

Maturation of the tumour from neuroblastoma, through ganglioneuroma to fibrosis has been documented, but progression may precede regression[37]. Patients with Stage IVS disease, as a group, have an excellent prospect for survival, regardless of treatment and more than 80% become long-term survivors[5]. An age less than 6 weeks and absence of skin involvement, however, seem adversely to affect survival in this group[38]. Death may result from the mechanical effect of massive hepatomegaly, chemotherapy effect or late disease progression/recurrence[36].

Histological

Some evidence suggests that patients with histologically differentiated tumours fare better than those whose tumours are poorly differentiated[9]. Shimada and colleagues[12] detailed several histologically determined prognostic variables that took account of the amount of stroma in the tumour (i.e. the amount of schwannian and supporting elements), the degree of tumour differentiation and nuclear morphology, as determined by the mitosis–karyorrhexis index (MKI). Stroma-rich tumours were additionally subcategorized into (a) well-differentiated, (b) intermixed and (c) nodular. Nodular tumours were regarded as unfavourable whereas the other two patterns were considered favourable.

Stroma-poor tumours were viewed as prognostically favourable or unfavourable depending on the MKI, degree of differentiation and the patient's age. For patients aged 1.5–5 years with stroma-poor tumours, MKI values greater than 100/5000 cells, or lack of differentiation, were considered unfavourable. In those over 5 years old, stroma-poor tumours were considered unfavourable. MKI values over 200 in patients younger than 1.5 years were regarded as unfavourable.

The time taken to assess some of the criteria (e.g. the MKI) and the current increasing reliance on small biopsy samples (or aspiration cytology) are some disadvantages of the Shimada system[34].

Biochemical

The ratio of VMA:HVA has been used as a prognostic index[39], higher values being predictive of a more favourable outcome. Since HVA is a precursor of VMA, tumours that elaborate more HVA are viewed as biochemically immature and as potentially more aggressive.

A raised serum enolase has been reported to correlate with advanced stage disease[34]. Advanced stage (III and IV) and raised values are reported to be associated with a worse outcome, compared with patients with advanced stage and low values. High serum levels of ferritin and chromogranin A are similarly linked with less favourable outcome[40].

Genetic/molecular markers

N-myc oncogene status is an influential predictor of outcome in patients with neuroblastoma[40]. Overexpression and/or amplification (more than three copies) of the N-myc oncogene is often found at diagnosis in patients with advanced stage disease and single copies of the gene are usually associated with Stages I, II and IVS disease. N-myc copy number in neuroblastoma is a stable tumour marker and is uninfluenced by time and site[41].

Patients with single copies of N-myc, irrespective of stage, generally respond well to conventional therapy. By contrast, those whose tumours have multiple copies tend to have a poor outlook[42]. N-myc gene amplification is reported to be related to double minutes and homogenous staining regions in neuroblastoma cells[43].

Tumour cell DNA content in neuroblastoma, as determined by flow cytometrical analysis, karyotyping or image analysis, is also recognized as an important prognostic parameter, especially in patients less than 18 months old[34,44]. An abnormal DNA content (aneuploidy or hyperdiploidy) links strongly with clinically favourable prognostic variables, such as an age less than 1 year, extra-adrenal location and clinical Stage I, II and IVS[45]. (This contrasts with aneuploid tumours in adults as they are generally associated with poor survival.)

Aneuploidy is associated with a greater prospect of survival, even in association with less favourable clinical variables. More neuroblastomas are aneuploid as opposed to diploid[45,46]; Cohn et al.[44] reported 62% of tumours to be aneuploid. Diploid tumours, by contrast, are associated with aggressive disease. Despite site of sampling, different tumour sites and tumour progression, DNA content of the neuroblastoma is reported to remain stable[46].

Abnormalities of the short arm of chromosome 1 correlate strongly with N-myc amplification, suggesting a genetic link between the two events[42,47]. The chromosome abnormality also strongly parallels diploidy and hypotetraploidy[42]. Conversely, structural chromosome abnormalities arise infrequently in association with aneuploidy[42].

A strong correlation is found between N-myc gene amplification and diploidy[42,44,48], although Cohn et al.[44] were only able to find diploidy in 60% of their N-myc amplified tumours.

REFERENCES

1. Dehner LP. Peripheral and central primitive neuroectodermal tumors. A nosologic concept seeking a consensus. Arch Pathol Lab Med. 1986;110:997–1005.
2. Marsden HB, Steward JB (eds). Tumours in children. Berlin, Heidelberg, New York: Springer; 1976:1.
3. Young JL, Miller RW. Incidence of malignant tumors in children. J Pediatr. 1975;86:254–8.
4. Kinnier Wilson LM. Neuroblastoma, its natural history and prognosis: a study of 487 cases. Br Med J. 1974;3:301–7.
5. Seeger RC, Siegal SE, Sidell N. Neuroblastoma: clinical perspectives, monoclonal antibodies, and retinoic acid. Ann Intern Med. 1982;97:873–84.
6. Adam A, Hocholzer L. Ganglioneuroblastoma of the posterior mediastinum: a clinicopathologic review of 80 cases. Cancer. 1981;47:373–81.
7. Brown RJ, Szymula NJ, Lore JM. Neuroblastoma of the head and neck. Arch Otolaryngol. 1978;104:395–8.
8. Punt J, Pritchard J, Pincott JR et al. Neuroblastoma: a review of 21 cases presenting with spinal cord compression. Cancer. 1980;45:3095–101.
9. Beckwith JB, Martin RF. Observations on the histopathology of neuroblastoma. J Pediatr Surg. 1968;3:106–10.
10. Brodeur GM, Seeger RC, Barrett A et al. International criteria for diagnosis, staging, and response to treatment in patients with neuroblastoma. J Clin Oncol. 1988;6:1874–81.
11. Triche TJ, Askin FB. Neuroblastoma and the differential diagnosis of small-, round-, blue-cell tumors. Hum Pathol. 1983;14:569–95.
12. Shimada H, Chatten J, Newton WA et al. Histopathologic prognostic

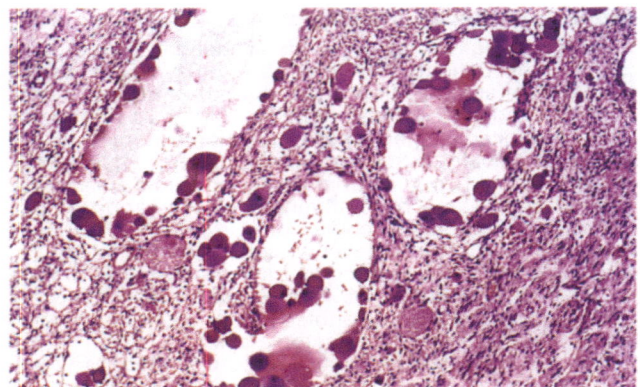

Fig. 5.11 Microcysts are present in this ganglioneuroma which was removed from the right retroperitoneum of a 7¹/₂-year-old boy. H&E × 75

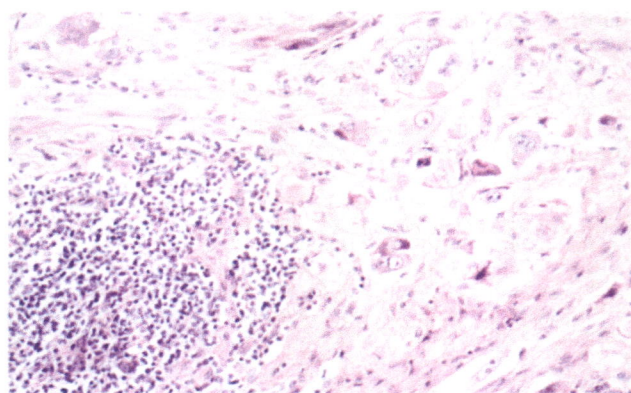

Fig. 5.12 A focus of lymphocytes is seen in a ganglioneuroma otherwise microscopically dominated by mature ganglion cells with a neurocollagenous background. Foci of lymphocytes should not be misinterpreted as neuroblasts. H&E × 185

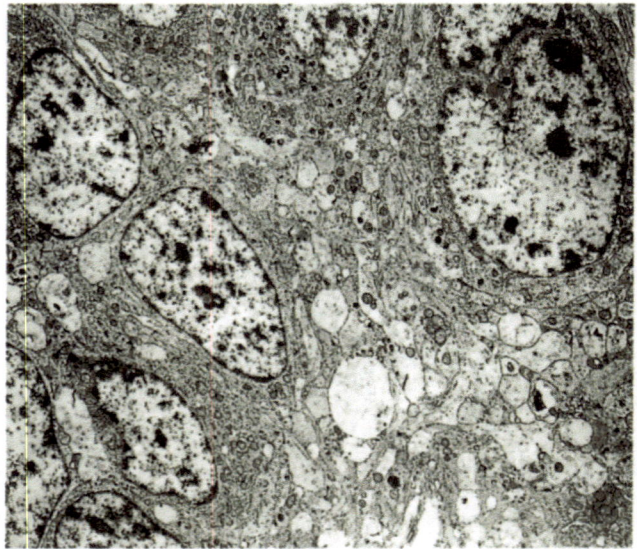

Fig. 5.13 Ultrastructural view of 'differentiating' neuroblastoma shows closely apposed interdigitating neurites in-between cells. × 4000

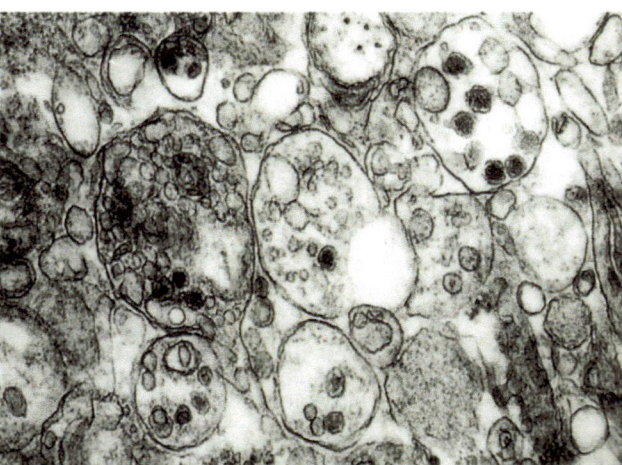

Fig. 5.14 Ultrastructural view of 'differentiating' neuroblastoma shows closely apposed neurites, several of which contain neurosecretory granules, and also clear vesicles. × 15 600

factors in neuroblastic tumors: definition of subtypes of ganglioneuroblastoma and age-linked classification of neuroblastomas. J Natl Cancer Inst. 1984;73:405–13.

13. Tobin R, Grippo RA. Pulmonary metastases in neuroblastoma. Am J R. 1982;138:75–8.

14. Mills AE, Bird AR. Bone marrow changes in neuroblastoma. Pediatr Pathol. 1986;5:225–34.

15. Oppedal BR, Storm-Mathison I, Kemshead JT, Brandtzaeg P. Bone marrow examination in neuroblastoma patients. A morphologic, immunocytochemical and immunohistochemical study. Hum Pathol. 1989;20:800–5.

16. Turkel SB, Itabashi HH. The natural history of neuroblastoma cells in the fetal adrenal gland. Am J Pathol. 1974;76:225–44.

17. Beckwith JB, Perrin EW. *In situ* neuroblastoma. Am J Pathol. 1963;43:1089–99.

18. Bolande RP. Benignity of neonatal tumors and the concept of cancer repression in early life. Am J Dis Child. 1971;122:12–14.

19. Knudson AG, Meadows AT. Regression of neuroblastoma IV-S; a genetic hypothesis. N Engl J Med. 1980;302:1254–5.

20. Stout AP. Ganglioneuroma of the sympathetic nervous system. Surg Gynecol Obstet. 1947;84:101–9.

21. Schweisguth O. Excretion of catecholamine metabolites in the urine of neuroblastoma patients. J Pediatr Surg. 1968;3:118–20.

22. Evans AE. Staging and treatment of neuroblastoma. Cancer. 1980;45:1799–802.

23. Kogut MD, Kaplan SA. Systemic manifestations of neurogenic tumors. J Pediatr. 1962;60:694–704.

24. Mendelsohn G, Eggleston JC, Olson JL, Said SI, Baylin SB. Vasoactive intestinal peptide and its relation to ganglion cell differentiation in neuroblastic tumors. Lab Invest. 1979;41:144–9.

25. Triche TJ. Neuroblastoma and other childhood neural tumors: a review. Pediatr Pathol. 1990;10:175–93.

26. Carter RL, Al-Sam SZ, Corbett RP, Clinton S. A comparative study of immunohistochemical staining for neuron-specific enolase, protein gene product 9.5 and S-100 protein in neuroblastoma, Ewing's sarcoma and other round cell tumours in children. Histopathology. 1990;16:461–7.

27. Shimada H, Aoyama C, Chiba T, Newton WA. Prognostic subgroups for undifferentiated neuroblastoma: immunohistochemical study with anti-S-100 protein antibody. Hum Pathol. 1985;16:471–6.

28. Misugi K, Misugi N, Newton WA. Fine structural study of neuroblastoma, ganglioneuroblastoma and phaeochromocytoma. Arch Pathol Lab Med. 1968;86:160–9.

29. Yokoyama M, Okada K, Tolue A, Takayasu H, Yamada R. Ultrastructural and biochemical study of neuroblastoma and ganglioneuroblastoma. Invest Urol. 1971;9:156–63.

30. Taxy JB. Electron microscopy in the diagnosis of neuroblastoma. Arch Pathol Lab Med. 1980;104:355–60.

31. Mackay B, Maasse SR, King OY, Butler JJ. Diagnosis of neuroblastoma by electron microscopy of bone marrow aspirates. Pediatrics. 1975;56:1045–9.

32. Reynolds CP, Smith RG, Frenkel EP. The diagnostic dilemma of the 'small round cell neoplasm'. Cancer. 1981;48:2088–94.

33. Bill AH. The regression of neuroblastoma. J Pediatr Surg. 1968;3:103–6.

34. Oppedal BR, Storm-Mathisen I, Lie SO, Brandtzaeg P. Prognostic factors in neuroblastoma. Clinical, histopathological and immunohistochemical features and DNA ploidy in relation to prognosis. Cancer. 1988;62:772–80.

35. D'Angio GJ, Evans AE, Koop CE. Special pattern of widespread neuroblastoma with a favourable prognosis. Lancet. 1971;1:1046–9.

36. Wilson PCG, Coppes MJ, Solh H. *et al.* Neuroblastoma stage IV-S: a heterogeneous disease. Med Pediatr Oncol. 1991;19:467–72.

37. Haas D, Ablin AR, Miller C, Zoger S, Matthay KK. Complete pathologic maturation and regression of stage IVS neuroblastoma without treatment. Cancer. 1988;62:818–25.

38. Stephenson SR, Cook BA, Mease AD, Ruymann FB. The prognostic significance of age and pattern of metastases in Stage IV-S neuroblastoma. Cancer. 1986;58:372–5.

39. Triche TJ. Round cell tumours in childhood: the application of newer techniques to the differential diagnosis. Perspect Pediatr Pathol. 1982;7:279–322.

40. Phillips WS, Stafford PW, Duvol-Arnold B, Ghosh BC. Neuroblastoma and the clinical significance of N-*myc* oncogene amplification. Surg Gynecol Obstet. 1991;172:73–80.

41. Brodeur GM, Hayes FA, Green AA et al. Consistent N-*myc* copy number in simultaneous or consecutive neuroblastoma samples from sixty individual patients. Cancer Res. 1987;47:4248–53.

42. Seeger RC, Brodeur GM, Sather H et al. Association of multiple copies of the N-*myc* oncogene with rapid progression of neuroblastoma. N Engl J Med. 1985;313:1111–16.

43. Hayashi Y, Kanda N, Inaba T et al. Cytogenetic findings and prognosis in neuroblastoma with emphasis on marker chromosome 1. Cancer. 1989;63:126–32.

44. Cohn SL, Rademaker AW, Salwen HR et al. Analysis of DNA ploidy and proliferative activity in relation to histology and N-*myc* amplification in neuroblastoma. Am J Pathol. 1990;136:1043–52.

45. Naito M, Iwafuchi M, Ohsawa Y et al. Flow cytometric DNA analysis of neuroblastoma: prognostic significance of DNA ploidy in unfavourable group. J Pediatr Surg. 1991;26:834–7.

46. Taylor SR, Blatt J, Costantino JP, Roederer M, Murphy RF. Flow cytometric DNA analysis of neuroblastoma and ganglioneuroma. A 10-year retrospective study. Cancer. 1988;62:749–54.

47. Fong CT, Dracopoli N, White PS et al. Loss of heterozygosity for the short arm of chromosome 1 in human neuroblastoma: correlation with N-*myc* amplification. Proc Natl Acad Sci USA. 1989;86:3753–7.

48. Look AT, Hayes A, Shuster JJ et al. Clinical relevance of tumor cell ploidy and N-*myc* gene amplification in childhood neuroblastoma: a pediatric oncology group study. J Clin Oncol. 1991;9:581–91.

Peripheral primitive neuroectodermal tumours other than neuroblastoma

6

These are extracranial neoplasms arising generally in soft tissues and displaying a primitive microscopic structure in which evidence of neural differentiation is demonstrated. The light microscopic features resemble those of many small-cell tumours, but more especially sympathetic neuroblastoma or Ewing's sarcoma[1]. Their precise origin is unclear, and they may arise from a pluripotential stem cell, either of embryonic neural crest or mesenchymal origin[2]. Entities that qualify for inclusion in this category continue to increase in number and complexity[1].

NEUROEPITHELIOMA (PERIPHERAL NEUROBLASTOMA)

Neuroepithelioma affects patients usually in the first two decades of life, although adults are sometimes involved. The soft tissues are the usual anatomical site[1], but the kidney and adrenal are rarely reported as primary locations[2,3]. Only exceptionally are catecholamine metabolites elaborated by the tumour[5] but the serum level of neuron-specific enolase may be raised.

Microscopically, the tumour cells are closely apposed with round-to-oval nuclei and a narrow rim of cytoplasm (Figure 6.1). Nucleoli are inconspicuous and mitotic activity is variable. Neural rosettes are commonly encountered and, while these are usually of the Homer—Wright type, Flexner-type rosettes are also seen occasionally (Figure 6.2)[4,6]. Fields of irregular interweaving or confluent pseudorosettes with corresponding cording and nesting of cells are also found (Figure 6.3)[7]. Ganglion cell differentiation is most unusual[4,6] and there may be angiomatoid areas (Figure 6.4).

Ultrastructural features[7] of neuroepithelioma include interdigitating cytoplasmic processes and lakes of intracytoplasmic glycogen (Figure 6.5); neurosecretory granules and neurotubules but, in many cases, intermediate filaments and junctional complexes are also observed.

Because of the apparent rarity of the neoplasm and lack of uniformity in therapeutic approach, prognosis is difficult to evaluate. The general view is that, despite an initial favourable response, the long-term outlook is bleak. 'Chest wall sarcoma of childhood with a good prognosis'[8] probably belongs to this category of neoplasm, suggesting that a poor outlook is not necessarily inevitable.

Cytogenetic study of some tumours demonstrates a reciprocal translocation (11;22)(q24;q12)[9]. The tumour cell cytoplasm often shows *en bloc* PAS positivity that facilitates a distinction from sympathetic neuroblastoma (Figure 6.6).

Askin's tumour (small-cell tumour of the thoracopulmonary region)

A malignant small-cell tumour arising in the soft tissue of the thoracopulmonary region of children and young adults was first reported by Askin et al.[10]. The precise histogenesis of the neoplasm at that time was unclear, and it was the application of ultrastructural and immunohistochemial studies some 7 years later that uncovered the neural nature of the neoplasm[11]. The thoracopulmonary tumour (Askin's tumour) is currently regarded as a clinicopathological variant of neuroepithelioma[5]. It is probably the most common malignant tumour of the chest wall among subjects less than 20 years of age[12]. Compared with extrathoracopulmonary neuroepithelioma, most reports document a female preponderance[5]. The average age of patients is 14 years[5,10]. Prior to its recognition as a distinct entity, many of these tumours were probably referred to as soft tissue variants of Ewing's sarcoma.

The growth arises in the chest wall and extends variably into the thoracic cavity, involving the pleura, peripheral lung, diaphragm, and even the mediastinum. Tumours are occasionally related to an intercostal nerve and secondary erosion of the ribs occurs in a small proportion of cases[5].

Grossly, the tumours are round, multinodular or lobulated and measure 2—14 cm in diameter. Encapsulation is absent and the cut surface is greyish-white with focal necrosis and haemorrhage.

The microscopic picture and antigenic profile are similar to those seen in extrathoracic neuroepithelioma[5]. Neural rosettes are demonstrated in a minority of cases[10,11]. Ten of the 15 cases reported by Linnoila et al.[11] also revealed PAS staining. The number of mitoses is variable. The presence of endothelial hyperplasia has been emphasized in one case[13]. The ultrastructure is similar to that found in similar tumours outside the thoracopulmonary region[5].

Immunopositivity for neuron-specific enolase has been reported in most series[5,11,13], and the tumours have also been reported to express other antigens, such as vimentin, S100-protein, GFAP[13] and CEA, cytokeratin and EMA[14]. Three microscopic patterns are recognized, including compact sheets of cells, a lobular pattern, and serpiginous bands of cells with intervening necrosis[5]. Any of these patterns may dominate.

Askin's tumour is associated with the reciprocal translocation (11;22)(q24;q12), similar to that seen in extrathoracic neuroepitheliomas[3]. Widespread or skeletal metastases are unusual in Askin's tumour.

DIFFERENTIAL DIAGNOSIS

Extracranial metastases from an occult central primitive neuroectodermal tumour should be considered in the differential diagnosis. However, it would be most unlikely for a central tumour to present in this way[7].

Primitive neuroectodermal tissue may form the dominant component of an immature ovarian teratoma and the remaining teratoma may be difficult to identify. Five examples of so-called monodermal teratomas composed of such tissue involving the ovaries of patients, whose ages ranged from 13 to 17 years, have been reported[15]. PNET-like foci are described in malignant peripheral neural sheath tumours in children and this component may dominate the histological picture[16]. The main consideration, however, lies in separating neuroepithelioma from neuroblastoma (Table 6.1).

MELANOTIC NEUROECTODERMAL TUMOUR OF INFANCY (MELANOTIC PROGONOMA; RETINAL ANLAGE TUMOUR; MELANOCYTIC NEUROECTODERMAL TUMOUR)

This is a rare pigmented tumour occurring usually in children less than 1 year old[21–23]. In more than 90% of cases, the neoplasm arises in the head and neck region, and the maxilla is most commonly involved[21]. Other

Table 6.1 Neuroblastoma vs. neuroepithelioma

	Neuroblastoma	Neuroepithelioma
Age	< 5 years	Older children and adolescents
Site	Adrenal/paraspinal	Peripheral
Spread	Early dissemination; bone/marrow	Locally aggressive; lungs[4]
Cell morphology	Tumour cells separated by pink fibrillary material; thick nuclear membranes; coarse chromatin	Tumour cells closely apposed; thin nuclear membranes; fine chromatin
	Frequent ganglion cell differentiation; Homer-Wright rosettes only; usually PAS negative[17]	Rare ganglion cell differentiation; Homer-Wright and Flexner-type rosettes; often en bloc PAS +ve[4]
Ultrastructure	Neural differentiation may be advanced. Lakes of glycogen rare	Only limited neural differentiation[4]. Lakes of glycogen often seen
Catecholamines	VMA, HVA raised in majority of cases	None (rare exceptions)[19]
Neurotransmitter enzyme	Adrenergic profile	Cholinergic profile[19]
Immunohisto-chemical	More uniform response to neural markers, β_2-microglobulin -ve, HSAN 1.2 +ve, S-100 protein +ve (focal). Vimentin −ve (some exceptions)	Capricious response to neural markers, β_2-microglobulin +ve[18], HSAN 1.2 -ve (or weakly positive)[19]. Usually vimentin +ve
Cytogenetic/molecular	Short arm deletion of chromosome 1 N-myc amplification MIC2 gene −ve	Reciprocal t(11;22)[19] c-myc amplification[19] MIC2 gene +ve[20]

less common sites include the mediastinum, epididymis, subcutaneous tissue and long bones[21]. Grossly, they are firm non-encapsulated circumscribed lobulated masses with a cut surface that varies from grey–white to dark brown and black[22].

Microscopically, the tumour recapitulates features of the early stage of retinal development[22]. This shows a biphasic pattern comprising undifferentiated neuroblastoma-like cells and epithelioid cells. The epithelioid cells contain fine granular pigment that stains positively for melanin[21]. The melanin-containing cells are often arranged to form acini that encompass clusters of neuroblastoma-like cells (Figure 6.7). Both cell types are also often arranged in sheets, nests or cords, separated by a prominent fibrocollagenous stroma (Figure 6.8). Ganglionic and neurite differentiation are unusual.

Immunohistochemically, the epithelioid and neuroblastoma-like cells express neuron-specific enolase; the epithelioid cells are also positive for vimentin and cytokeratin, but are negative for S-100 protein[22,23].

The majority of patients are cured by wide local excision. There is a 15% recurrence risk after surgery and, microscopically, the recurrences are virtually identical to the original tumour. Catecholamine levels are elevated in a few cases[22]. Overt malignant behaviour has been reported in some instances[21,22].

ECTOMESENCHYMOMA

This tumour has so far been described only in children[24–26], and, as the name implies, the histology includes neuroectoderm and mesenchyme. The basis of this unusual coexistence is the reputed capacity of the embryological neural crest tissue to produce mesenchyme (so-called 'ectomesenchyme'). The mesenchyme most often shows sarcomatous or leiomyomatous differentiation (Figure

6.9); neuroblastomatous (Figure 6.10) or ganglioneuroblastomatous tissue usually represents the ectodermal component. The two elements (mesenchymal and ectodermal) invariably merge imperceptibly.

OLFACTORY NEUROBLASTOMA (ESTHESIONEUROBLASTOMA)

Although the majority of these tumours have been reported in adults, children are occasionally affected[27,28]. The neoplasm resembles conventional neuroblastoma, histologically and ultrastructurally. Involvement of older patients, lack of ganglion cell differentiation and the occasional demonstration of epithelial elements[29] attest to its 'non-neuroblastomatous' nature.

PERIPHERAL MEDULLOEPITHELIOMA

This is an extremely rare tumour usually arising in the cerebral or intraocular compartments. Neoplasms with similar features are rarely reported to arise from the peripheral nerve[30]. The chief microscopic component is neuroepithelium, frequently arranged to form embryonic medullary plate or neural tube.

INTRA-ABDOMINAL DESMOPLASTIC SMALL-CELL TUMOUR WITH DIVERGENT DIFFERENTIATION

These neoplasms are included here provisionally as their relationship to primitive neuroectodermal tumours is as yet unclear. The tumours have been variously designated 'desmoplastic small-cell tumour with divergent differentiation'[31], and 'intra-abdominal desmoplastic small round-cell tumour'[32]. The largest series so far reported has been by Gerald et al.[33]. According to this report, tumour behaviour is aggressive and the survival rate is poor. Males are strongly represented[33]. The age range is 8–38 years, with a mean of 18.6 years.

Most of the tumours were large and associated with multiple nodules attached to the peritoneal surface. The microscopic picture sharply outlines clusters of small round cells separated by cellular myxoid stroma (Figure 6.11). Cell necrosis is common, especially within the larger islands of tumour. Mild-to-moderate amounts of intracytoplasmic glycogen may be demonstrated on PAS staining. The growth pattern is typically invasive. The tumours consistently display a complex immunohistochemical profile[31–34] that includes epithelial, neural, myogenic and mesenchymal antigens. The histogenesis is unknown. The relationship of this neoplasm to the 'polyphenotypic small-cell tumour of childhood' reported by Swanson et al. is unclear.

The microscopic differential diagnosis includes mesothelioma, extrarenal rhabdoid tumour and Ewing's sarcoma[35]. The tumours reported by Variend et al.[34] were similar but additionally showed glandular structures and neural rosettes (Figure 6.12); they were viewed as primitive neuroectodermal tumours on the basis of neural differentiation.

REFERENCES

1. Dehner LP. Peripheral and central primitive neuroectodermal tumors. A nosologic concept seeking a consensus. Arch Pathol Lab Med. 1986;110:997–1005.
2. Dehner LP. Whence the primitive neuroectodermal tumor? Arch Pathol Lab Med. 1990;114:16–17.
3. Seemayer TA, Thelmo WL, Bolande RP, Wiglesworth FW. Peripheral neuroectodermal tumours. Perspect Pediatr Pathol. 1975;2:151–72.
4. Marina NM, Etcubanas E, Parham DM, Bowman LC, Green A. Peripheral primitive neuroectodermal tumour (peripheral neuroepithelioma) in children. A review of the St. Jude experience and

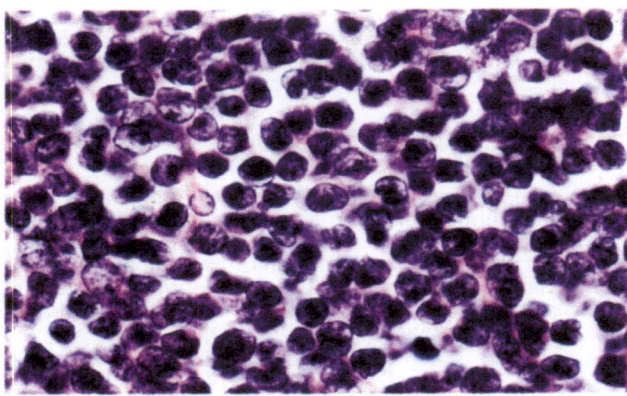

Fig. 6.1 Neuroepithelioma. This shows a non-rosetting poorly differentiated histology that is indistinguishable from other small-cell tumours. Immunohistochemically, the tumour marked positively with neural markers and the patient's age and anatomical location were incompatible with a diagnosis of neuroblastoma. H&E × 750

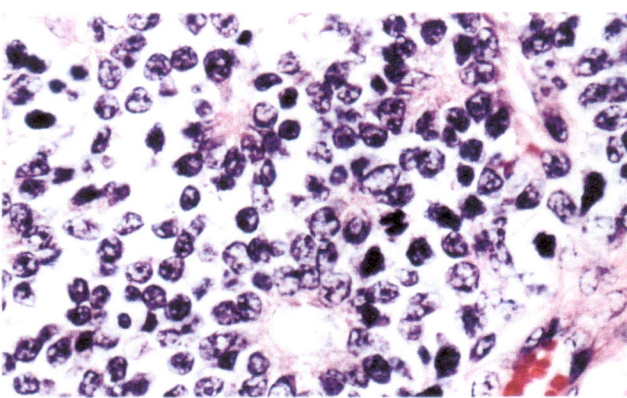

Fig. 6.2 Askin's tumour. Microscopy shows a small-cell tumour with a mixture of Homer Wright and Flexner-type rosettes. Following presentation with a small pleural effusion, radiology and exploratory surgery showed an extensively necrotic tumour involving the chest wall of a 12-year-old boy. H&E × 560

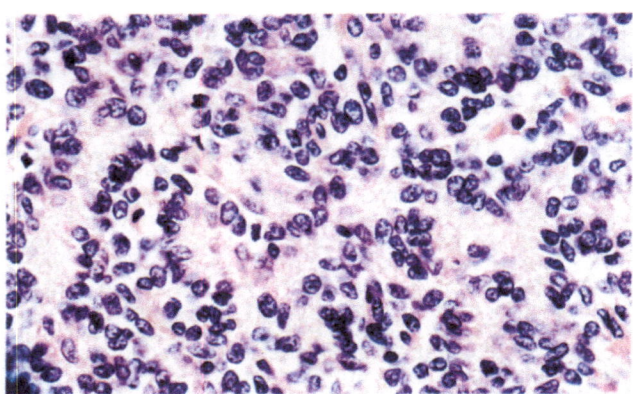

Fig. 6.3 Intraabdominal neuroepithelioma shows indistinct interweaving or confluent rosettes. Nuclei are vesicular and the cytoplasm is ill-defined and wispy. H&E × 480

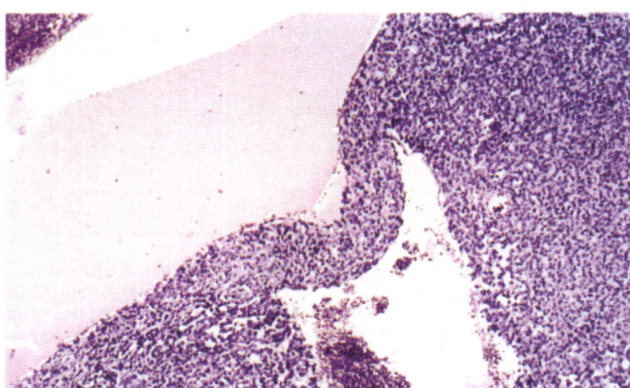

Fig. 6.4 Askin's tumour. Large vascular spaces are a prominent feature in this microscopic field of Askin's tumour. Same tumour as in Figure 6.2. H&E × 75

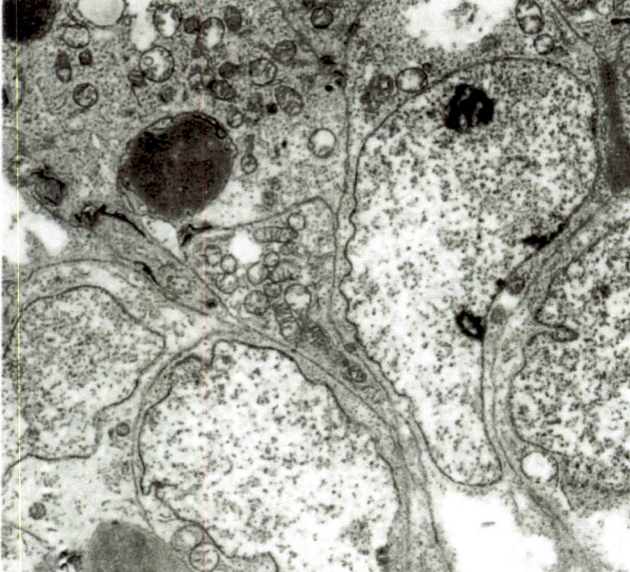

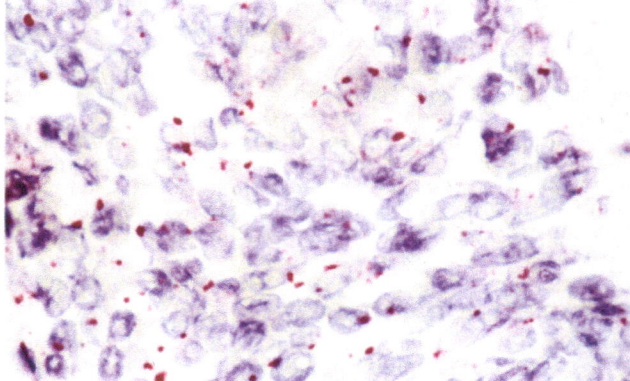

Fig. 6.6 Askin's tumour. A PAS reaction exhibits intracytoplasmic block-like positivity in many cells; the material was diastase-sensitive. × 750

Fig. 6.5 Askin's tumour. Ultrastructure shows a central patch of intertwined cytoplasmic processes and lakes of intracytoplasmic glycogen. A rare neurosecretory granule is seen. Same tumour as in Figure 6.4. × 50 000

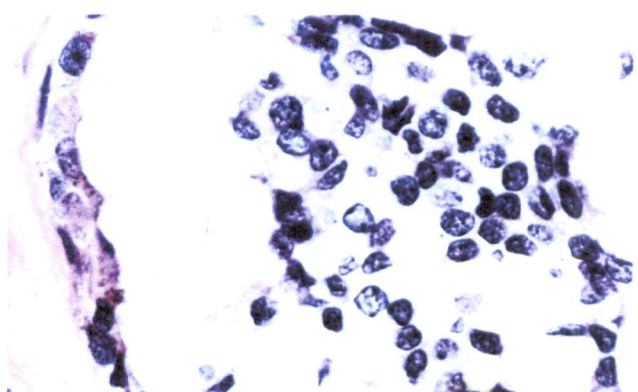

Fig. 6.7 Melanotic progonoma. A glandular structure lined by pigmented cuboidal epithelium containing a cluster of neuroblast-like cells is a common microscopic feature. The patient was a 4-year-old girl who presented with a rapidly growing mass in the maxilla. H&E × 750

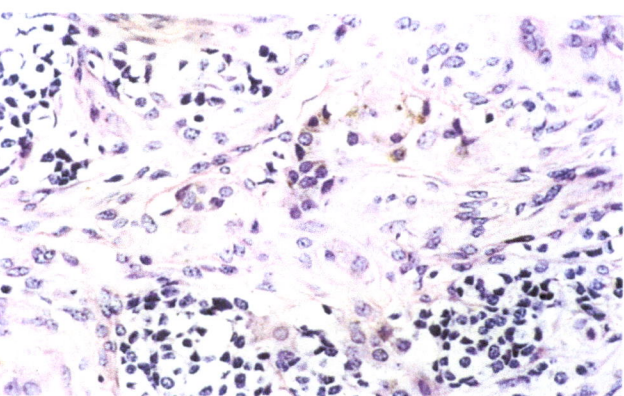

Fig. 6.8 Melanotic progonoma. This microscopic view shows a more haphazard arrangement of neuroblast-like cells and pigmented cuboidal epithelium. Same tumour as in Figure 6.7. H&E × 300

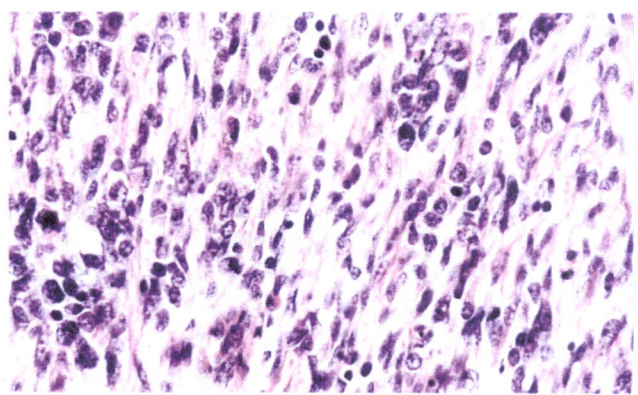

Fig. 6.9 Ectomesenchymoma. A spindle-cell pattern predominates in this microscopic field. The tumour arose in the anterior abdominal wall of an 8-month-old girl. H&E × 300

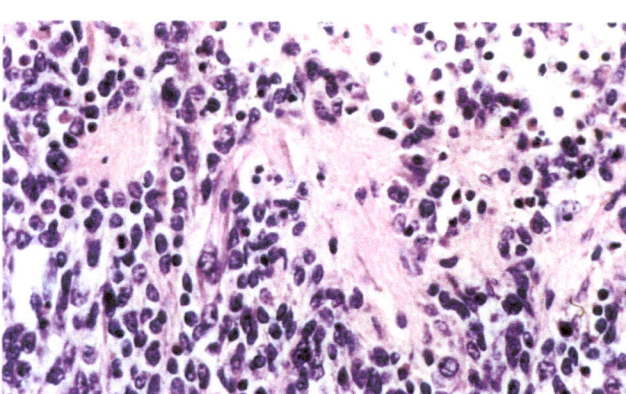

Fig. 6.10 Ectomesenchymoma. Neural rosettes are conspicuous in this microscopic field. Same tumour as in Figure 6.9. H&E × 300

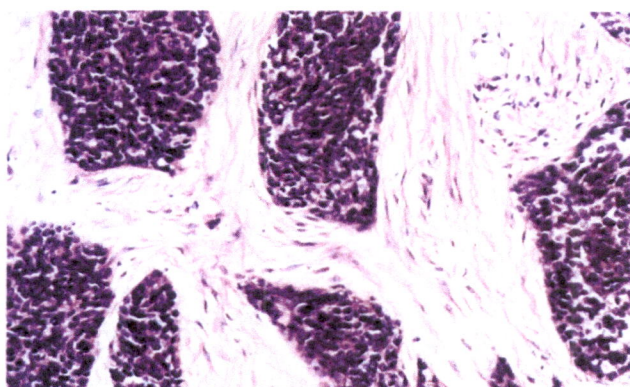

Fig. 6.11 Desmoplastic small round cell tumour. Microscopy shows lobules of closely packed small oval and spindle-shaped cells separated by copious myxofibrous stroma. The tumour arose in the pelvis of a 13-year-old boy. H&E × 185

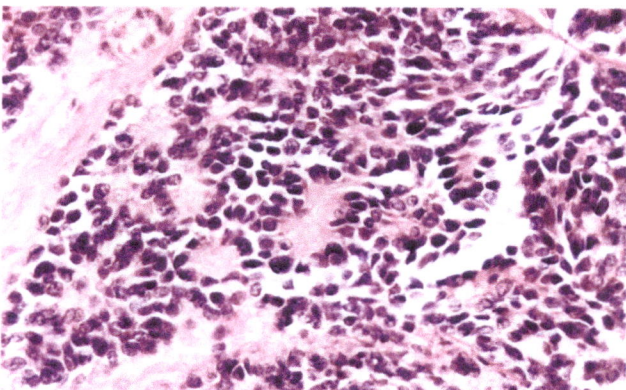

Fig. 6.12 Desmoplastic small round cell tumour. Same tumour as depicted in preceding figure shows prominent neural rosettes. H&E × 300

controversies in diagnosis and management. Cancer. 1989;64: 1952-60.

5. Coffin CM, Dehner LP. Peripheral neurogenic tumours of the soft tissue in children and adolescents: a clinicopathologic study of 139 cases. Pediatr Pathol. 1989;9:387-407.

6. Schmidt D, Harms D, Burdach S. Malignant peripheral neuroectodermal tumours of childhood and adolescence. Virchows Arch (Pathol Anat). 1985;406:351-65.

7. Voss BL, Pysher TJ, Humphrey GB. Peripheral neuroepithelioma in childhood. Cancer. 1984;54:3059-64.

8. Barson AJ, Ahmed A, Gibson AAM, MacDonald AM. Chest wall sarcoma of childhood with a good prognosis. Arch Dis Childh. 1978;53:882-9.

9. Whang-Peng J, Triche TJ, Knutsen T, Miser J, Douglass EC, Israel MA. Chromosome translocation in peripheral neuroepithelioma. N Engl J Med. 1984;311:584-5.

10. Askin FB, Rosai J, Sibley RK, Dehner LP, McAlister WH. Malignant small cell tumor of the thoracopulmonary region in childhood. A distinctive clinicopathologic entity of uncertain histogenesis. Cancer. 1979;43:2438-51.

11. Linnoila RI, Tsoko M, Triche TJ, Marangos PJ, Chandra RS. Evidence for neural origin and PAS-positive variants of the malignant small cell tumour of thoracopulmonary region ('Askin tumor'). Am J Surg Pathol. 1986;10(2):124-33.

12. Shamberger RC, Grier HE, Weinstein HJ, Perez-Atayde AR, Tarbell NJ. Chest wall tumors of infancy and childhood. Cancer. 1989;63:774-85.

13. Gonzalez-Crussi F, Wolfson SL, Misugi K, Nakajima T. Peripheral neuroectodermal tumors of the chest wall in childhood. Cancer. 1984;54:2519-27.

14. Fujii Y, Hongo T, Nakagawa Y et al. Cell culture of small round cell tumour originating in the thoracopulmonary region. Evidence for derivation from a primitive pluripotent cell. Cancer. 1989;64:43-51.

15. Aquirre P, Scully RE. Malignant neuroectodermal tumor of the ovary, a distinctive form of monodermal teratoma. Report of five cases. Am J Surg Pathol. 1982;6:283-92.

16. Meis JM, Enzinger FM, Martz KL, Neal JA. Malignant peripheral nerve sheath tumors (malignant Schwannomas) in children. Am J Surg Pathol. 1992;16:694-707.

17. Yunis EJ, Agostini RM, Walpusk JA, Hubbard JD. Glycogen in neuroblastomas. A light- and electron-microscopic study of 40 cases. Am J Surg Pathol. 1979;3:313-23.

18. Donner L, Triche TJ, Israel MA, Seeger RC, Reynolds CP. A panel of monoclonal antibodies which discriminate neuroblastoma from Ewing's sarcoma, rhabdomyosarcoma, neuroepithelioma, and hematopoietic malignancies. Prog Clin Biol Res. 1985;175:347-66.

19. Triche TJ. Neuroblastic and other childhood neural tumors: a review. Pediatr Pathol. 1990;10:175-93.

20. Ambros IM, Ambros PF, Strehl S, Kovar H, Gadner H, Salzer-Kuntschik M. MIC2 is a specific marker for Ewing's sarcoma and peripheral primitive neuroectodermal tumors. Cancer. 1991;67:1886-93. .

21. Young S, Gonzalez-Crussi F. Melanotic neuroectodermal tumor of the foot. Report of a case with multicentric origin. Am J Clin Pathol. 1985;84:371-8.

22. Pettinato G, Manivel C, d'Amore ESG, Jaszcz W, Gorlin RJ. Melanotic neuroectodermal tumor of infancy. A reexamination of a histogenetic problem based on immunohistochemical, flow cytometric, and ultrastructural study of 10 cases. Am J Surg Pathol. 1991;15:233-45.

23. Stirling RW, Powell G, Fletcher CDM. Pigmented neuroectodermal tumour of infancy: an immunohistochemical study. Histopathology. 1988;12:425-35.

24. Naka A, Matsumoto S, Shirai T, Itoh T. Ganglioneuroblastoma associated with malignant mesenchymoma. Cancer. 1975;36:1050-6.

25. Karcioglu Z, Someren A, Mathes SJ. Ectomesenchymoma. A malignant tumor of migratory neural crest (ectomesenchyme) remnants showing ganglionic, schwannian, melanocytic and rhabdomyoblastic differentiation. Cancer. 1977;39:2486-96.

26. Cozzutto C, Comelli A, Bandelloni R. Ectomesenchymoma. Report of two cases. Virchows Arch (Pathol Anat). 1982;398:185-95.

27. Kadish S, Goodman M, Wang CC. Olfactory neuroblastoma. A clinical analysis of 17 cases. Cancer. 1976;37:1571-5.

28. Mills EM, Frierson HF. Olfactory neuroblastoma. A clinicopathological study of 21 cases. Am J Surg Pathol. 1985;9:317-27.

29. Ng HK, Poon WS, Poon CY, South JR. Intracranial olfactory neuroblastoma mimicking carcinoma: Report of two cases. Histopathology. 1988;12:393-403.

30. Nakamura Y, Becker LE, Mancer K, Gillespie R. Peripheral medulloepithelioma. Acta Neuropathol (Berl). 1982;57:137-42.

31. Gerald WL, Rosai J. Desmoplastic small cell tumour with divergent differentiation. Pediatr Pathol. 1989;9:177-83.

32. Gonzalez-Crussi F, Crawford SE, Sun CCJ. Intraabdominal desmoplastic small-cell tumors with divergent differentiation. Observations on three cases of childhood. Am J Surg Pathol. 1990;14:633-42.

33. Gerald WL, Miller HK, Battifora H, Miettinen M, Silva EG, Rosai J. Intra-abdominal desmoplastic small round-cell tumor. Report of 19 cases of a distinctive type of high-grade polyphenotypic malignancy affecting young individuals. Am J Surg Pathol. 1991;15:499-513.

34. Variend S, Gerrard M, Norris PD, Goepel J. Intraabdominal neuroectodermal tumour of childhood with divergent differentiation. Histopathology. 1991;18:45-51.

35. Layfield LJ, Lenarsky C. Desmoplastic small cell tumors of the peritoneum coexpressing mesenchymal and epithelial markers. Am J Clin Pathol. 1991;96:536-43.

Ewing's sarcoma

7

OSSEOUS EWING'S SARCOMA

In 1921, James Ewing[1] described a primary malignant tumour of bone in which he emphasized the perivascular arrangement of the tumour cells. A wide age range is affected but the neoplasm predominates in the second decade. It is the second most common malignant tumour of bone in children. The most common affected sites are the pelvis and femur and there is a modest male predominance. Babies and toddlers are affected in 2% of cases[2]. The most frequent symptoms are pain and swelling.

Macroscopically, the tumour is often very friable and frequently discloses necrosis and degeneration[3–5]. The friability is attributed to lack of any appreciable supporting stroma in the tumour, a feature readily demonstrated on staining sections for reticulin. The cortical bone is often invaded (Figure 7.1) and an extraosseous mass may arise at some distance from the tumour epicentre[6].

The prototype histology is best seen in those areas of the tumour that are optimally preserved. In such areas, the cells have a uniform appearance, being of moderate size, with round-to-oval nuclei and vesicular nuclei (Figure 7.2). Nuclear membranes are distinct and nucleoli are inconspicuous. Mitoses are recognizable in most tumours but are not especially common. Cell boundaries are ill-defined and the cytoplasm may be granular, clear or vacuolated, probably reflecting the presence of glycogen removed through conventional fixation and processing.

A proportion of tumours display cells with small dark angulated nuclei and scalloped cytoplasmic borders (Figure 7.3). These cells, often referred to as 'secondary cells', occur singly or in groups. A degenerative phenomenon has been proposed for their origin[7,8]. Rosettes are often reported in Ewing's sarcoma, but usually no distinction has been made between neural rosettes and the so-called apoptotic pseudorosettes[9]. Strong PAS-positive diastase-sensitive staining for glycogen in the tumour cell cytoplasm is demonstrated frequently; the positivity may be en bloc (Figure 7.4) or finely dispersed within the cytoplasm. Glycogen is usually sparse or even absent in the 'secondary cell'. The demonstration of glycogen is influenced by the type of fixation; fixation in alcohol or frozen section preparations produces optimal results. Silver impregnation outlines connective tissue and blood vessels, with little tendency for the fibres to insinuate between individual tumour cells (Figure 7.5)[5,6]. Formation of vascular lakes or sinuses ('vascular variant'), geographical necrosis with perivascular sparing, metaplastic bone or cartilage formation are other recognized histological characteristics[10]. Cytogenetically, the tumour displays a distinctive reciprocal (11:22) translocation (Figure 7.6)[11,12].

Diffuse, lobular, filigree and trabecular patterns are recognized histologically[3,4]. The lung, bone, bone marrow and regional lymph nodes represent the common metastatic sites, but cerebral metastases are recognized increasingly with longer survival[4].

Clinically, radiologically and even microscopically, Ewing's sarcoma may masquerade as osteomyelitis[13,14]. The histological differential diagnosis includes small-cell osteosarcoma[15] and mesenchymal chondrosarcoma (polyhistiocytoma)[16,17]. Cytoplasmic glycogen is found in the cells of both these tumours but a careful search will usually reveal osteoid or chondroblastic differentiation respectively, although difficulties may arise when only small samples of tissue are available.

The small-cell variant of osteosarcoma comprises up to 4% of all osteosarcomas; it is a high-grade tumour with an anatomical distribution similar to conventional osteosarcoma[18]. Three histological patterns have been reported: Ewing's-like, lymphoma-like and spindle celled. Of these, the Ewing's-like pattern was the most common. A silver impregnation showed individual tumour cells to be encompassed by reticulin. The average age of the patients with the small-cell variant of osteosarcoma was 14.8 years[18].

HISTOGENESIS OF EWING'S SARCOMA OF BONE

The histogenesis of the tumour is still controversial and derivation from the endothelial cell[1], primitive mesenchyme[19] and myelogenous tissue[20] has been postulated. Accumulating evidence suggests, however, that the tumour is of neuroectodermal origin. But whether this applies to all cases of osseous Ewing's sarcoma is still unclear. Data supporting a neural basis for Ewing's sarcoma are wide-ranging:

(a) Jaffe et al.[9] described primary bone tumours with morphological evidence of neural differentiation. These were referred to as primitive neuroectodermal tumours of bone and had been previously called Ewing's sarcoma.

(b) The reciprocal (11:22) translocation, also found in neuroepithelioma and Askin's tumour, has been reported in osseous Ewing's sarcoma[11,12].

(c) Some ultrastructural studies of Ewing's sarcoma have emphasized neural features[21].

(d) Moll et al.[22] recently reported among Ewing's sarcomas a complex immunophenotype that included positivity for neurofilament protein.

(e) The MIC2 gene is expressed in large amounts in Ewing's sarcoma and PNETs[23].

EXTRAOSSEOUS VARIANT OF EWING'S SARCOMA

A soft tissue tumour showing similar microscopic features to those of Ewing's sarcoma of bone (Figure 7.7) has been reported[24–26]. The features include the presence of 'secondary cells', intracytoplasmic glycogen' (Figure 7.8) and the distribution of reticulin around lobules rather than individual tumour cells. Extraosseous (or soft tissue) Ewing's sarcoma is usually deep-seated. As in osseous Ewing's sarcoma, there is a slight male predominance although patients with the extraosseous variant tend to be older, with a median age of 20 years. Common sites of the tumour include the chest wall, paravertebral regions and lower extremities (Figure 7.9).

The tumour shows aggressive behaviour and, following surgical excision, there is a high rate of local recurrence. The best chance of survival seems to be offered by

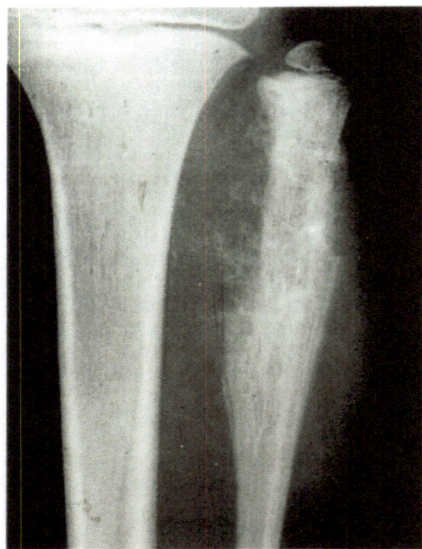

Fig. 7.1 X-ray shows Ewing's sarcoma involving the upper fibula. The patient was a 6-year-old girl who presented with local pain and swelling

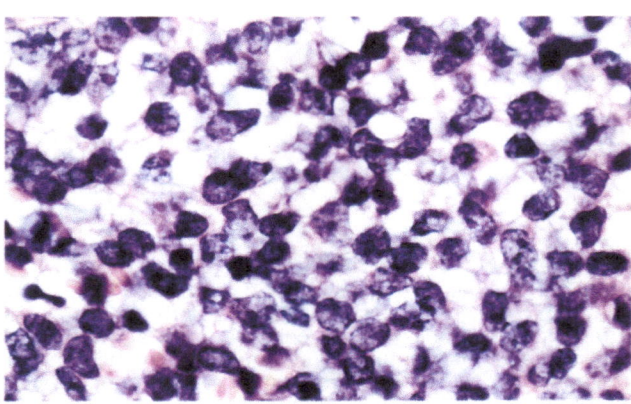

Fig. 7.2 High-magnification view of osseous Ewing's sarcoma shows small tumour cells with oval-to-round vesicular nuclei and scant often clear cytoplasm with ill-defined cytoplasmic boundaries. H&E × 750

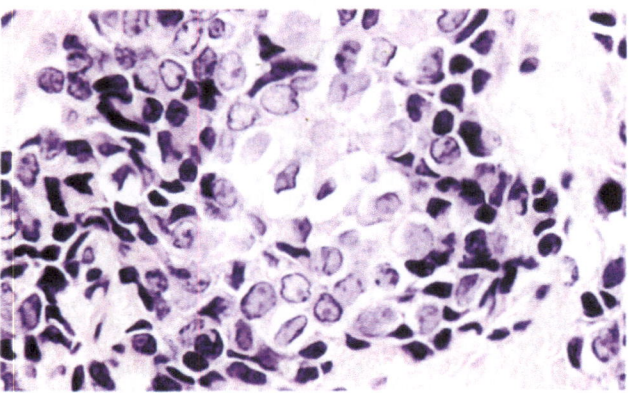

Fig. 7.3 Osseous Ewing's sarcoma shows a number of 'secondary cells' characterized by small dark angulated nuclei. H&E × 750

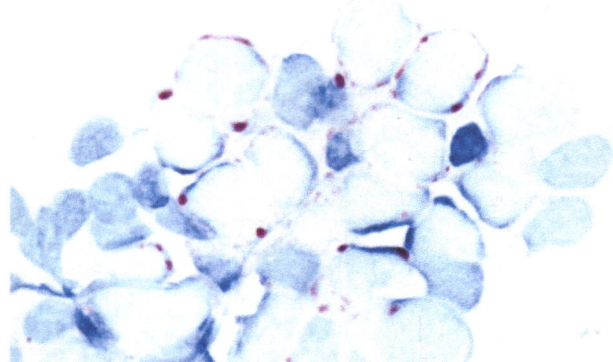

Fig. 7.4 Cytological preparation from osseous Ewing's sarcoma stained with PAS shows strong intracytoplasmic punctate positivity around several nuclei. PAS × 810

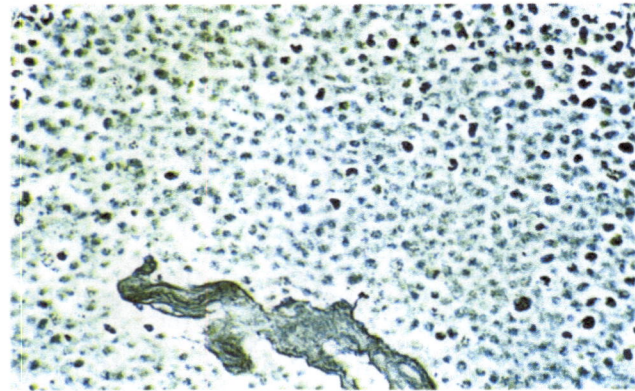

Fig. 7.5 Osseous Ewing's sarcoma demonstrates absence of reticulin fibres around individual tumour cells. Reticulin is limited to a vascular structure in the lower part of the field. Gomori reticulin × 300

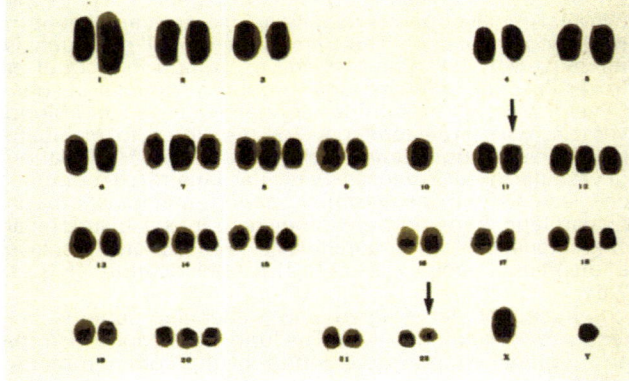

Fig. 7.6 Chromosome karyotype of Ewing's sarcoma shows a characteristic t(11,22); several non-specific trisomies are also evident

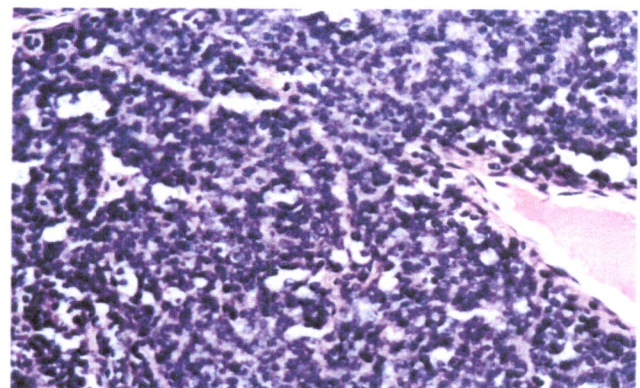

Fig. 7.7 Soft tissue Ewing's tumour shows an undifferentiated small-cell tumour pattern. The microscopic picture is difficult to segregate from undifferentiated rhabdomyosarcoma which is the main consideration in the differential diagnosis. H&E × 240

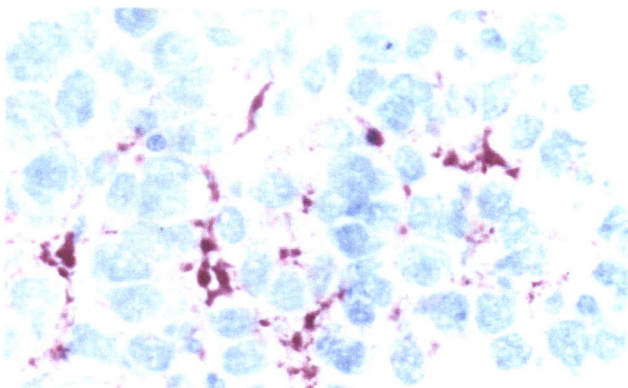

Fig. 7.8 Same tumour as shown in Figure 7.7, reveals prominent intracytoplasmic punctate PAS positivity. (Undifferentiated rhabdomyosarcoma, an important differential diagnosis, is not expected to show this degree of PAS positivity) PAS × 750

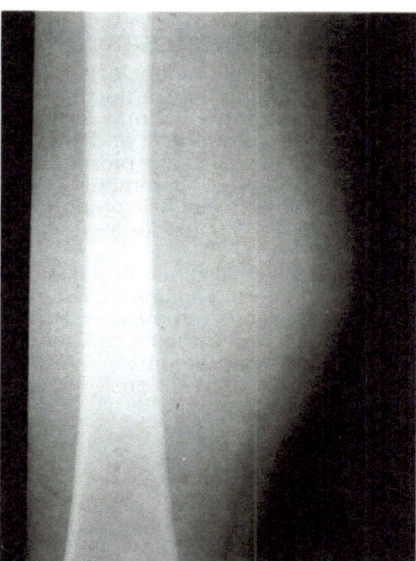

Fig. 7.9 A soft tissue mass is outlined on X-ray of the right thigh of a 12-year-old girl who presented with a swelling in the area. The underlying bone is uninvolved. Widespread pulmonary nodules were demonstrated on computerized tomography. The tumour was diagnosed microscopically as soft-tissue Ewing's sarcoma (see Figures 7.7 and 7.8)

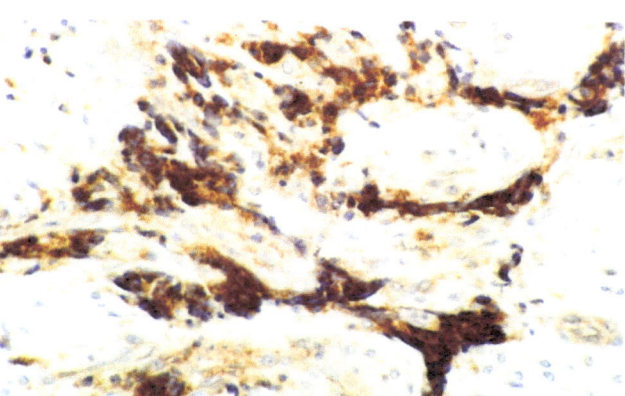

Fig. 7.10 Poorly preserved Ewing's sarcoma expresses strong cytoplasmic positivity for β_2-microglobulin in paraffin section on immunohistochemistry. × 300

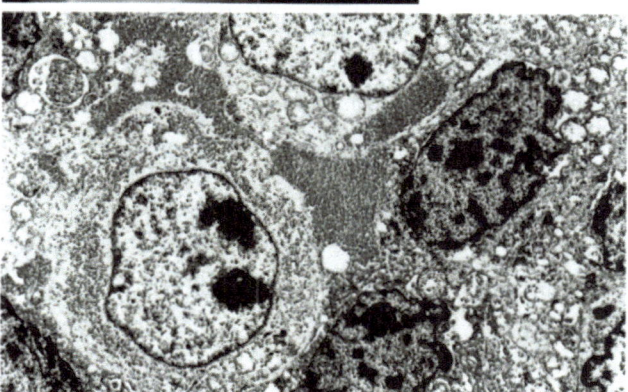

Fig. 7.11 Ultrastructure of osseous Ewing's tumour shows nuclei with generally smooth outlines and one or two conspicuous nucleoli. Pools of glycogen are demonstrated in moderate amounts of cytoplasm that is otherwise poorly populated with organelles. × 4300

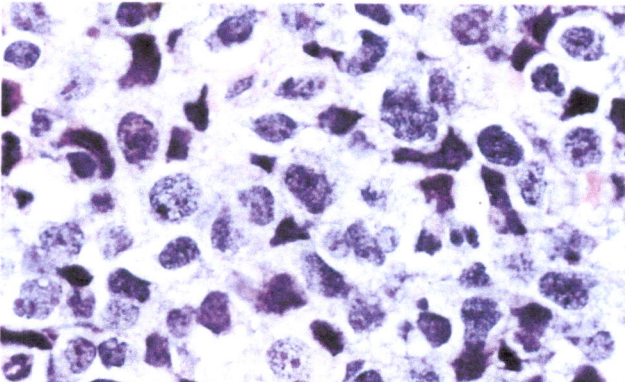

Fig. 7.12 Large-cell variant of osseous Ewing's sarcoma shows tumour cells with large pleomorphic nuclei. Many of the tumour cells show clear cytoplasm and several 'secondary cells' are also seen. (The cytoplasm disclosed punctate PAS positivity.) H&E × 750

multimodality therapy including surgery, radiotherapy and chemotherapy[26]. General agreement exists that the paravertebral 'round-cell' tumours in children reported by Tefft et al.[27] are examples of extraosseous Ewing's sarcoma. It is also increasingly apparent that many of the soft tissue Ewing's sarcomas previously reported to affect the chest wall were examples of Askin's tumour (see Chapter 6). Extraosseous Ewing's sarcoma may show neural rosettes in conventional sections, neuron-specific enolase and S-100 protein on immunohistochemistry, and neurosecretory granules on ultrastructure[26], supporting the neuroectodermal nature of some, and possibly all, such tumours.

The differential diagnosis of soft tissue Ewing's sarcoma includes undifferentiated (primitive) rhabdomyosarcoma and synovial sarcoma.

IMMUNOHISTOCHEMISTRY OF OSSEOUS AND EXTRAOSSEOUS EWING'S SARCOMA

The tumour cells are immunoreactive for vimentin but negative for desmin and for endothelial markers (Factor VIII-related antigen and UEAI)[28]. The tumours also mark positively for a range of neural markers[29,30]. Culture cell lines of osseous and extraosseous tumours demonstrate strong affinity for antibodies to β_2-microglobulin and HLA-ABC[31]. β_2-microglobulin is expressed by osseous Ewing's sarcoma in paraffin section (Figure 7.10). Ewing's sarcoma demonstrates surface antigens that are related to neuroectoderm lineage[32], and a complex immunophenotype (vimentin, keratin and neurofilament protein) was detailed by Moll et al.[22].

Table 7.1 Common features in neuroepithelioma and Ewing's sarcoma suggest a common lineage

	Neuroepithelioma	Extraosseous ES
Clinical	Similar age distribution and anatomical location	
Light microscopy	Undifferentiated tumour ± neural features Glycogen +	Undifferentiated tumour ± neural features[45] Glycogen +[30]
Ultrastructure	Neural differentiation	Neural differentiation (±)[45]
Biochemical	CAT activity	CAT activity[44]
Cytogenetic	t(11;22) MIC2 gene +	t(11;22)[46] MIC2 gene +[23]
Molecular	Similar pattern of oncogene expression[44]	
Experimental		In vitro induction of neural differentiation[36]

CAT = choline acetyl transferase

ULTRASTRUCTURE OF EWING'S SARCOMA

Electron microscopy has been an important tool in the diagnosis of Ewing's sarcoma[7,8,33,34]. Ultrastructure confirms the undifferentiated nature of the cells. The cells are ovoid to polygonal in shape and the nuclear outlines are usually smooth, with one or two conspicuous nucleoli. Nuclear chromatin is finely dispersed but marginated along the nuclear membrane and the paucity of cytoplasm is confirmed. Intracytoplasmic organelles are limited to a few mitochondria and profiles of endoplasmic reticulum. Free ribosomes and polyribosomes, on the other hand, are fairly numerous. Deposits of cytoplasmic glycogen are a striking feature (Figure 7.11)[7,33]. Preparations from paraffin-embedded tissue may fail to reveal glycogen due

to prior dissolution during conventional fixation and processing.

Primitive cell–cell attachments are commonly encountered[35] and intracytoplasmic microfilaments (6–7 nm), a Golgi apparatus, dense bodies and lipid droplets are occasionally found. Extracellular matrix is generally absent. The 'secondary cell' shows condensed chromatin and vacuolated cytoplasmic processes insinuating between other cells.

Neurosecretory granules, cytoplasmic processes and neurotubules have been demonstrated in osseous Ewing's sarcoma on ultrastructure[21,30], and similar features are seen in extraosseous Ewing's sarcoma[30]. By these criteria, Ushigome et al. reclassified their cases from osseous and extraosseous Ewing's sarcoma to PNETs. Cavazzana et al.[36] observed neurofilaments, microtubules and dense core secretory granules in cell culture lines of Ewing's sarcoma following neural induction with cyclic AMP.

Extraskeletal Ewing's sarcoma has an ultrastructural appearance indistinguishable from osseous ES[35,37–39]. Ewing's sarcoma and alveolar rhabdomyosarcoma have similar ultrastructural features[19], but ultrastructural examination has been used to separate extraskeletal Ewing's sarcoma from primitive rhabdomyosarcoma[35].

LARGE-CELL VARIANT OF EWING'S SARCOMA

An uncommon atypical or large-cell variant of Ewing's sarcoma shows a nuclear irregularity and a nuclear size about twice that seen in conventional Ewing's sarcoma (Figure 7.12)[40,41]. Nucleoli are prominent and mitotic activity is increased. 'Secondary cells' are present and cytoplasmic glycogen is observed commonly. The anatomical location, age distribution and male preponderance is similar to that seen in conventional Ewing's sarcoma.

Soft-tissue Ewing's sarcoma may also manifest a large-cell variant[24], and Rud et al.[26] reported a large-cell variant in 26% of their cases of extraosseous tumours. This form of Ewing's sarcoma may be mistaken for large-cell lymphoma or the small-cell variant of osteosarcoma[40]. A similar appearance may be induced in conventional Ewing's sarcoma by radiotherapy or chemotherapy[41].

PROGNOSIS IN EWING'S SARCOMA

Tumours arising in the pelvis and proximal extremities[3,42] and metastatic disease at the time of diagnosis[10] are factors associated with a lower survival rate. Patients with typical Ewing's sarcoma fare better than patients with atypical variants or those with neural variants of the tumour[10]. No important difference in survival is reported between patients with extraosseous and osseous lesions[10]. The filigree histological pattern[3] and microscopic tumour invasion of the sarcoplasm of skeletal muscle[43] has been reported to confer poor prognosis.

NOTE ADDED IN PROOF

The antigen p 30/32^{mic2} is demonstrated on the cells of Ewing's sarcoma and primitive neuroectodermal tumour using the monoclonal antibody HBA-71 (Dehner LP. Primitive neuroectodermal tumour and Ewing's sarcoma. Am J Surg Pathol. 1993;17:8–13).

REFERENCES

1. Ewing J. Diffuse endothelioma of the bone. Proc New York Pathol Soc. 1921;21:17–18.
2. Siegal GP, Schoppe J, Foulkes M, Kissane JM, Askin FB. Ewing's sarcoma in babies and toddlers; a clinicopathological report from

the Intergroup Ewing's Sarcoma Study Group (Abstract). Lab Invest. 1983;48:13P.

3. Kissane JM, Askin FB, Foulkes M, Stratton LB, Shirley SF. Ewing's sarcoma of bone: clinicopathologic aspects of 303 cases from the Intergroup Ewing's Sarcoma Study. Hum Pathol. 1983;14:773–9.

4. Kissane JM, Askin FB, Nesbit ME Jr et al. Sarcomas of the bone in childhood: pathologic aspects. Cancer Inst Monogr. 1981;56: 29–41.

5. Lichtenstein L, Jaffe HL. Ewing's sarcoma of bone. Am J Pathol. 1947;23:43–77.

6. Dahlin DC, Coventry MB, Scanlon PW. Ewing's sarcoma: a critical analysis of 165 cases. J Bone Jt Surg. 1961;43A:185–92.

7. Povysil C, Matejovsky A. Ultrastructure of Ewing's tumour. Virchows Arch (Pathol Anat). 1977;374:303–16.

8. Mahoney JP, Alexander RW. Ewing's sarcoma. A light- and electron-microscopic study of 21 cases. Am J Surg Pathol. 1978;2: 283–98.

9. Jaffe R, Santamaria M, Yunis EJ et al. The neuroectodermal tumor of bone. Am J Surg Pathol. 1984;8:885–98.

10. Hartman KR, Triche TJ, Kinsella TJ, Miser JS. Prognostic value of histopathology in Ewing's sarcoma. Cancer. 1991;67:163–71.

11. Aurias A, Rimbaut C, Buffe D, Dubousset J, Mazabraud A. Chromosomal translocations in Ewing's sarcoma. N Engl J Med. 1983;309:496–7.

12. Turc-Carel C, Philip I, Berger MP, Philip T, Lenoir GM. Chromosomal translocation in Ewing's sarcoma. N Engl J Med. 1983;309:497–8.

13. Nance CL, Roberts WM, Miller GR. Ewing's sarcoma mimicking osteomyelitis. South Med J. 1967;60:1044–50.

14. Cabanela ME, Franklin HS, Beabout JW, Dahlin DC. Osteomyelitis appearing as neoplasms: a diagnostic problem. Arch Surg. 1974;109:68–72.

15. Sim FH, Unni KK, Beabout JW, Dahlin DC. Osteosarcoma with small cells simulating Ewing's tumour. J Bone Jt Surg. 1979;61A:207–15.

16. Salvador AH, Beabout JW, Dahlin DC. Mesenchymal chondrosarcoma – observation in 30 new cases. Cancer. 1971;28:605–15.

17. Jacobson SA. Polyhistiocytoma: a malignant tumor of bone and extraskeletal tissue. Cancer. 1977;40:2116–30.

18. Ayala AG, Ro JY, Raymond AK et al. Small cell osteosarcoma: a clinicopathologic study of 27 cases. Cancer. 1989;64:2162–73.

19. Churg A, Ringus J. Ultrastructural observations on the histogenesis of alveolar rhabdomyosarcoma. Cancer. 1978;41:1355–61.

20. Kadin ME, Bensch KG. On the origin of Ewing's tumor. Cancer. 1971;27:257–73.

21. Schmidt D, Mackay B, Ayala AG. Ewing's sarcoma with neuroblastoma-like features. Ultrastruct Pathol. 1982;3:143–51.

22. Moll R, Lee I, Gould VE et al. Immunohistochemical analysis of Ewing's tumors. Am J Pathol. 1987;127:288–304.

23. Ambros IM, Ambros PF, Strehl S, Kovar H, Gadner H, Salzer-Kuntschik M. MIC2 is a specific marker for Ewing's sarcoma and peripheral primitive neuroectodermal tumors. Cancer. 1991;67: 1886–93.

24. Angervall L, Enzinger FM. Extraskeletal neoplasm resembling Ewing's sarcoma. Cancer. 1975;36:240–51.

25. Soule EH, Newton W Jr, Moon TE, Tefft M. Extraskeletal Ewing's sarcoma. Cancer. 1978;42:259–64.

26. Rud NP, Reiman HM, Pritchard DJ, Frassica FJ, Smithson WA. Extraosseous Ewing's sarcoma. Cancer. 1989;64:1548–53.

27. Tefft M, Vawter GF, Mitus S. Paravertebral 'round-cell' tumours in children. Radiology. 1969;92:1501–9.

28. Miettinen M, Lehto VP, Virtanen I. Histogenesis of Ewing's sarcoma. An evaluation of intermediate filaments and endothelial cell markers. Virchows Arch (Pathol Anat). 1982;41:277–84.

29. Carter RL, Al-Sam SZ, Corbett RP, Clinton S. A comparative study of immunohistochemical staining for neuron-specific enolase, protein gene product 9.5 and S-100 protein in neuroblastoma, Ewing's sarcoma and other round cell tumours in children. Histopathology. 1990;16:461–7.

30. Ushigome S, Shimoda T, Takaki K et al. Immunocytochemical and ultrastructural studies of the histogenesis of Ewing's sarcoma and putatively related tumors. Cancer. 1989;64:52–62.

31. Donner L, Triche TJ, Israel MA, Seeger RC, Reynolds CP. A panel of monoclonal antibodies which discriminate neuroblastoma from Ewing's sarcoma, rhabdomyosarcoma, neuroepithelioma, and hematopoietic malignancies. Prog Clin Biol Res. 1985;175:347–66.

32. Lipinski M, Braham K, Philip I et al. Neuroectoderm-associated antigens on Ewing's sarcoma cell lines. Cancer Res. 1987;47:183–7.

33. Llombart-Bosch A, Blanche R, Peydro-Olaya A. Ultrastructural study of 28 cases of Ewing's sarcoma: typical and atypical forms. Cancer. 1978;41:1362–73.

34. Hou-Jensen K, Priori E, Dmochowski L. Studies on ultrastructure of Ewing's sarcoma of bone. Cancer. 1972;29:280–6.

35. Dickman PS, Triche TJ. Extraosseous Ewing's sarcoma versus primitive rhabdomyosarcoma. Diagnostic criteria and clinical correlation. Hum Pathol. 1986;17:881–93.

36. Cavazzana AO, Miser JS, Jefferson J, Triche TJ. Experimental evidence for a neural origin of Ewing's sarcoma of bone. Am J Pathol. 1987;127:507–18.

37. Wigger HJ, Salazar GH, Blanc WA. Extraskeletal Ewing's sarcoma. An ultrastructural study. Arch Pathol Lab Med. 1977;101:446–9.

38. Meister P, Gokel JM. Extraskeletal Ewing's sarcoma. Virchows Arch (Pathol Anat). 1978;378:173–9.

39. Navas-Palacios JJ, Aparicio-Duque R, Valdes MD. On the histogenesis of Ewing's sarcoma. An ultrastructural immunohistochemical and cytochemical study. Cancer. 1984;53:1882–901.

40. Nascimento AG, Unni KK, Pritchard DJ, Cooper KL, Dahlin DC. A clinicopathological study of 20 cases of large-cell (atypical) Ewing's sarcoma of bone. Am J Clin Pathol. 1980;4:29–36.

41. Llombart-Bosch A, Blanche R, Peydro-Olaya A. Round cell sarcomas of bone and their differential diagnosis (with particular emphasis on Ewing's sarcoma and reticulosarcoma). Hum Pathol. 1982;17:113–45.

42. Phillips RF, Higginbotham NL. The curability of Ewing's endothelioma of bone in children. J Pediatr. 1967;70:391–7.

43. Stratton B, Askin FB, Kissane JM. Intramyofiber skeletal muscle invasion in Ewing's sarcoma of the bone: clinicopathological observations from the Intergroup Ewing's Sarcoma Study. Am J Pediatr Hematol Oncol. 1982;4:231–5.

44. McKeon C, Thiele CJ, Ross RA et al. Indistinguishable patterns of protooncogene expression in two distinct but closely related tumors: Ewing's sarcoma and neuroepithelioma. Cancer Res. 1988;48: 4307–11.

45. Shimada H, Newton WA, Soule EH, Qualman SJ, Aoyama C, Maurer HM. Pathologic features of extraosseous Ewing's sarcoma. A report from the Intergroup Rhabdomyosarcoma Study. Hum Pathol. 1988;19:442–53.

46. Whang-Peng J, Triche TJ, Knuten T, Miser J, Douglass EC, Israel MA. Chromosome translocation in peripheral neuroepithelioma. N Engl J Med. 1984;311:584–5.

Histiocytic disorders

8

This is a complex group of reactive and neoplastic disorders that originate generally from at least two different subsets of immune accessory cell: (a) the dendritic cell system (DCS) and (b) the mononuclear phagocyte system (MPS)[1-3]. Immunohistochemistry and electron microscopy are often important in their differentiation[4].

The dendritic cells are non-phagocytic and express S-100 protein and also, to a variable extent, thymic antigen (CD1)[1]. Immunoreactivity for lysozyme and α_1-antichymotrypsin is usually absent and Birbeck granules are demonstrated by ultrastructural examination. In addition to the Langerhans cell, the DCS includes indeterminate cells, interdigitating reticulum cells, follicular dendritic cells and the veiled cell[1]. Histiocytosis X or Langerhans cell histiocytosis is the most important disorder related to this cell system.

Table 8.1 Histiocytic disorders

Langerhans cell histiocytosis
Congenital self-healing reticulohistiocytosis
Juvenile xanthogranuloma
Benign cephalic histiocytosis
Familial haemophagocytic lymphohistiocytosis
Reactive haemophagocytic syndrome
Sinus histiocytosis with massive lymphadenopathy
Malignant histiocytosis
Regressing atypical histiocytosis
'Malignant histiocytosis' associated with leukaemia and lymphoma

The MPS comprises phagocytic macrophages that express lysozyme and α_1-antichymotrypsin; they lack S-100 protein and the thymocyte-related antigen (CD1), and Birbeck granules are not seen ultrastructurally. The cells are derived from promonocytes and undergo differentiation into monocytes in the peripheral blood, prior to migrating into tissues. The haemophagocytic lymphohistiocytoses (familial haemophagocytic lymphohistiocytosis and reactive haemophagocytic syndrome) are some histiocytic disorders associated with the MPS[5]. Sinus histiocytosis with massive lymphadenopathy (Rosai–Dorfman disease) exhibits an antigenic profile representative of both immune accessory cell[6].

LANGERHANS CELL HISTIOCYTOSIS (HISTIOCYTOSIS X)

The term histiocytosis X was introduced by Lichtenstein in 1953[7] in an attempt to integrate the three clinical syndromes (Letterer–Siwe disease, Schüller–Christian syndrome and eosinophilic granuloma of bone) into a single pathological entity.

Histiocytosis X occurs throughout the world, and boys are twice as often affected as girls[1]. Recent evidence convincingly implicates the Langerhans dendritic cell of the epidermis as the cell of origin of histiocytosis X[1,2]; i.e. histiocytosis X probably represent localized or disseminated proliferation of the Langerhans cell[1,2]. An indigenous cell of the epidermis and squamous mucosa, the Langerhans cell shows dendritic processes and occupies the basal layer. Histiocytosis X is thus more accurately referred to as Langerhans cell histiocytosis (or Langerhans granulomatosis), and the term is preferentially used throughout the remainder of the chapter. The stimulus for the proliferation of the Langerhans cell is unknown, and attempts to isolate a causative agent have so far proved unsuccessful[8]. A disorder of immune regulation has been implicated, but this is unproven. There is no convincing evidence that the disease is neoplastic. In children, the skeleton and the skin are the sites most commonly involved[1,2,8]. (This contrasts with adults, in whom the lung is most commonly involved.)

Microscopically, the single most important diagnostic feature of Langerhans cell histiocytosis is the morphology of the lesional cell[9]. This is a large cell (15–30 μm) with fairly abundant, faintly eosinophilic, finely vacuolated cytoplasm. The nucleus is indented or reniform with a groove or cleft across the nuclear membrane (reminiscent of a 'coffee bean') (Figure 8.1). Nucleoli are generally single and conspicuous. Mitoses are unusual. Phagocytic activity is rare. Giant cells containing five or six nuclei are often seen, especially in osseous lesions.

In the more established lesions, the Langerhans cell is commonly part of a polymorphous infiltrate that includes lymphocytes, macrophages, neutrophils and eosinophils. Necrosis is common in such lesions. Plasma cells are unusual, but eosinophils may be so numerous as to mask the underlying lesion and Charcot–Leyden crystals may be prominent[9]. There are no differences in the microscopic appearance of the Langerhans cell between the localized and disseminated forms of the disease.

The Langerhans cell displays immunoreactivity for S-100 protein (Figure 8.2), the monoclonal antibody for the thymocyte-related antigen (CD1) (Figure 8.3), HLA-DR (Ia) and peanut agglutinin[8]. Immunohistochemistry for CD1 requires frozen tissue. The cells are negative for lysozyme. The ultrastructure of the histiocytes demonstrates the so-called Birbeck (or X) granule which is a straight or curved pentalaminary rod of variable length, often vesicular at one end, frequently resembling a racquet[1] (Figure 8.4). Currently their function is unknown. They are located mostly in the peripheral part of the cell cytoplasm, adjacent to the plasma membrane from which they appear to arise. The granules seem to be present in all cases but the number of cells containing granules varies greatly[1]. Their number within cells has been linked to cellular maturity, larger numbers being associated with immaturity. They are described in other types of dendritic cells[10] as well as in some neoplastic conditions[11]. Birbeck granules may resemble other cytoplasmic organelles.

Nezelof[9] drew attention to the variable histological picture related to different phases of the lesion:

(a) Lesions composed chiefly or exclusively of Langerhans cells represent the proliferative stage (Figure 8.5);

(b) The granulomatous stage is characterized by necrotic areas, lymphocytes and polymorphs (especially eosinophils), in addition to Langerhans cells (Figure 8.6);

(c) Accumulation of lipid in the histiocytic cytoplasm and prominence of fibrous tissue characterize the xanthogranulomatous stage (Figure 8.7).

The causes of death in patients with Langerhans cell histiocytosis include superadded infection, respiratory failure and drug-related complications[12].

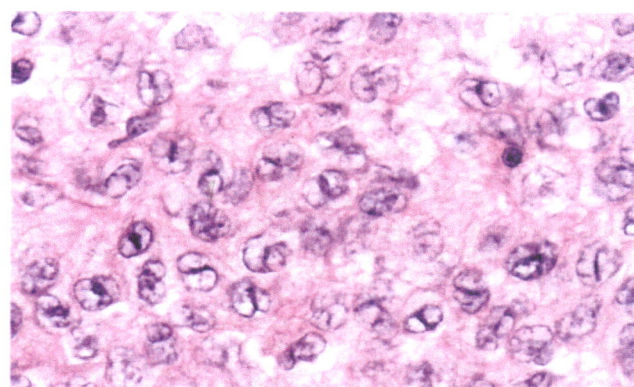

Fig. 8.1 A high-power view of constituent cells in Langerhans cell histiocytosis displays the characteristic cellular morphology. The cytoplasm is abundant, ill-defined, eosinophilic and granular. The nuclei are vesicular and irregular with frequent linear folding. (Note the resemblance to coffee beans.) H&E × 750

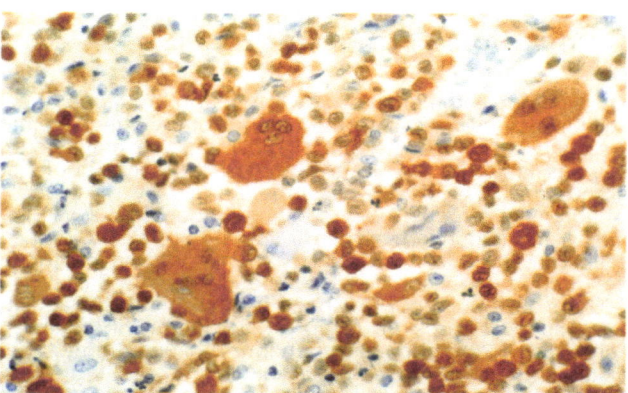

Fig. 8.2 Eosinophilic granuloma of the skull showing many Langerhans cells and multinucleate giant cells; both cell types express S-100 protein on immunohistochemistry. S-100 protein × 300

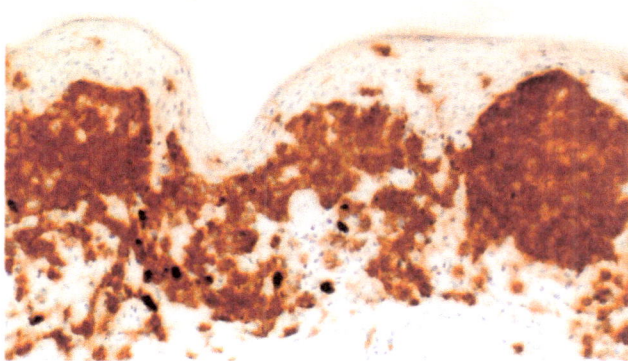

Fig. 8.3 Immunohistochemistry for CD1 (T6) carried out on a frozen section of skin reveals strong positivity in the cytoplasm of the lesional cells, mainly occupying the papillary dermis. Occasionally positive reacting cells are also seen in the epidermis. CD1 × 75

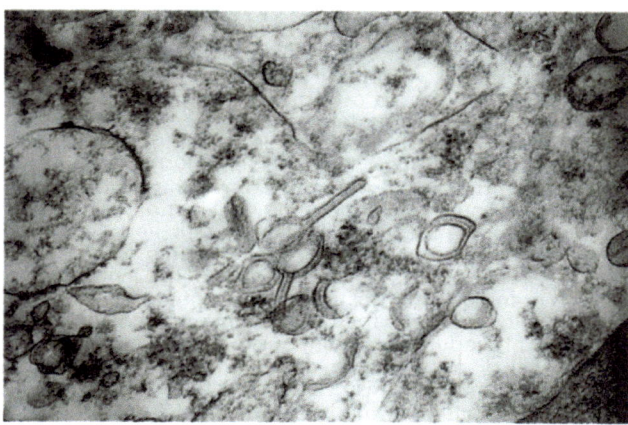

Fig. 8.4 An electron micrograph shows pentalaminar Birbeck granules in the cytoplasm in a Langerhans cell. The cell formed part of Langerhans cell histiocytosis that was discovered incidentally in the thymus at autopsy in a 7-month old boy. × 56 000

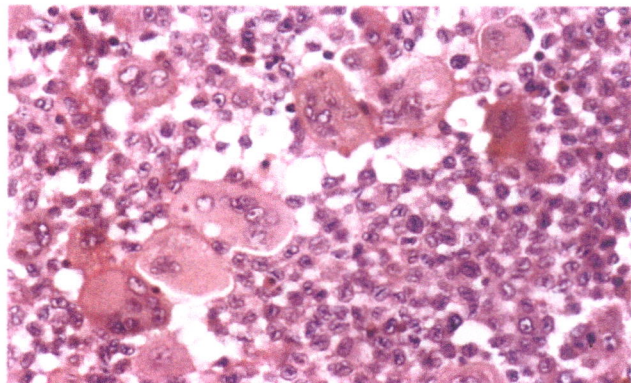

Fig. 8.5 The microscopy of this osseous lesion is dominated by Langerhans cells and multinucleated giant cells; little if any reactive component is present. This type of cellular pattern is sometimes referred to as 'proliferative'. H&E × 300

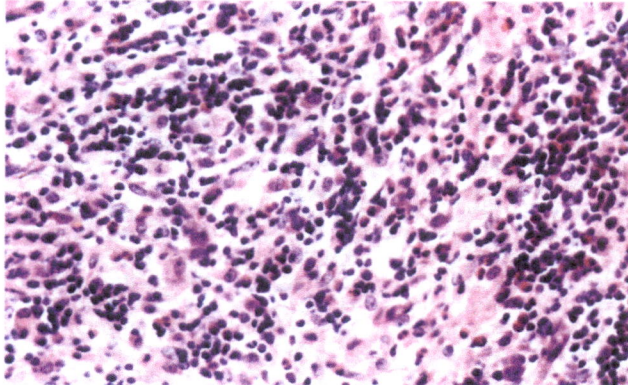

Fig. 8.6 An eosinophilic granuloma curetted from the mastoid region shows the Langerhans cells to be virtually masked by an inflammatory infiltrate rich in eosinophils and lymphocytes. H&E × 300

INVOLVEMENT OF SPECIFIC SITES BY LANGERHANS CELL HISTIOCYTOSIS

Bone

The skeleton is the most common location for Langerhans cell histiocytosis[2]. Pain and swelling over the affected area are the usual symptoms; pathological fractures may occur. Lesions limited to bone are referred to as eosinophilic granulomas. The osseous lesions are usually solitary[2,13]. Children are affected more commonly than adults, with a peak age incidence between 5 and 10 years. Radiologically, an irregular lytic area with or without cortical destruction is observed in the medulla (Figure 8.8).

Bone lesions tend to affect haemopoietically active sites, such as the skull (Figure 8.9), femur, ribs, pelvis, vertebrae and mandible in children[9]; accordingly, the distal extremities are seldom involved.

Microscopically, osseous involvement illustrates typically the evolutionary changes described above[9], the end-result of which may be difficult to gauge unless preceded by a diagnostic biopsy.

Loosening of the teeth often accompanies involvement of the maxilla or mandibula[1]. Ear disease occurs with or without localized temporal bone involvement (eosinophilic granuloma)[14], and the more common clinical manifestation is aural discharge. Less frequently temporal bone swelling is the first sign. Non-osseous aural disease usually accompanies systemic disease, affects a younger age and correlates with poor prognosis[14].

Haemosiderin may be conspicuous in osseous lesions, which also often display large numbers of multinucleate giant cells (Figure 8.10). The older lesions with foam cells, fibrosis and inflammatory cells may be difficult to distinguish from healing osteomyelitis. Plasma cells are, however, unusual in Langerhans cell histiocytosis, and immunohistochemistry for S-100 protein and CD1 are useful in separating the two entities (Figures 8.2, 8.3). In the older lesions, foam cells do not usually demonstrate Birbeck granules on ultrastructural investigation[1].

Surgical curettage is the only treatment usually necessary; the procedure simultaneously provides tissue for histological diagnosis. Low-dose X-ray therapy may be necessary, as curettage is contraindicated when the vertebrae and ischium are involved[12].

Additional osseous lesions may arise after curettage, or there may be progression to a disseminated disease; while this is uncommon, it is heralded by an increase in size of an osseous lesion on X-ray[13]. In a follow-up study of 43 patients with monostotic disease, 11% went on to develop additional lesions[13].

Skin

The skin is the second most common site and the scalp is particularly susceptible, corresponding probably to the abundance of epidermal Langerhans cells normally found at this site[1]. Exclusive dermal involvement is extremely uncommon and involvement of the skin usually occurs as part of disseminated disease.

Clinically, the lesions may be macular, maculopapular (Figure 8.11), petechial or even vesicular; less commonly, they are eczematoid or seborrhoeic (Figure 8.12).

Microscopically, the papillary dermis is the site of histiocytic proliferation (Figure 8.13). The epidermal basement membrane is frequently disrupted and exocytosis of the lesional cells into the epidermis is common. Giant cells tend to be uncommon in skin lesions[1]; secondary superficial ulceration may occur.

The differential diagnosis includes juvenile xanthogranuloma, urticaria pigmentosa, graft vs. host disease, histiocytoid haemangioma and congenital self-healing reticulohistiocytosis[8].

Lymph nodes

Lymph nodes are involved in several ways[8]:

(a)   The sole site of involvement – primary eosinophilic granuloma of lymph node.
(b)   Involvement of a lymph node within a field of lymphatic drainage from another site, e.g. bone, lung.
(c)   Part of disseminated disease.
(d)   An incidental finding in malignant lymphomas.

Primary eosinophilic granuloma of lymph node is rare and occurs predominantly in children and young adults. Of the 30 cases reported by Motoi et al.[15], 30% were under 13 years of age. One or several lymph nodes may be affected simultaneously. Focal involvement of the node, infiltration of the capsule and surrounding tissue, and necrosis are features that help to distinguish primary involvement from disseminated disease[15].

In common with other examples of unifocal disease, exclusive involvement of the lymph node carries a good prognosis[15].

A picture indistinguishable from Langerhans cell histiocytosis has been described in lymph nodes coexisting with Hodgkin's disease and non-Hodgkin's lymphoma[16]. All six patients reported were adults. Whether the two lesions were related or fortuitous was not satisfactorily resolved.

The differential diagnosis of lymph nodal Langerhans cell histiocytosis includes dermatopathic lymphadenopathy, sinus histiocytosis with massive lymphadenopathy (Rosai–Dorfman disease), mycobacterial infection, lipogranulomas with eosinophilia[8] and Hodgkin's disease[17].

Liver

Involvement of the liver usually causes hepatomegaly and is always part of disseminated disease[1]. Jaundice is usually the first sign. Four basic patterns of hepatic involvement are recognized:

(a)   Infiltration and proliferation of histiocytes within the portal triads accompanied by fibrosis;
(b)   Lymph node involvement at the porta hepatis causing extrahepatic biliary obstruction;
(c)   Protracted cholestasis that may be accompanied by portal hypertension[18];
(d)   Hepatotoxic effects of chemotherapy.

In relation to (c), intraoperative cholangiography demonstrates patency of the extrahepatic bile ducts and distortion of the intrahepatic bile ducts. Histologically, there is fibrous expansion of the portal triads in association with bile ductular proliferation, but bile stasis is usually sparse. The demonstration of histiocytic infiltration in the liver is exceptional.

Lung

The lung may be involved as part of disseminated disease or may be the only site affected; the latter tends to occur in young adults[8,12]. The patient may be asymptomatic or manifest symptoms, such as cough, dyspnoea and cyanosis. The formation of bullae is common, and clinical presentation with pneumothorax is well recognized. Fibrosis is a late finding and may lead to bronchiectasis ('honeycomb' lung) (Figure 8.14) and chronic cor pulmonale. Very few Langerhans cells are found in association with the late fibrotic stage.

Spleen and haemopoietic tissue

Splenomegaly is rare at first presentation[9], and splenic involvement is either part of disseminated disease or secondary to portal hypertension associated with hepatic portal fibrosis. The association of anaemia–leucopenia–thrombocytopenia indicates marrow involvement or treatment-induced hypoplasia[9].

Gastrointestinal tract

Involvement of the intestinal tract is increasingly reported but the bowel is rarely affected in isolation[19]. Depending on the level and extent of the disease, patients may present with intestinal malabsorption or diarrhoea. The microscopic differential diagnosis includes Crohn's disease, chronic granulomatous disease of childhood, malakoplakia and mycobacterial disease secondary to *Mycobacterium avium–intracellulare*[20].

Central nervous system

Information on morphological involvement of the central nervous system is virtually non-existent[1]. Recognized clinical sequelae include diabetes insipidus, which is usually permanent, although easy to control[12]. The morphological lesion associated with diabetes insipidus is poorly understood[1].

Thymus

Isolated involvement of the thymus is rarely reported. The histopathology is similar to lesions occurring elsewhere[8]. Thymic involvement may occur with or without symptoms, the former being associated with respiratory obstruction. The prognosis for isolated thymic involvement is good[8].

CLINICAL VARIANTS OF LANGERHANS CELL HISTIOCYTOSIS

Localized and disseminated forms of the disease are an important distinction in terms of prognosis[2,12]. Disseminated disease can be divided into acute, subacute and chronic, although there is considerable overlap.

The acute disseminated type is equivalent to Letterer–Siwe disease in the older terminology[2]; it predominates in infancy and is associated with a poor outcome. After clinical remission it is not unusual for the acute disseminated type to evolve into a subacute or chronic form[12].

The chronic disseminated form equates with Hand–Schüller–Christian disease, now preferably designated multiple focal eosinophilic granuloma. The condition characteristically affects older children or young adults, and classically refers to the clinical triad of lytic lesions involving the cranial bones, exophthalmos and diabetes insipidus; although, in reality, this combination rarely occurs in isolation and is often associated with extracranial manifestations. As previously indicated, localized Langerhans cell histiocytosis has a predilection for the bones, lung and lymph node.

PROGNOSIS OF LANGERHANS CELL HISTIOCYTOSIS

Prognosis in Langerhans cell histiocytosis takes account of a number of clinical parameters. Adverse prognostic factors include an age less than 12 months, multiple organ involvement and associated organ dysfunction[9]. The prognosis is particularly poor in newborn infants with multiorgan involvement[21].

Several attempts have been made to link prognosis with histological features, but results have been variable. A recent study[22] failed to predict outcome on the basis of microscopic appearances.

Bone marrow involvement without osteolysis is associated with poor outcome[9], contrasting with the favourable outcome of eosinophilic granuloma.

CONGENITAL SELF-HEALING RETICULOHISTIOCYTOSIS (CSHR) (CONGENITAL SELF-HEALING HISTIOCYTOSIS; RETICULOHISTIOCYTOMA OF HASHIMOTO AND PRITZKER)

Congenital self-healing reticulohistiocytosis (CSHR) is a rare histiocytic disorder that has many features in common with Langerhans cell histiocytosis[23]. Clinically, the condition is characterized by a cutaneous eruption of firm brown or violaceous nodules. Any part of the body may be affected but the mucous membranes are spared. The eruption is virtually always present at birth (or soon after) and the lesions are limited to the skin[23,24]. Systemic manifestations are absent[23]. The sexes are affected with equal frequency. Spontaneous regression can be expected within 6–12 months. The lesions are usually multiple and the overlying skin may be eroded or ulcerated[23]. Histologically, the lesions are indistinguishable from Langerhans cell histiocytosis[25] and the histiocytes also express S-100 and CD1. Birbeck granules are demonstrated ultrastructurally in 10–20% of the cells[25].

CSHR should be segregated from congenital Langerhans cell histiocytosis with systemic involvement as the latter condition is associated with a dismal prognosis[21].

JUVENILE XANTHOGRANULOMA (NAEVOXANTHOENDOTHELIOMA)

Juvenile xanthogranuloma (JXG) generally affects infants and young children and may present at birth[26]. Less often it is found in adolescents and young adults. The male : female ratio is about 4 : 1. About 80% of lesions are solitary. Small nodules, at first pink and tense and later becoming yellow and wrinkled, is the usual clinical picture. The size of the lesions ranges from 1 mm to a few centimetres. The facial and truncal skin are mostly affected[26,27]. The natural course is one of spontaneous regression, generally without scarring. The genital mucosa and eye are rarely affected[2].

Microscopically, the dermis is typically involved but the lesion may extend into the subcutis[27]. The epidermis is spared but is often flattened. The lesion shows a mixture of mature histiocytes, foamy macrophages, Touton-type giant cells, fibroblast-like cells, small blood vessels and varying numbers of inflammatory cells (Figure 8.15). The cell constituents lack nuclear atypism and pleomorphism; mitoses are rare. Interstitial fibrosis is common and may impart a vague storiform pattern, and haemosiderin may be present.

The cellular composition is variable and various microscopic patterns are described: xanthomatous, xanthogranulomatous, fibrohistiocytic, or a combination[26]. Of these, the xanthogranulomatous pattern is most common.

The differential diagnosis includes Langerhans cell histiocytosis, xanthomas associated with hyperlipidaemia, dermatofibroma and reticulohistiocytoma[27]. JXG is sometimes seen in association with von Recklinghausen's disease[2].

Immunoreactivity for S100-protein has been variously reported as positive[26] and negative[27,28]. Langerhans granules have not been demonstrated ultrastructurally[2]. Immunoreactivity for lysozyme is usually present[27].

A deep variant of JXG is occasionally described[29,30]. This is located in the subcutaneous tissue and muscle and the overlying skin is uninvolved. Compared with the cutaneous form of JXG, the deep variant shows greater circumscription, more cellular monotony and less Touton-

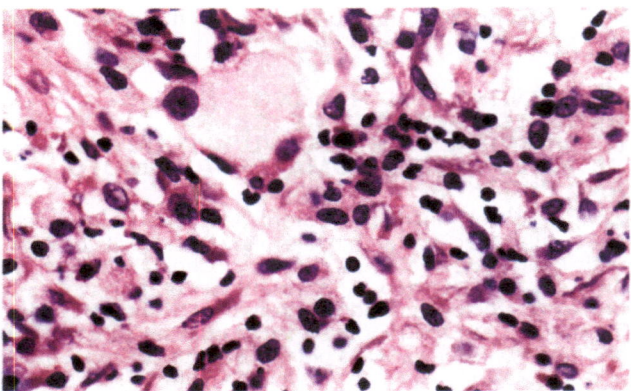

Fig. 8.7   The histology of this lesion shows greater cellular heterogeneity; the infiltrate comprises fibroblasts, lymphocytes and eosinophils, as well as several foamy macrophages. This is the usual picture of Langerhans cell histiocytosis in a phase of resolution. The patient, a 10-year-old girl, presented with a swelling in the right parietal bone of the skull; curettage was curative. H&E × 480

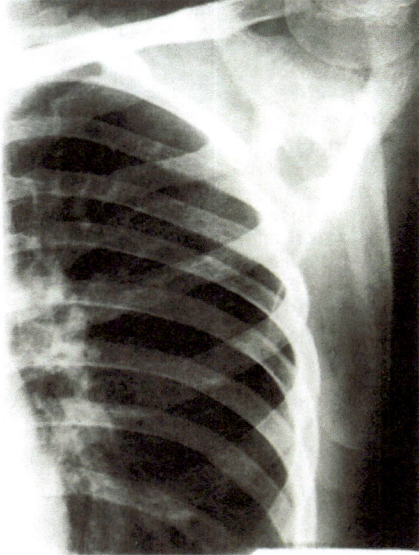

Fig. 8.8   X-ray of the left hemithorax shows a lytic lesion involving the upper part of the scapula in a 13-year-old boy who had complained of shoulder pain

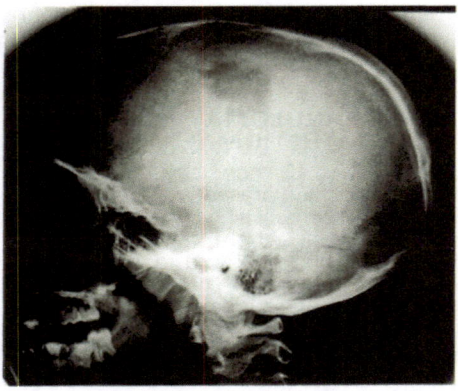

Fig. 8.9   X-ray of skull shows a sharply outlined lytic lesion in the parietal area of the skull. The lesion was curetted and, on microscopy, showed a cellular infiltrate that included many Langerhans cells

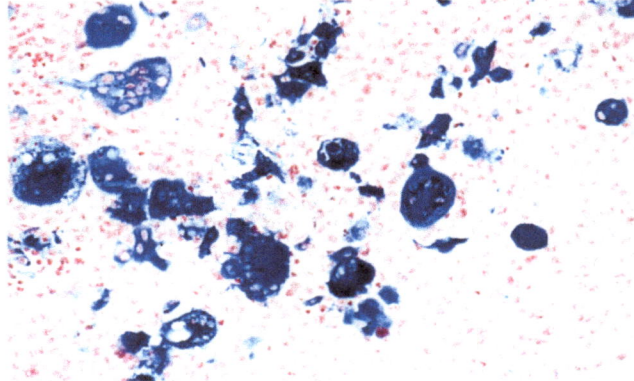

Fig. 8.10   Skull lesion showing large numbers of mononuclear and multinucleate Langerhans cells that are markedly siderotic. Perl's reaction × 185

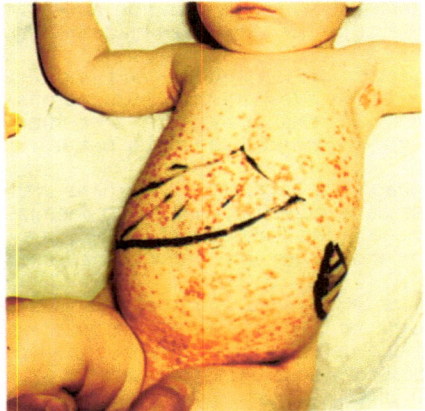

Fig. 8.11   A maculopapular rash is present on the trunk of this 10-month-old female infant who also had hepatosplenomegaly. A diagnosis of Langerhans cell histiocytosis was made on a skin biopsy

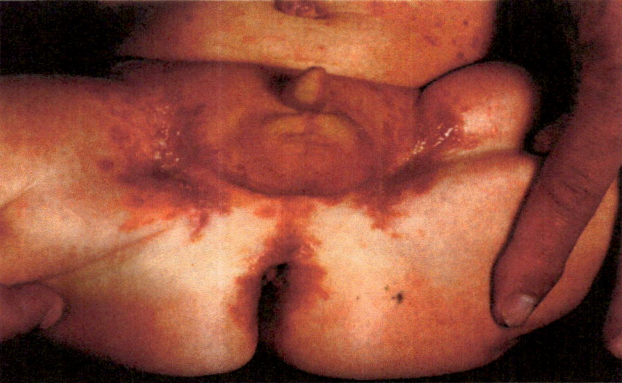

Fig. 8.12   This male infant shows an intertriginous rash in the perineum and around the scrotum. The distribution of the rash helps to distinguish Langerhans cell histiocytosis from a napkin eruption; the latter generally involves the skin over anatomical protuberances

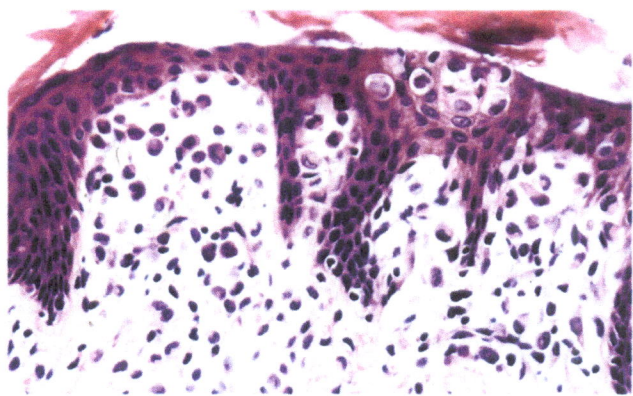

Fig. 8.13 The papillary dermis contains an infiltrate of large cells showing abundant granular eosinophilic cytoplasm and vesicular nuclei. A few eosinophils are also present. The lesional cells have infiltrated the epidermis. The patient was a 5-month-old boy who presented with a hard lump in the left temporal region of the skull and a truncal maculopapular rash. H&E × 300

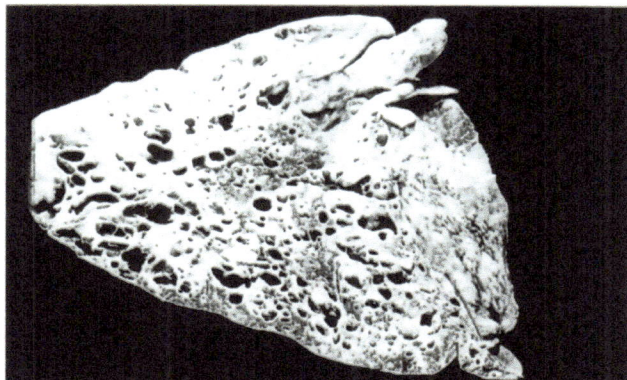

Fig. 8.14 Post-mortem lung from a 3-year-old child who died with disseminated Langerhans cell histiocytosis shows bronchiectasis

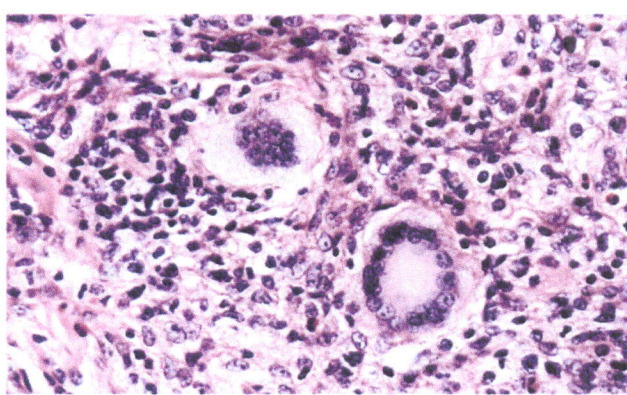

Fig. 8.15 Microscopy of juvenile xanthogranuloma displays two Touton-type giant cells surrounded by a mixture of foam cells, fibroblasts and a scatter of lymphocytes. H&E × 300

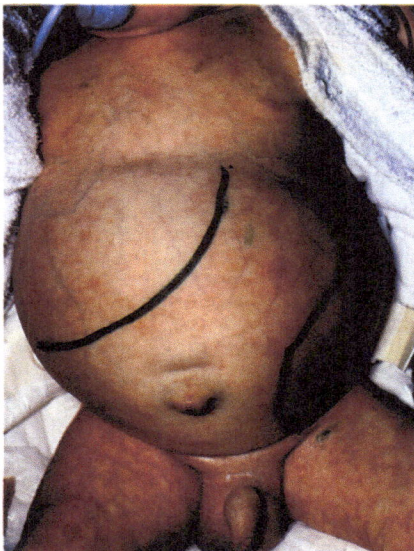

Fig. 8.16 Marked hepatosplenomegaly is outlined on the abdominal wall of this 6-week-old boy in whom a liver biopsy confirmed a diagnosis of familial haemophagocytic lymphohistiocytosis

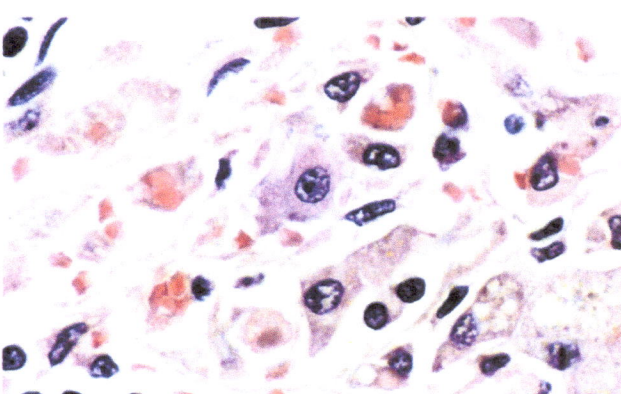

Fig. 8.17 Familial haemophagocytic lymphohistiocytosis. High-power microscopic view of liver to show composition of the cellular infiltrate at the edge of a portal triad. Several mature histiocytes have ingested red blood cells. A child of a consanguineous relationship, he presented at the age of 2 months with a 3-week history of rash over the scalp and right groin. H&E × 750

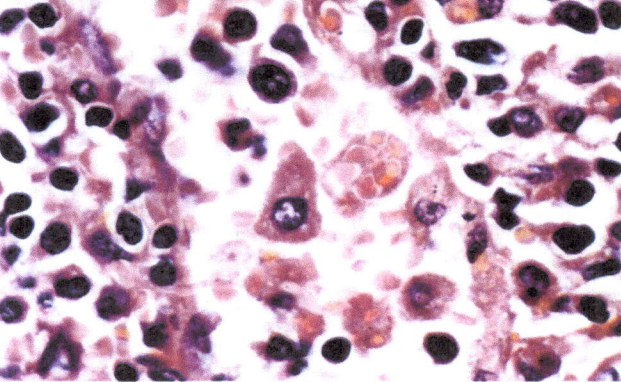

Fig. 8.18 Familial haemophagocytic lymphohistiocytosis. Microscopic view of splenic tissue shows histiocytes phagocytosing erythrocytes within a dilated sinus. H&E × 750

type giant cells. Because of their deep location, the lesions are likely to be confused with a malignant process.

BENIGN CEPHALIC HISTIOCYTOSIS

This is a benign self-limiting 'non-X' non-lipid histiocytic disorder clinically manifest as a yellowish papular eruption involving the skin of the head, neck and shoulders, rarely the thighs and buttocks[31,32]. The eruption usually commences in the second half-year after birth. The infants are otherwise healthy.

Microscopically, circumscribed cellular infiltrates predominate in the upper dermis. The infiltrate is composed chiefly of histiocytes with an oval, elongate or bean-shaped nucleus. Cytoplasm is abundant, pale and ill-defined. There is a variable admixture of lymphocytes and a few giant cells may be found.

The differential diagnosis includes juvenile xanthogranuloma, urticaria pigmentosa, generalized eruptive histiocytoma and Langerhans cell histiocytosis. Electron microscopically, membrane-bound dense bodies and/or worm-like bodies (comma-shaped bodies) are usually found in the cytoplasm[31,32]. The worm-like bodies are non-specific as they are also found in other histiocytoses[31]. Birbeck granules have not been described in benign cephalic histiocytosis.

FAMILIAL HAEMOPHAGOCYTIC LYMPHOHISTIOCYTOSIS (CONGENITAL HAEMOPHAGOCYTIC RETICULOSIS; FAMILIAL ERYTHROPHAGOCYTIC LYMPHOHISTIOCYTOSIS; FAMILIAL LYMPHOHISTIOCYTOSIS)

Familial haemophagocytic lymphohistiocytosis (FHL) is a rare condition first described by Farquhar and Claireaux in 1952[33]. Infants are usually affected in the first few months after birth; the upper age limit for the disease is unclear. The diagnosis is strongly supported by parental consanguinity or a positive family history[34]. The condition affects both sexes with equal frequency. Cases reported previously as familial Letterer–Siwe probably belong to this group[35].

Prolonged fever and hepatosplenomegaly (Figure 8.16) are almost universally present[36]. Other features include lymphadenopathy, irritability, pallor, oedema, petechial haemorrhages and a transient maculopapular rash. Jaundice is usually a late manifestation. Cerebral symptoms occasionally dominate the clinical picture[37]. Osseous involvement does not occur[36].

Investigations reveal progressive pancytopenia (anaemia, neutropenia and thrombocytopenia), liver dysfunction, coagulopathy and hyperlipidaemia. Hypofibrinogenaemia occurs in the majority of cases[36]. The cerebrospinal fluid contains increased protein and lymphocytes[38].

The usual microscopic picture is a diffuse histiocytic infiltrate showing erythrophagocytosis, accompanied by an infiltrate of cytologically benign lymphocytes (Figure 8.17)[38]. Erythrophagocytosis may be difficult to identify in ante-mortem tissues. The histiocytes are generally mature and are often masked by the lymphocytic infiltrate. All organs are affected, most notably the liver, spleen (Figure 8.18), lymph nodes (Figure 8.19), bone marrow and central nervous system (Figure 8.20).

In the liver, the portal triads are expanded by the lymphohistiocytic infiltrate that often extends focally into the adjoining lobular parenchyme (somewhat reminiscent of chronic aggressive hepatitis) (Figure 8.21). Kupffer cells are unduly prominent and reactive; extramedullary haemopoiesis is common. In the majority of cases, the bone marrow shows erythroid hyperplasia; haemophagocytosis is generally inconspicuous in this location[38].

Immunohistochemically, the histiocytes in FHL are reactive for α_1-antichymotrypsin and lysozyme; there is no reactivity for S-100 protein and CD1[39], and Birbeck granules are not demonstrated ultrastructurally[38,39]. The lymphocyte population is predominantly of T-cell derivation[39].

The stimulus for the histiocytic proliferation in this condition is unclear, although dysfunction of both humoral and cellular limbs of the immune system has been implicated. The outcome is nearly always fatal[36], and death usually follows a combination of infection, haemorrhage and neurological involvement[36]. Extensive bacteriological and virological studies are important to exclude an infection-associated histiocytic disorder[36,38]; however, the clinical course of FHL is frequently complicated by infections[35].

REACTIVE HAEMOPHAGOCYTIC SYNDROME (VIRUS-ASSOCIATED HAEMOPHAGOCYTIC SYNDROME; INFECTION-ASSOCIATED HAEMOPHAGOCYTIC SYNDROME)

Reactive haemophagocytic syndrome (RHS) is a multi-system histiocytic proliferation characterized by prominent haemophagocytosis[40,41]. It is associated with a wide range of infections[42], most notably viral, many of which belong to the herpes group (cytomegalovirus, Epstein–Barr virus, varicella zoster and herpes virus). Clinically, RHS is characterized by fever, hepatosplenomegaly, lymphadenopathy, skin eruption and pulmonary infiltrates[42]. Pancytopenia and coagulation disorders occur commonly. In Risdall's original series, six of the 19 patients died in the acute episode; the remainder recovered within 2–8 weeks[40].

The diagnosis of RHS is most readily made on examination of the bone marrow aspirate or trephine biopsy; this reveals a proliferation of well-differentiated histiocytes displaying conspicuous phagocytosis, admixed with lymphoid cells. The phagocytosed elements include intact or degenerate red blood cells, platelets, and haemopoietic cells. Lymph nodes, liver and splenic red pulp are also commonly involved and show a similar microscopic picture.

Patients with RHS may have no pre-existing illness while others have drug-related immunosuppression[40]. RHS may complicate haemic malignancies (including malignant lymphoma), bolstering the view that the syndrome is an expression of an immune paralysis for a specific infection. An instance of familial RHS has been recorded[42].

RHS has been reported in fatal EBV infection, as a sporadic event or in association with X-linked lymphoproliferative syndrome[43]. Chen et al.[44] report an aggressive form of the disease in Taiwan associated with a high mortality in previously well young children; evidence of Epstein–Barr virus infection was observed in a large proportion of the patients.

POSSIBLE RELATIONSHIP BETWEEN FAMILIAL HAEMOPHAGOCYTIC LYMPHOHISTIOCYTOSIS (FHL) AND REACTIVE HAEMOPHAGOCYTIC SYNDROME (RHS)

Many clinical, haematological and biochemical parameters are shared by FHL and RHS[45]. Both entities, for example, share the following clinical features: fever, hepatosplenomegaly, pancytopenia, CSF pleocytosis, hypofibrinogenaemia, hypertriglyceridaemia and evidence of preceding viral infection. A disseminated visceral infiltrate of lymphoid and erythrophagocytic histiocytes are common to both conditions[46]. However, macrophages associated with the two conditions are reported to show antigenic differences[47], although the investigators admit to difficulties in clinically separating the two entities.

SINUS HISTIOCYTOSIS WITH MASSIVE LYMPHADENOPATHY (SHML) (ROSAI–DORFMAN DISEASE; CYTOPHAGIC SINUS HISTIOCYTOSIS)

This is a rare histiocytic disorder occurring predominantly in the first two decades[48]. Yale University School of Medicine in the United States holds a national Registry that has provided valuable insight into the condition[49].

A wide age range is reported for this disease, with a mean age of onset of 20.6 years. Children are commonly affected and the Yale University Registry includes a case of congenital disease. The number of white patients with this condition has probably been underestimated[49].

Painless but prominent bilateral cervical lymphadenopathy is the usual mode of presentation, but, in some 30% of patients, lymphadenopathy occurs at other sites. The affected lymph nodes may be quite enormous and produce symptomatic compression of contiguous structures. Symptoms such as fever, malaise and weight loss are common, and anaemia, leukocytosis, and elevated ESR are often seen; polyclonal hypergammaglobulinaemia is a consistent feature.

Extranodal manifestations are reported to occur in 43% of cases[49], although these authors concede that such cases are probably over-represented in the Yale University Registry. Among the extranodal sites, the skin is involved most commonly and the upper respiratory tract, salivary glands, orbit, bone and testes are other locations that may be affected.

Histologically, the marginal and medullary sinuses of the lymph nodes are markedly distended by large numbers of histiocytes that display copious foamy pale eosinophilic cytoplasm and round vesicular nuclei (Figure 8.22). Mitoses are rare. The histiocytes are accompanied by lymphocytes, neutrophils and plasma cells. A characteristic finding is the presence of large numbers of well-preserved lymphocytes within the histiocytic cytoplasm (Figure 8.23), referred to as lymphocytophagocytosis or emperipolesis. Multinucleate histiocytes are encountered occasionally. The medullary cords are often expanded by numerous plasma cells (Figure 8.24). Reactive germinal centres are infrequent. The microscopy is similar in extranodal and nodal disease[50].

The histiocytes mark positively for S-100 protein, in addition to lysozyme, α_1-antitrypsin and α_1-antichymotrypsin, representing features of both the dendritic cell and mononuclear phagocyte[6].

The aetiology and pathogenesis of the condition are poorly understood, although some patients demonstrate immune dysfunction[6]. A protracted clinical course has been reported[50], and a small group is known to develop a fatal form of the disease[49,51].

In the great majority of cases, the condition is benign and surgical excision is usually curative; alternatively, the enlarged lymph nodes subside spontaneously. The differential diagnosis should include a storage disorder or one of the other histiocytic syndromes.

MALIGNANT HISTIOCYTOSIS (HISTIOCYTIC MEDULLARY RETICULOSIS)

Malignant histiocytosis affects adults predominantly, but a small number of cases involve children[52,53]. Hepatosplenomegaly and peripheral lymphadenopathy, reflecting multisystem involvement, is the usual clinical presentation and jaundice and constitutional disturbance are common. There is progressive involvement of bone marrow and peripheral blood. The prognosis is poor.

Microscopically, an infiltrate of immature and mature histiocytes, exhibiting erythrophagocytosis, is usually accompanied by lymphocytes and polymorphs (particularly eosinophils). Erythrophagocytosis is more often seen in the mature (reactive) histiocytes. The malignant cells are pleomorphic with hyperchromatic nuclei, prominent nucleoli and scant cytoplasm. Mitotic figures are common and frequently atypical.

The tumour cells express the following antigens: lysozyme (muramidase), α_1-antitrypsin, α_1-antichymotrypsin and Ia-antigen; and, enzyme histochemically, there is positivity for acid phosphatase, adenosine triphosphatase and acid α-naphthylacetate esterase.

Recently, the number of cases of malignant histiocytosis confidently diagnosed has been declining, and many such cases are now recognized as large-cell lymphoma or reactive haemophagocytic syndrome[54,55]. T-cell receptor and immunoglobulin gene arrangement studies provide additional evidence that many cases of 'malignant histiocytosis' are, in fact, T-cell lymphoma[56].

REGRESSING ATYPICAL HISTIOCYTOSIS

This is a rare nodulo-ulcerative condition of the skin characterized by spontaneous regression and recurrence. One of the cases reported originally by Flynn et al. was that of a 10-year-old girl[57]. Microscopy shows a neoplastic proliferation of atypical mononuclear and multinucleated histiocytic cells with associated erythrophagocytosis, against a background of fibrosis and mixed inflammatory infiltrate. The current view is that these tumours are probably examples of Ki-1 lymphoma[58].

'MALIGNANT HISTIOCYTOSIS' ASSOCIATED WITH T-CELL LEUKAEMIA AND LYMPHOMA

A malignant histiocytosis-like picture may develop as a preterminal event in patients with acute lymphoblastic leukaemia[59–61]. Children and adults are affected. Rosner and Grunwald[59] reviewed 17 patients with this disorder and found that the interval between leukaemotherapy and the onset of the malignant histiocytosis-like picture varied between 1.5 months and 7 years.

Clinically, the syndrome is marked by pancytopenia and rapid organ enlargement, and in most cases leukaemia was of T-cell type. Bar one, all the patients reported by Rosner and Grunwald[59] died with widespread multi-organ involvement. A possibly related disorder associated with T-cell lymphoma has been described in adults[62,63].

Argument is presented that these disorders are in fact examples of reactive haemophagocytic syndrome[63]. Pathogenetic theories include:

(a) A common stem cell for the lymphoma and histiocytic component;
(b) Oversecretion of lymphokines by the T-cell lymphoma[63].

HISTIOCYTIC LYMPHOMA

See Chapter 4.

REFERENCES

1. Favara BE, McCarthy RC, Mierau GW. Histiocytosis X. Hum Pathol. 1983;14:663–76.
2. Nezelof C, Barbey S. Histiocytosis: nosology and pathobiology. Pediatr Pathol. 1985;3:1–41.
3. Headington JT, Cerio R. Dendritic cells and the dermis. Am J Dermatopathol. 1990;12:217–220.
4. The Writing Group of the Histiocyte Society. Histiocytosis syndromes in children. Lancet. 1987;1:208–9.
5. Goldberg J, Nezelof C. Lymphohistiocytosis: a multi-factorial syndrome of macrophage activation. Clinicopathological study of 38 cases. Hematol Oncol. 1986;4:275–89.

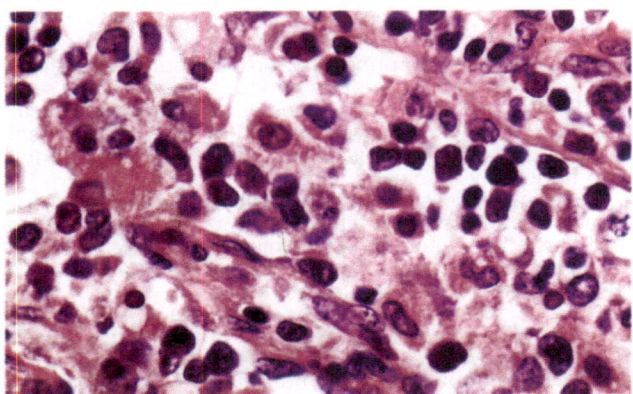

Fig. 8.19 Medullary sinus of cervical lymph node from an infant with familial haemophagocytic lymphohistiocytosis contains several mature histiocytes and lymphocytes; erythrophagocytosis is not conspicuous. H&E × 750

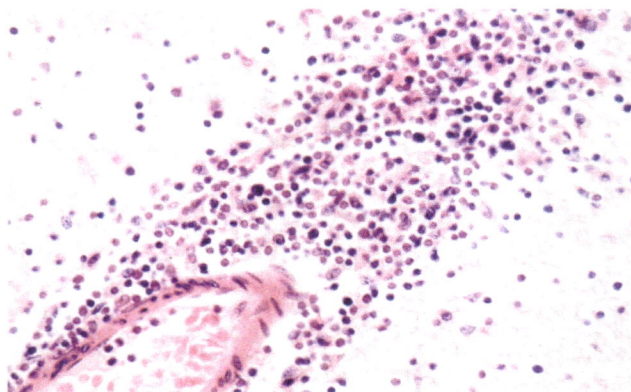

Fig. 8.20 Histology of brain tissue shows a perivascular infiltrate of lymphocytes and mature histiocytes in a boy aged 4 years with familial haemophagocytic lymphohistiocytosis who died with multisystem disease. H&E × 300

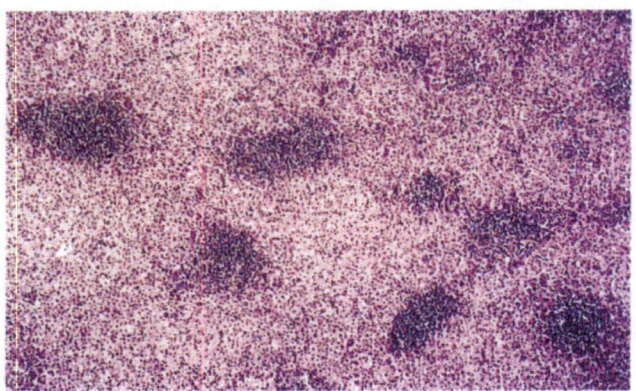

Fig. 8.21 Familial haemophagocytic lymphohistiocytosis. Low-magnification view of liver biopsy from a 5-month-old boy shows regular expansion of the portal traids by a dense cellular infiltrate; the appearance is reminiscent of aggressive chronic hepatitis. H&E × 48

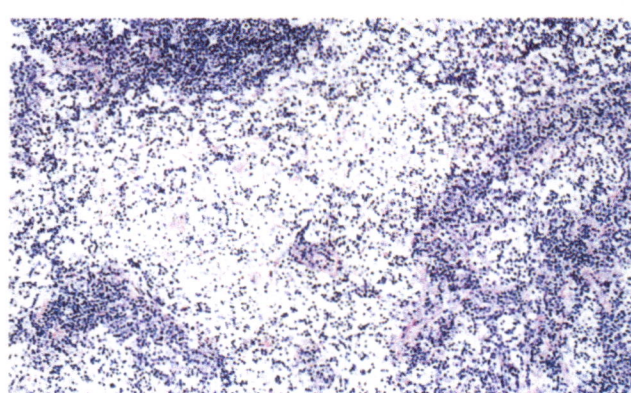

Fig. 8.22 Rosai–Dorfman disease. The lymph node shows marked expansion of the medullary sinuses. The patient was a 9-year-old Caucasian girl who presented with massive cervical lymphadenopathy. H&E × 75

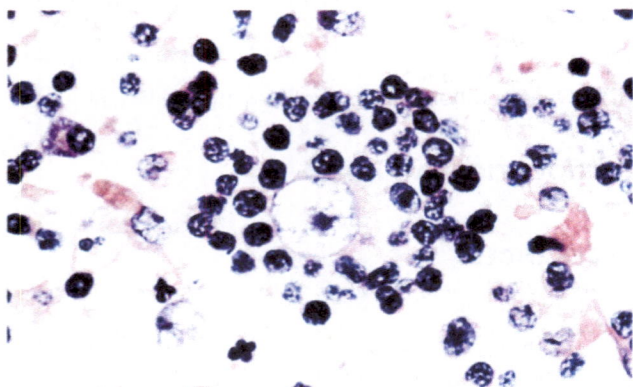

Fig. 8.23 Rosai–Dorfman disease. A large histiocyte within an expanded sinus shows prominent lymphophagocytosis. H&E × 840

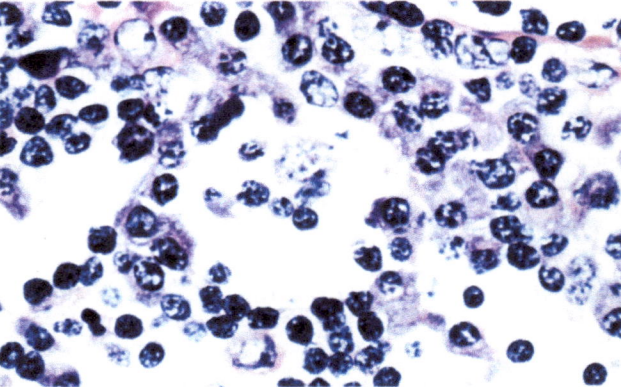

Fig. 8.24 Rosai–Dorfman disease. Plasma cells form a prominent component of the cellular infiltrate involving the medullary tissue of an affected lymph node. H&E × 750

6. Maennle DL, Grierson HL, Gnarra DG, Weisenburger DD. Sinus histiocytosis with massive lymphadenopathy: a spectrum of disease and dysfunction. Pediatr Pathol. 1991;11:399–412.
7. Lichtenstein L. Histiocytosis X. Integration of eosinophilic granuloma of bone, 'Letterer–Siwe disease', and 'Schuller–Christian disease' as related manifestations of a single nosologic entity. Arch Pathol. 1953;56:84–102.
8. Jaffe R. Pathology of histiocytosis X. Perspect Pediatr Pathol. 1987;9:4–47.
9. Nezelof C. Histiocytosis X: histological and histogenetic study. Perspect Pediatr Pathol. 1979;5:153–78.
10. Steinman RM. Dendritic cells. Transplantation. 1981;31:151–5.
11. Webster SM, Beabout JW, Unni KK, Dahlin DC. Langerhans' cell granulomatosis (histiocytosis X) of bone in adults. Am J Surg Pathol. 1982;6:413–26.
12. Basset F, Nezelof C, Ferrans VJ. The histiocytoses. Pathol Annu. 1983;18:27–78.
13. McCullough CJ. Eosinophilic granuloma of bone. Acta Orthop Scand. 1980;51:389–98.
14. McCaffrey TV, McDonald TJ. Histiocytosis X of the ear and temporal bone: review of 22 cases. Laryngoscope. 1979;89:1735–42.
15. Motoi M, Helbron D, Kaiserling E, Lennert K. Eosinophilic granuloma of lymph nodes – a variant of histiocytosis X. Histopathology. 1980;4:585–606.
16. Kjeldsberg CR, Kim H. Eosinophilic granuloma as an incidental finding in malignant lymphoma. Arch Pathol Lab Med. 1980;104:137–40.
17. Reid H, Fox H, Whittaker JS. Eosinophilic granuloma of lymph nodes. Histopathology. 1977;1:31–7.
18. Leblanc A, Hadchouel M, Jehan P, Odievre M, Alagille D. Obstructive jaundice in children with histiocytosis X. Gastroenterology. 1981;80:134–9.
19. Egeler RM, Schipper MEI, Heymans HSA. Eur J Pediatr. 1980;149:325–9.
20. Dehner LP. Gastrointestinal tract. In: Dehner LP. editor. Pediatric surgical pathology, 2nd edn. Baltimore: Williams & Wilkins; 1987:360.
21. Tamura T, Umetsu M, Motoya H, Yokoyama S. Congenital Letterer–Siwe disease associated with protein losing enteropathy. Eur J Pediatr. 1980;135:77–80.
22. Risdall RJ, Dehner LP, Duray P, Kobrinsky N, Robison L, Nesbit ME. Histiocytosis X (Langerhans' cell histiocytosis). Arch Pathol Lab Med. 1983;107:59–63.
23. Alexis JB, Poppiti RJ, Turbat-Herrera E, Smith MD. Congenital self-healing reticulohistiocytosis. Report of a case with 7-year follow-up and review of the literature. Am J Dermatopathol. 1991;13:189–94.
24. Dehner LP, Bamford JT, McDonald EC. Spontaneous regression of congenital cutaneous histiocytosis X: Report of a case with discussion of nosology and pathogenesis. Pediatr Pathol. 1983;1:99–106.
25. Kanitakis J, Zambruno G, Schmitt D, Cambazard F, Jacquemier D, Thivolet J. Congenital self-healing histiocytosis (Hashimoto-Pritzker). An ultrastructural and immunohistochemical study. Cancer. 1988;61:508–16.
26. Tahan RT, Pastel-Levy C, Bhan AK, Mihn MC. Juvenile xanthothogranuloma. Clinical and pathologic characterization. Arch Pathol Lab Med. 1989;113:1057–61.
27. Sonoda T, Hashimoto H, Enjoji M. Juvenile xanthogranuloma. Clinicopathologic analysis and immunohistochemical study of 57 patients. Cancer. 1985;56:2280–6.
28. Seo S, Whan Min K, Mirkin D. Juvenile xanthogranuloma. Arch Pathol Lab Med. 1986;110:911–15.
29. Janney CG, Hurt MA, Santa Cruz DJ. Deep juvenile xanthogranuloma. Subcutaneous and intramuscular forms. Am J Surg Pathol. 1991;15:150–9.
30. White W, Garen P. Juvenile xanthogranuloma of the paravertebral soft tissue in infancy: a report of two cases. Pediatr Pathol. 1991;11:105–13.
31. Gianotti F, Caputo R, Ermacora E, Gianni E. Benign cephalic histiocytosis. Arch Dermatol. 1986;122:1038–43.
32. Barsky BL, Lao I, Barsky S, Rhee HL. Benign cephalic histiocytosis. Arch Dermatol. 1984;120:650–5.
33. Farquhar JW, Claireaux AE. Familial haemophagocytic reticulosis. Arch Dis Child. 1952;27:519–25.
34. Henter JI, Elinder G, Ost A and the FHL Study Group of the Histiocyte Society. Diagnostic guidelines for hemophagocytic lymphohistiocytosis. Semin Oncol. 1991;18:29–33.
35. Spritz RA. The familial histiocytoses. Pediatr Pathol. 1985;3:43–57.
36. Janka GE. Familial hemophagocytic lymphohistiocytosis. Eur J Pediatr. 1983;140:221–30.
37. Henter JI, Elinder G. Cerebromeningeal haemophagocytic lymphohistiocytosis. Lancet. 1992;339:104–7.
38. Gilbert EF, ZuRhein GM, Webster SM et al. Familial hemophagocytic lymphohistiocytosis: report of four cases in two families and review of the literature. Pediatr Pathol. 1985;3:59–92.
39. Wieczorek R, Greco MA, McCarthy K, Bonetti F, Knowles DM. Familial erythrophagocytic lymphohistiocytosis: immunophenotypic, immunohistochemical, and ultrastructural demonstration of the relation to sinus histiocytes. Hum Pathol. 1986;17:55–63.
40. Risdall RJ, McKenna RW, Nesbit ME, Krivit W, Balfour HH, Simmons RL, Brunning RD. Virus-associated hemophagocytic syndrome. A benign histiocytic proliferation distinct from malignant histiocytosis. Cancer. 1979;44:993–1002.
41. McKenna RW, Risdall RJ, Brunning RD. Virus associated hemophagocytic syndrome. Hum Pathol. 1981;12:395–8.
42. Arya S, Hong R, Gilbert EF. Reactive haemophagocytic syndrome. Pediatr Pathol. 1985;3:129–41.
43. Mroczek EC, Weisenburger DD, Lipscomb Grierson H, Markin R, Purtilo DT. Fatal infectious mononucleosis and virus-associated hemophagocytic syndrome. Arch Pathol Lab Med. 1987;111:530–5.
44. Chen RL, Su IJ, Lin KH. Fulminant childhood hemophagocytic syndrome mimicking histiocytic medullary reticulosis. Am J Clin Pathol. 1991;96:171–6.
45. McClain K, Gehrz R, Grierson H, Purtillo D, Filipovich A. Virus-associated histiocytic proliferations in children. Am J Ped Hemat/Oncol. 1988;10:196–205.
46. Goldberg J, Nezelof C. Lymphohistiocytosis: a multi-factorial syndrome of macrophagic activation. Clinico-pathological study of 38 cases. Hematol Oncol. 1986;4:275–89.
47. Buckley PJ, O'Laughlin S, Komp DM. Histiocytes in familial and infection-induced/idiopathic hemophagocytic syndromes may exhibit phenotypic differences. Pediatr Pathol. 1992;12:51–66.
48. Rosai J, Dorfman RF. Sinus histiocytosis with massive lymphadenopathy: a newly recognized benign clinicopathological entity. Arch Pathol. 1969;87:63–70.
49. Foucar E, Rosai J, Dorfman R. Sinus histiocytosis with massive lymphadenopathy (Rosai–Dorfman disease): review of the entity. Semin Diagnost Pathol. 1990;7:19–73.
50. Foucar E, Rosai J, Dorfman RF. Sinus histiocytosis with massive lymphadenopathy. Ear, nose and throat manifestations. Arch Otolaryngol. 1978;104:687–93.
51. Buchino JJ, Byrd RP, Kmetz DR. Disseminated sinus histiocytosis with massive lymphadenopathy. Its pathological aspects. Arch Pathol Lab Med. 1982;106:13–16.
52. Zucker JM, Caillaux JM, Vanel D, Gerard-Marchant R. Malignant histiocytosis in childhood. Clinical study and therapeutic results in 22 cases. Cancer. 1980;45:2821–9.
53. Jurco S, Starling K, Hawkins E. Malignant histiocytosis in childhood: morphological considerations. Hum Pathol. 1983;14:1059–65.
54. Chan JKC, Ng CS, Hui PK, et al. Anaplastic large cell Ki-1 lymphoma. Delineation of two types. Histopathology. 1989;15:11–34.
55. Ishii E, Hara T, Okumura J, et al. Malignant histiocytosis in infants: surface marker analysis of malignant cells in two cases. Med Ped Oncol. 1987;15:102–8.
56. Weiss LM, Trela MJ, Cleary ML, Turner RR, Warnke RA, Sklar J. Frequent immunoglobulin and T-cell receptor gene rearrangements in 'histiocytic' neoplasms. Am J Pathol. 1985;121:369–73.
57. Flynn KJ, Dehner LP, Gajl-Peczalska KJ, Dahl MV, Ramsay N, Wang N. Regressing atypical histiocytosis: a cutaneous proliferation of atypical neoplastic histiocytes with unexpectedly indolent biological behaviour. Cancer. 1982;49:959–70.
58. Dehner LP. Case 5. Ki-1 lymphoma. Pediatr Pathol. 1991;11:183–90.
59. Rosner F, Grunwald HW. Association of T cell acute lymphoblastic leukaemia and histiocytic medullary reticulosis. Am J Med. 1984;77:910–14.
60. Chen TK, Nesbit ME, McKenna R, Kersey JH. Histiocytic medullary reticulosis in acute lymphocytic leukaemia of T cell origin. Am J Dis Child. 1976;130:1262–4.
61. Yin Liu JA, Kumaran TO, Marsh GW, Rossiter M, Catovksy D. Complete recovery of histiocytic medullary reticulosis-like syndrome in a child with acute lymphoblastic leukemia. Cancer. 1983;51:200–2.
62. Jaffe ES, Costa J, Fauci AS, Cossman J, Tsokos M. Malignant lymphoma and erythrophagocytosis simulating malignant histiocytosis. Am J Med. 1983;75:741–9.
63. Chan EYT, Pi D, Chan GTC, Todd D, Ho FCS. Peripheral T-cell lymphoma presenting as hemophagocytic syndrome. Hematol Oncol. 1989;7:275–85.

Germm cell tumours

9

The incidence of germ cell neoplasms in children and adolescents is difficult to estimate from epidemiological data[1]. Females are mostly affected, but this is mainly due to the frequency of ovarian involvement[2]. The histogenesis of germ cell tumours remains controversial and theories include derivation from totipotent germ cells, origin from yolk sac and totipotent embryonic cells, and 'fetus-in-fetu'[3].

Germ cell tumours composed of tissues from all three germ cell layers (ectoderm, mesoderm and endoderm) are referred to as teratomas. They may also present in the form of a pure germ cell tumour (yolk sac tumour, embryonal carcinoma, dysgerminoma or choriocarcinoma). Germ cell tumours showing a combination of teratoma and pure germ cell component are referred to as mixed teratomas.

A spectrum of differentiation and organization exists in teratomas which, in its most advanced form, is referred to as 'fetus-in-fetu'[4]; these teratomas resemble a human fetus to the extent of revealing axialization and metameric segmentation.

Germ cell tumours are remarkable, not only for their complex microscopic structure, but also for their diversity in location and biological behaviour. The gonads and the sacrococcygeal region are the most common sites[2,5,6], and an asymptomatic mass is the most common presentation. Clinical features are often related to compression of adjacent structures[2].

Teratomas are subdivided into benign, immature (depending on the degree of differentiation of constituent somatic tissues) and malignant. Malignancy depends on the inclusion of a pure germ cell component[1]. Benign teratomas comprise mature (or fully differentiated) tissues, while immature teratomas show variable proportions of embryonal/fetal tissues. Neuroglial tissue is the most common mature component, while primitive neuroectoderm is the most common expression of immaturity[5]. Less frequently encountered immature components include primitive mesenchyme, fetal cartilage, myoblastic tissue, immature renal and hepatic tissue. In practice, immature elements usually occur in combination with mature somatic structures. A teratoma composed purely of immature structures is uncommon in childhood. About 80% of childhood teratomas are benign (mature and immature)[6].

A pure germ cell component, such as yolk sac tumour, embryonal carcinoma, dysgerminoma or choriocarcinoma, occurs in isolation or as a component of a mature or immature teratoma. In children, the most frequent pure germ cell component (pure and mixed) is yolk sac tumour[7,8]. Malignant germ cell tumours usually spread to the lungs, liver, regional lymph nodes and central nervous system; less frequently, they involve bone, but bone marrow *per se* and other sites are only rarely affected[9].

The gross appearance of teratomas often predicts their histological make-up[3]; thus mature teratomas are well-demarcated, encapsulated and cystic, contrasting with malignant neoplasms that are usually more solid in appearance. Germinomas are soft, friable and granular, while areas of haemorrhage and necrosis characterize embryonal carcinoma and choriocarcinoma.

Standard classifications of germ cell tumours in adults are difficult to apply to a paediatric population because embryonal carcinoma, germinoma and choriocarcinoma are far less commonly found in children. The classification proposed by Kooijman[10] seems appropriate for this age group (Table 9.1). The immature component is graded 1–3 depending on the amount that is present.

Table 9.1 Classification of childhood germ cell tumours

I	Germinoma
II	Endodermal sinus tumour
III	Embryonal carcinoma
IV	Choriocarcinoma
V	Combinations of I–IV
VI	Teratoma
	A Mature
	B Immature (1–3)
	C Mature or immature teratoma combined with neoplastic tissue from groups I–IV

YOLK SAC TUMOUR (ENDODERMAL SINUS TUMOUR, INFANTILE EMBRYONAL CARCINOMA, YOLK SAC CARCINOMA, TEILUM TUMOUR, INFANTILE ORCHIOBLASTOMA)

This is the most common type of pure germ cell tumour found in children[5,8]. It is highly malignant and has a distinctive microscopic appearance with differentiation towards extraembryonic structures.

The testes and ovaries are the sites most commonly affected. For the first 2 years after birth, it constitutes the most common form of testicular tumour. Extragonadal locations include the vagina, sacrococcygeal area, pelvis, retroperitoneum, anterior mediastinum and pineal area; these are also the common sites for other germ cell neoplasms[1].

Gross specimens show large soft greyish–tan mucoid masses[1]. Microscopically, yolk sac tumour expresses variable cellular patterns[14], including reticular (Figure 9.1), polyvesicular vitelline (Figure 9.2), pseudopapillary (Figure 9.3) and solid (Figure 9.4) patterns[1,11]. Coexistence of these patterns in the same tumour in varying combination is commonly seen, one pattern frequently dominating. The polyvesicular vitelline pattern is characterized by glandular spaces lined by flattened, cuboidal or columnar cells and separated by a myxoid stroma containing spindle and stellate cells.

Structures comprising a central blood vessel covered by a mantle of tumour cells, projecting into an ill-defined sinus, are referred to as Schiller–Duval bodies, endodermal sinuses or 'glomeruloid' bodies (Figure 9.5). They are diagnostic of yolk sac tumour but are found only in some 50–75% of neoplasms[1]. They arise most commonly in association with the pseudopapillary pattern.

Intracellular and extracellular PAS-positive diastase-resistant hyaline globules are another important microscopic feature (Figure 9.6)[7], and are found most often in association with the reticular pattern. ('Hyaline globules' are also seen as a feature of undifferentiated (embryonal) sarcoma of the liver; see Chapter 1.) Significant numbers of mitoses and cellular atypia are generally lacking in yolk sac tumour, and foci of haemorrhage and necrosis are seldom encountered. Calcification is rarely observed.

A mesenchymal component composed of spindle and

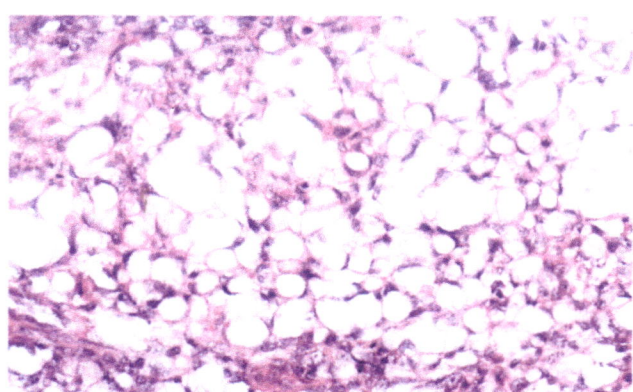

Fig. 9.1 A reticular pattern of yolk sac tumour is demonstrated. H&E × 185

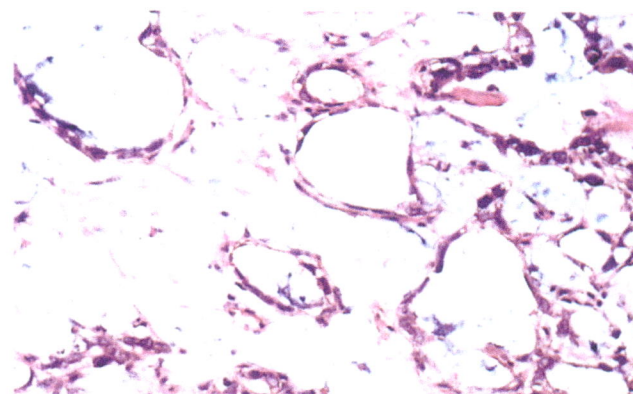

Fig. 9.2 This microscopic field of a yolk sac tumour shows a polyvesicular vitelline pattern. H&E × 185

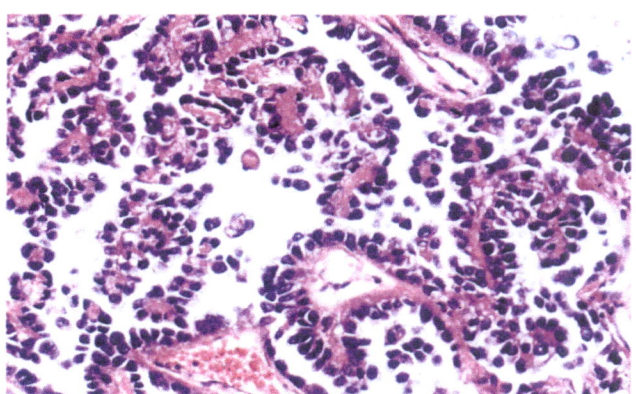

Fig. 9.3 A pseudopapillary pattern of a yolk sac tumour. This 13-month-old boy had widespread involvement of the peritoneal cavity; a portion of the tumour was removed for microscopic diagnosis. H&E × 185

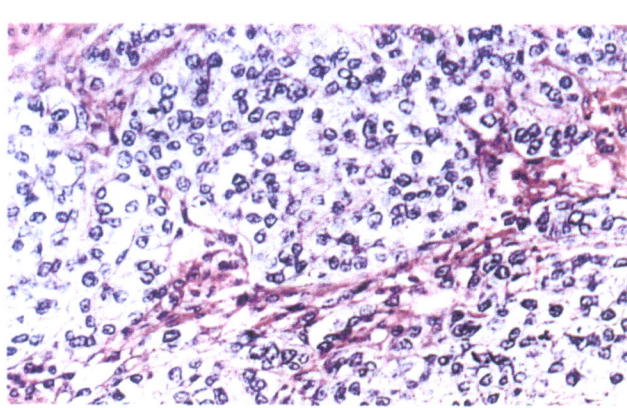

Fig. 9.4 A solid pattern of yolk sac tumour is demonstrated in this microscopic field. H&E × 185

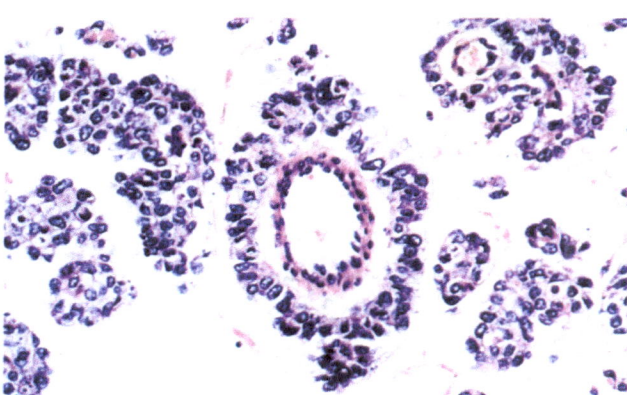

Fig. 9.5 Yolk sac tumour demonstrates a large Schiller–Duval body in the centre of the field. H&E × 300

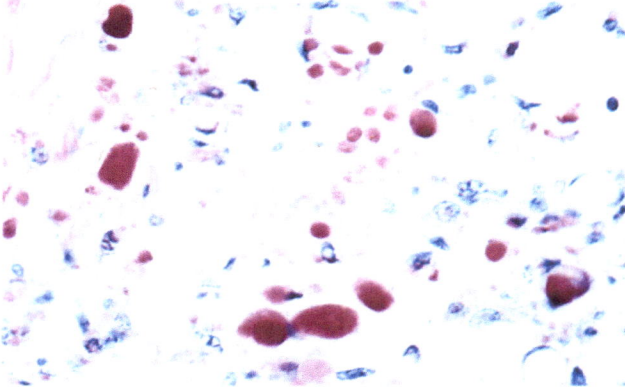

Fig. 9.6 Eosinophilic globules in a yolk sac tumour are seen most commonly in association with the reticular pattern. The globules which are strongly PAS positive may be intracytoplasmic, or they may lie free between cells. PAS × 336

stellate cells containing thin-walled blood vessels is often present; it is set in a myxoid background which stains positively with alcian blue (Figure 9.7), the positivity decreasing with hyaluronidase predigestion.

Truong et al.[11] investigated tumour tissue immunohistochemically from seven patients with mediastinal yolk sac tumour and found that all of the tumours stained positively for alpha-fetoprotein and α_1-antitrypsin; the positivity was mainly confined to the epithelium. A smaller number of tumours was positive for carcinoembryonic antigen and keratin. Only some of the hyaline globules marked positively with α_1-antitrypsin and alpha-fetoprotein. β-HCG was not expressed by the tumour cells in any of their cases[11], although Harms and Jänig[8] found single and small clusters of β-HCG-positive giant cells in some yolk sac tumours.

Yolk sac tumour may arise in isolation, occur as part of a mixed teratoma (Figure 9.8), or is mixed with other pure germ cell tumours (e.g. embryonal carcinoma, dysgerminoma, choriocarcinoma). In a mixed teratoma, the amount of yolk sac tumour varies from minute to being the dominant element[12].

Patients with yolk sac tumour invariably have a raised serum level of alpha-fetoprotein (AFP), an important diagnostic marker[12]. There is good correlation between the quantity of tumour and the level of serum AFP. AFP has a half-life of 4 days and, consequently, is useful for monitoring the course of the disease. Following complete surgical extirpation, the level of serum AFP should revert to normal within a period equivalent to its half-life; if not, residual or occult disease should be suspected. Embryologically, AFP is elaborated by the yolk sac and its derivatives, including the liver and gastrointestinal tract; hence, it is not surprising to find a clinically raised serum level occasionally associated with a teratoma containing intestinal glandular tissue[13].

The single most important factor in prognosis is the completeness of surgical excision, and this is probably the basis for the excellent outlook for tumours of the testis. This contrasts with yolk sac tumours occurring at other sites, especially those involving the pineal–hypothalamic site[1]. A correlation does not seem to exist between prognosis and histological pattern[14].

Metastases occur via the lymphatic and haematogenous routes. Recurrence following resection of a primary mature or immature teratoma may be composed entirely of yolk sac tumour[2,14,15]. A raised AFP at the time of diagnosis of an immature teratoma is said to be predictive of such recurrence[16]. Several explanations have been advanced for this phenomenon[16], including malignant change in an originally benign tumour; malignant growth in pluripotential cells remaining from the first diagnosis; sampling error of the resected material at initial diagnosis; and presence of a second primary tumour. Yolk sac tumour may express itself microscopically solely as mesenchymal tissue (i.e. without an epithelial component)[17]; this is especially likely to follow chemotherapy.

EMBRYONAL CARCINOMA

Embryonal carcinoma is traditionally separated into 'adult-type' and 'infantile-type'; the latter is more commonly referred to as yolk sac tumour[1]. Nowadays the term embryonal carcinoma generally applies to the 'adult-type'. Histologically, embryonal carcinoma is represented by sheets of cells that are larger than those found in yolk sac tumour (Figure 9.9). Nucleoli are prominent with nuclear pleomorphism, overlapping nuclei and frequent mitoses[7]. Haemorrhage and necrosis are common[7]. The tumour cells react positively for placental alkaline phosphatase[18] and Ki-1 (CD30)[19].

Embryonal carcinoma shares certain features with yolk sac tumour including a 'papillary pattern' (Figure 9.10) and the ability to elaborate AFP[7] and placental alkaline phosphatase[18]. The histological patterns of yolk sac tumour and embryonal carcinoma may coexist. In contrast to yolk sac tumour, embryonal carcinoma tends to occur in late adolescence or young adulthood. A similar survival rate has been reported for children with embryonal carcinoma and yolk sac tumour[14].

GERMINOMA

Germinoma may involve the gonads or extragonadal sites. Seminoma is the recommended terminology when the testis is affected; the same tumour affecting the ovary is referred to as dysgerminoma. When the neoplasm arises at other sites germinoma is the usual appellation[1].

Extragonadal sites for germinoma include the retroperitoneum, anterior mediastinum and the pineal area. Germinoma may occur in pure form or admixed with other germ cell elements. Germinoma has been reported to comprise some 10% of germ cell tumours in childhood[8].

Testicular seminomas in children are very rare; their presence should raise the possibility of mixed gonadal dysgenesis or pseudohermaphroditism[1]. Anterior mediastinal germinomas are generally confined to adolescents and young adults. Dysgerminoma of the ovary is the most common form of pure germinoma in the first two decades of life[1].

Solid sheets, aggregates and linear profiles of large cells with central round and vesicular nuclei typify the microscopic picture (Figure 9.11)[1,20]. Two or three nucleoli are usually present. The cytoplasm is clear to granular and contains moderate-to-abundant glycogen as demonstrated on PAS positivity/diastase lability (Figure 9.12). Fibrous septation, lymphoid tissue and a granulomatous reaction (Figure 9.13) are reactive changes frequently found. These occur in varying proportions and may be so conspicuous as to obscure the underlying tumour. The monotonous cytology and the monolayering of tumour cells are important distinguishing features[7]. The tumour cells express strong diffuse membrane-bound positivity for placental alkaline phosphatase[18,21].

Germinoma is among the most radiosensitive of neoplasms and there is an excellent prospect for long-term survival[1].

CHORIOCARCINOMA

Choriocarcinoma may arise as a gestational or non-gestational neoplasm. Gestational neoplasms originate from the trophoblast and metastasize rarely in utero to the fetus, presenting as multiple visceral lesions[22]. Both forms of choriocarcinoma are exceptionally uncommon, the non-gestational type more so. Choriocarcinoma is associated with a poor prospect for survival and elevated titres of human chorionic gonadotrophin (β-HCG) are recorded in many cases[20].

Non-gestational choriocarcinoma may occur in pure form or as part of a malignant mixed teratoma and, as with other germ cell neoplasms, may affect the gonads or extragonadal sites. The latter includes the retroperitoneum, anterior mediastinum or intracranium.

Microscopically, the tumour is composed of multinucleated syncytiotrophoblastic-like cells (Figure 9.14) and mononuclear cytotrophoblastic-like cells (Figure 9.15). Vascularity is prominent and haemorrhage and necrosis are common.

Scattered syncytiotrophoblast-like cells have been reported in ovarian dysgerminoma[20] and ovarian embryonal carcinoma[23]; they do not influence prognosis and should not be used as a basis for the diagnosis of choriocarcinoma[20].

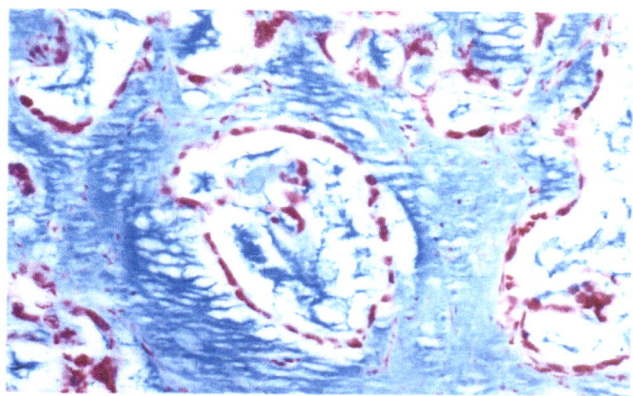

Fig. 9.7 Polyvesicular vitelline pattern of yolk sac tumour in which the mesenchymal component is mucoid and shows a markedly positive Alcian blue reaction. Alcian blue counterstained with neutral red × 185

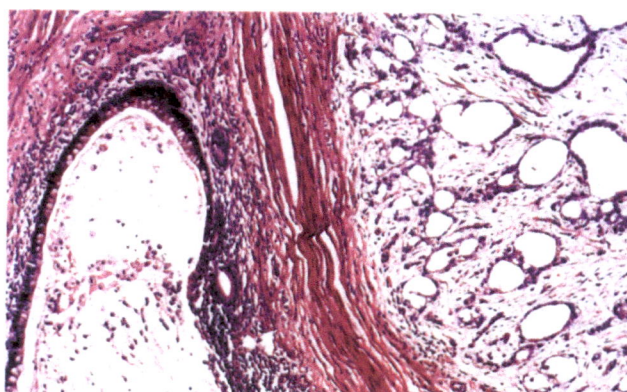

Fig. 9.8 Polyvesicular vitelline pattern of yolk sac tumour is shown alongside a large glandular structure. This combination represents a mixed teratoma. H&E × 75

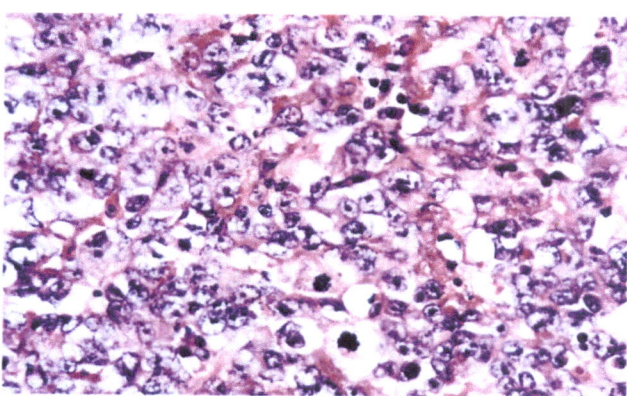

Fig. 9.9 Embryonal carcinoma showing a solid pattern with overlapping of the tumour cells. Cellular anaplasia and mitotic activity are more evident than is usually seen in yolk sac tumour. This tumour was part of a mixed teratoma which also featured seminoma and various differentiated glandular structures. H&E × 300

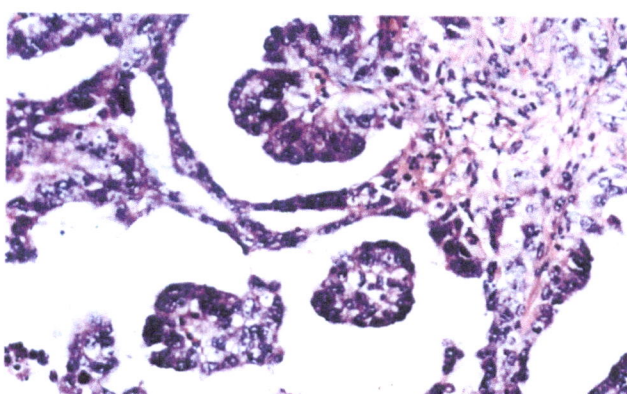

Fig. 9.10 Pseudopapillary pattern of embryonal carcinoma is demonstrated. The pattern is reminiscent of yolk sac tumour but cellular anaplasia and increased mitotic activity in embryonal carcinoma are helpful distinguishing features. H&E × 185

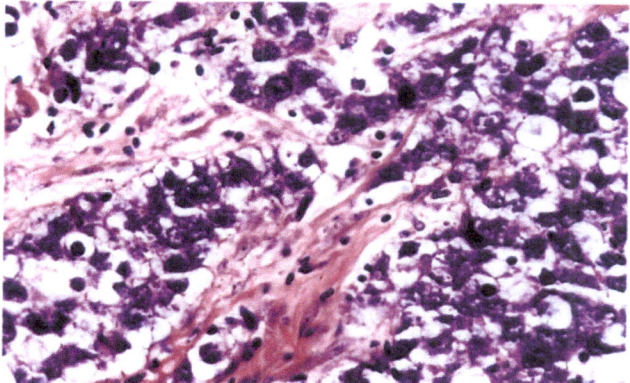

Fig. 9.11 Ovarian dysgerminoma shows large cells with central round vesicular nuclei and prominent nucleoli. The cytoplasm is clear to granular. A few lymphocytes are intermixed. H&E × 300

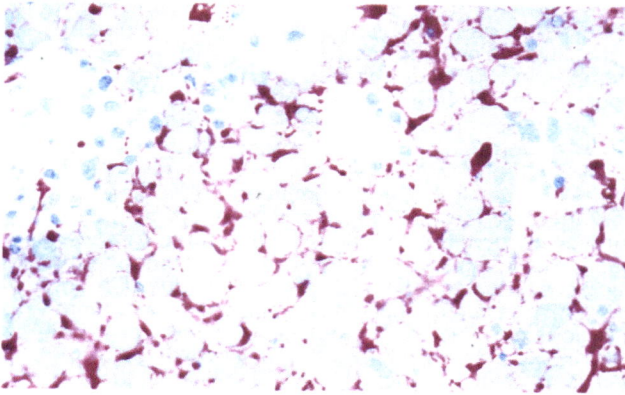

Fig. 9.12 Due to their high content of intracytoplasmic glycogen, dysgerminomas are frequently markedly positive on PAS staining. PAS; frozen section × 300

SACROCOCCYGEAL TERATOMA

This is the most common anatomical location for teratoma in childhood[1,24]. Sacrococcygeal teratoma occurs three times more frequently in girls than in boys[25]. The great majority of tumours are present at birth or are detected in the neonatal period. Plain radiographs show focal calcification or even teeth in 20–50% of cases[25]. Associated congenital anomalies commonly involve the vertebrae, genitourinary tract and anorectum[26]; these have been ascribed to developmental aberration secondary to tumour growth *in utero*. Older infants generally have smaller tumours.

Four major growth patterns are recognized[27]: (a) postsacral, (b) tumours with roughly equal postsacral and presacral proportions, (c) asymmetrical 'dumbell' tumours with predominantly presacral growth, and (d) wholly intrapelvic neoplasms. The postsacral tumours are the most common[27].

Intrapelvic tumours are associated with an increased incidence of malignancy, presumably related to delay in clinical diagnosis. Postsacral tumours usually show a midline sessile or pedunculated growth between the legs; extension may occur into one buttock. The skin surface may be tense, smooth or wrinkled, hyperkeratotic, atrophic, haemangiomatous, ulcerated or naevoid (Figure 9.16)[15,25].

Larger lesions may cause fetal hydrops, obstruct delivery, or may rupture at birth resulting in exsanguinating haemorrhage[25]. Macroscopically, benign sacrococcygeal tumours are usually encapsulated or well-circumscribed (Figure 9.17). The cut surface is often cystic, the cysts containing serous fluid, mucus, cheesy material, opaque coagulum or haemorrhage and fetal parts of variable complexity may be recognizable. A solid cut surface generally correlates with malignancy.

The coccyx must be surgically removed with the tumour to ensure complete resection[6] and a positive attempt should be made by the pathologist to identify this structure in the resected material. However, absence of the coccyx has been noted in association with some tumours[25].

Microscopic examination in the majority of cases shows the constituent tissues to be fully differentiated. These include glia, intestine, cartilage, choroid plexus, pancreas and bronchial mucosa, although virtually any tissue may be represented[3]. The most common component is mature neuroglial tissue, present in more than 90% of tumours (Figure 9.18). In nearly 50% of cases, it represents the predominant element.

Primitive neuroectoderm is the most common expression of immaturity[25,28], and, while disturbing in appearance, does not usually imply malignant potential[28]. Typically, this shows sheets of small hyperchromatic cells (reminiscent of neuroblastoma) (Figure 9.19) and/or neuroepithelial tubules (Figure 9.20). Immunohistochemically, the primitive neuroectoderm is non-reactive for alpha-fetoprotein. Other immature components include cartilage (Figure 9.21), primitive mesenchyme, myoblastic tissue (Figure 9.22) and primitive hepatic parenchyma (Figure 9.23). Renal blastema with glomeruloid and tubular elements, resembling Wilms' tumour, have also been described and may form a large component of a sacrococcygeal teratoma[29,30]. These latter tumours are not known to recur or metastasize[28,31] and consequently a judicious approach to therapy is advocated.

Yolk sac tissue may be present in varying proportion and is the most frequently encountered malignant component in sacrococcygeal tumours[6,28]. This germ cell component is rarely found in sacrococcygeal tumours removed at or soon after birth[32]; their prevalence increases markedly with an increasing interval after birth.

Thus the following features adversely affect prognosis:

(a) greater age at diagnosis, (b) the presence of a substantial presacral or intrapelvic component, and (c) the inclusion of a yolk sac component[15]. The size of the sacrococcygeal tumour does not appear to influence prognosis, apart from imposing a greater surgical hazard. Familial examples of sacrococcygeal 'teratoma' with autosomal dominant inheritance have been described in association with presacral masses, sacral defects and anal stenosis[25].

Myelomeningocele, enteric cysts, tail gut cysts, dermoid cysts and sinuses, sacral lipomas and lipomeningomyeloceles are other lesions that may occupy a postsacral location[25].

TERATOMAS OF THE HEAD AND NECK (EXTRACRANIAL)

Approximately 5% of teratomas in children involve the craniocervical region[24]. The orbit, nasopharynx, oropharynx, face and the cervicothyroid area are the usual sites. Most are located in the cervicothyroid area[15]. They are anatomically closely related to the thyroid but an actual origin in the gland is usually difficult to demonstrate; clinically, they may be mistaken for lymphangioma or cystic hygroma[15].

The great majority of tumours are clinically manifest at birth[24,33] and, in this respect, are reminiscent of sacrococcygeal tumours. Respiratory and feeding difficulties often accompany teratomas of the naso- and oropharynx; polyhydramnios, non-immune fetal hydrops and dystocia are other complications. In view of the complex anatomical relationship, there is a low rate of surgical resectability. Tumours in the oral cavity often take origin in the basicranium and, in the older literature, were referred to collectively as 'epignathi'.

The majority of the tumours show a mature histological appearance and behave in a benign fashion. However, immature somatic structures are frequently observed but, in the young, do not appear to impart aggressive potential[24]. Yolk sac tumours are occasionally found as part of a mixed teratoma or as a pure germ cell neoplasm[24,33]. According to Dehner *et al.*[33] germinomatous and choriocarcinomatous patterns have not been reported in cervicocranial (extracranial) teratomas. Of the 16 cases of head and neck teratomas reported by Lack[24], two arose in the orbit.

OVARIAN TERATOMA

The ovary is second only to the sacrococcygeal area as the most common site for the occurrence of childhood teratomas[1,15]. Clinical presentation is often precipitated by haemorrhage or torsion. The presenting age is usually between 9 and 11 years[1]. The majority of ovarian teratomas are unilateral, the right and left ovary being affected with equal frequency. In children, about 60–70% of ovarian teratomas are mature and cystic[1], and are usually referred to as ovarian dermoids. These are composed of a single cystic locule occupying a large portion of the ovary and containing copious quantities of lardaceous material and hair (Figure 9.24). A calcified nodule in the wall of the cyst is a frequent finding (Figures 9.25, 9.26).

Microscopically, the cyst is lined by squamous epithelium with underlying adnexal structures, in association with mature elements, such as adipose tissue, cartilage, neuroglial tissue together with multiple cysts lined by a variety of epithelia (Figure 9.27).

Other ovarian teratomas are mainly solid, showing smaller cysts that contain serous, mucinous, cheesy or even haemorrhagic material. The solid areas are soft, grey and 'encephaloid' in appearance; haemorrhage and necrosis are common. Extensive sampling for microscopy

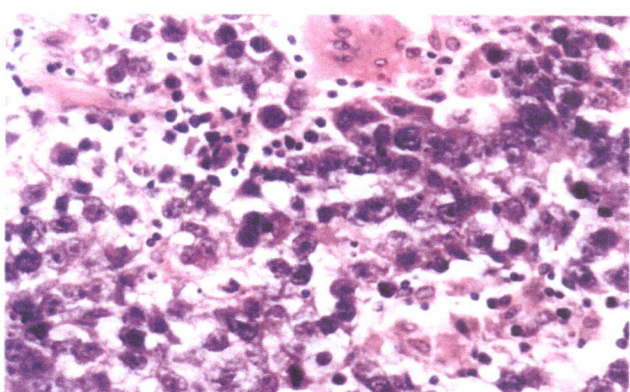

Fig. 9.13 Ovarian dysgerminoma shows two ill-defined histiocytic granulomas as part of a more complex histological picture. H&E × 300

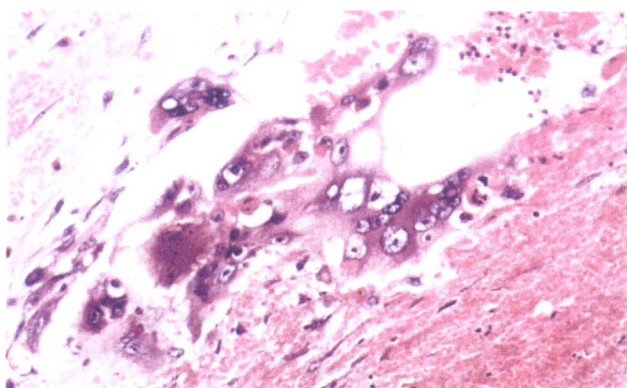

Fig. 9.14 Choriocarcinoma shows as its principal features large syncytiotrophoblastic cells accompanied by haemorrhage and necrosis. This was a histological component in a large right ovarian tumour removed from an 11-year-old girl; other components included yolk sac tumour and mature glandular structures. The resected mass weighed 3 kg. H&E × 300

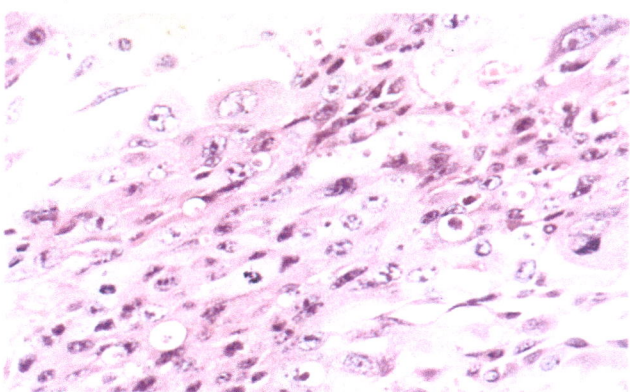

Fig. 9.15 Cytotrophoblastic cells form the dominant feature in this microscopic view of choriocarcinoma. Same tumour as in preceding figure. H&E × 300

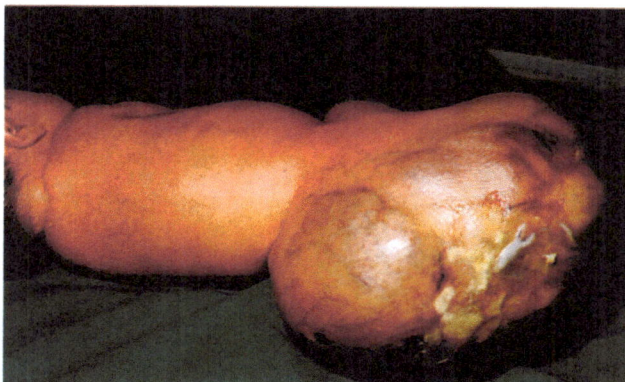

Fig. 9.16 Gross appearance of a large post-sacral sacrococcygeal teratoma in a newborn. The overlying skin shows marked vascularity and ulceration

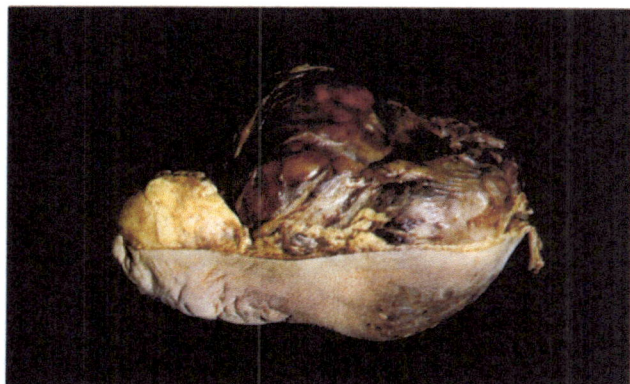

Fig. 9.17 Gross appearance of sacrococcygeal teratoma resected from a 3-day-old girl. The deep surface of the tumour is well demarcated. The specimen weighed 465 g and measured 16 × 10 × 6 cm

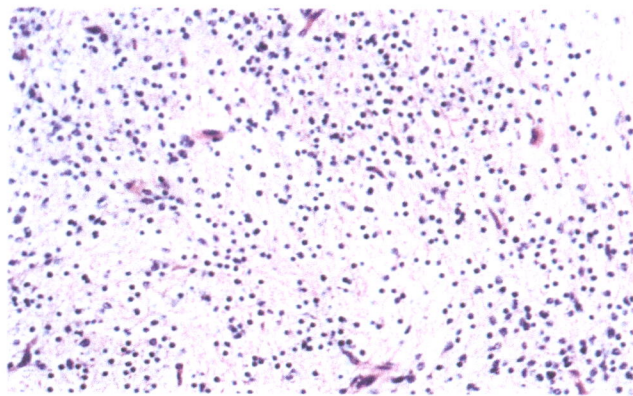

Fig. 9.18 Mature neuroglial tissue is the most common tissue component found in benign teratomas. H&E × 185

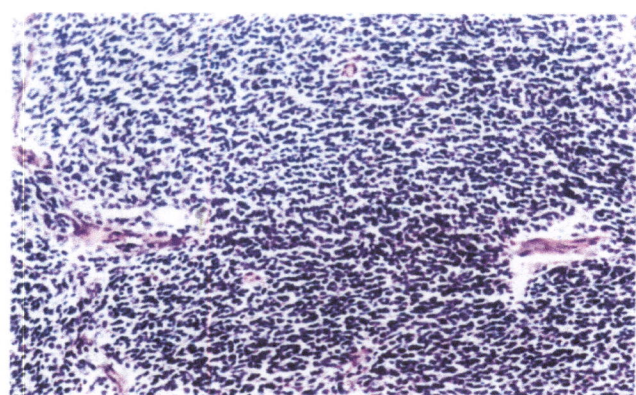

Fig. 9.19 Immature neuroglial material is the most common type of immature tissue found in teratomas. H&E × 185

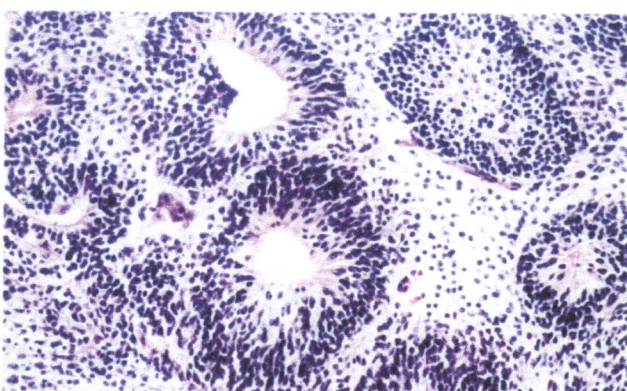

Fig. 9.20 Neuroglial canals occur commonly in association with immature neuroglial tissue. H&E × 185

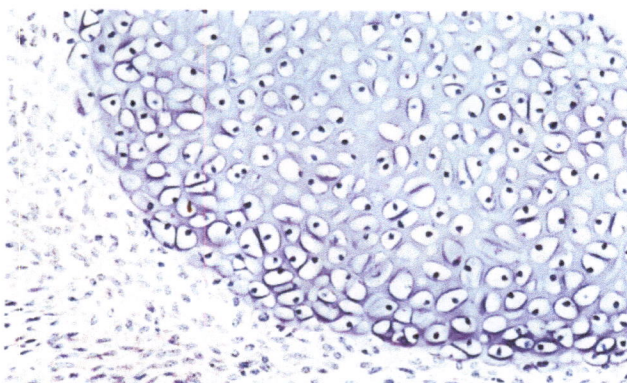

Fig. 9.21 Embryonal cartilage is demonstrated as an immature component in a sacrococcygeal teratoma. H&E × 185

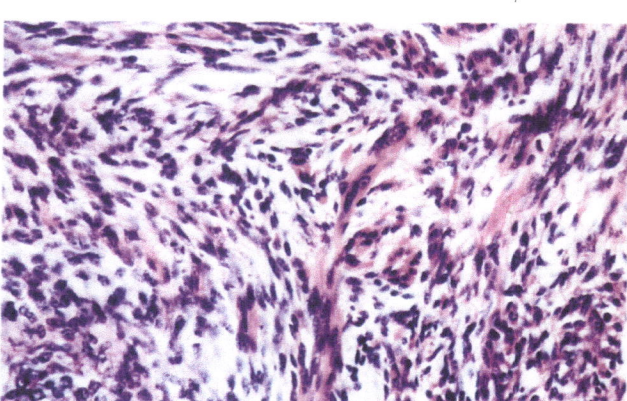

Fig. 9.22 Immature myogenic tissue is present in this teratoma removed from a newborn female. H&E × 300

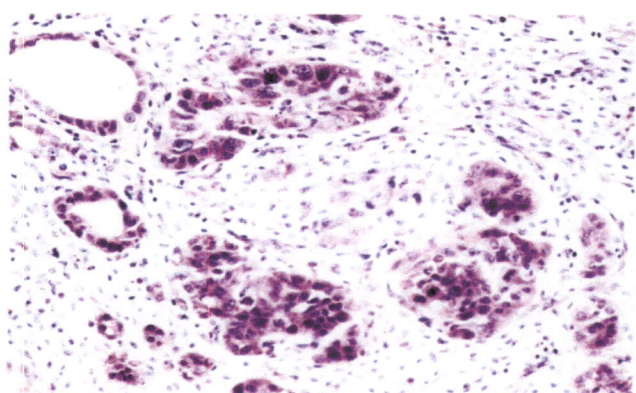

Fig. 9.23 Embryonic liver tissue in a teratoma probably explained the marked elevation of the serum alpha-fetoprotein level found prior to surgery. Immunohistochemically, the tissue was markedly positive for alpha-fetoprotein. Liver is rarely encountered as a component of a teratoma. H&E × 185

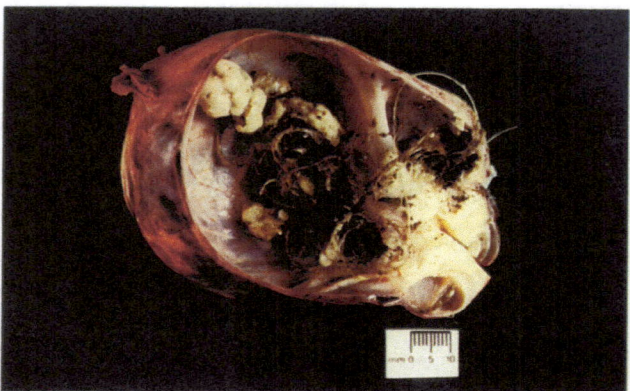

Fig. 9.24 An opened dermoid cyst of the ovary shows cheesy content and hair in the cyst lumen

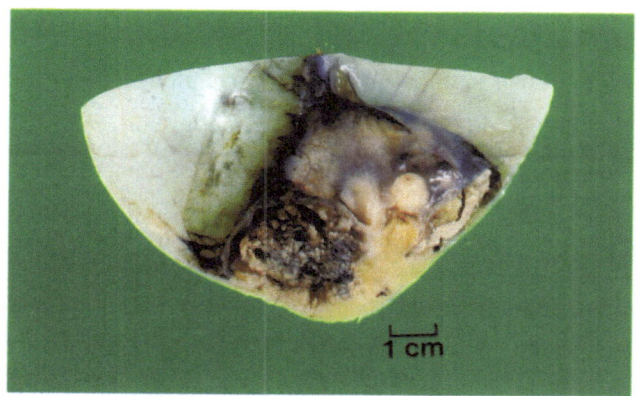

Fig. 9.25 The cut surface of this ovarian teratoma was mainly cystic. Part of the wall contains a large nodule, a common feature of ovarian dermoids. The patient was 3 years old; the excised specimen weighed 425 g

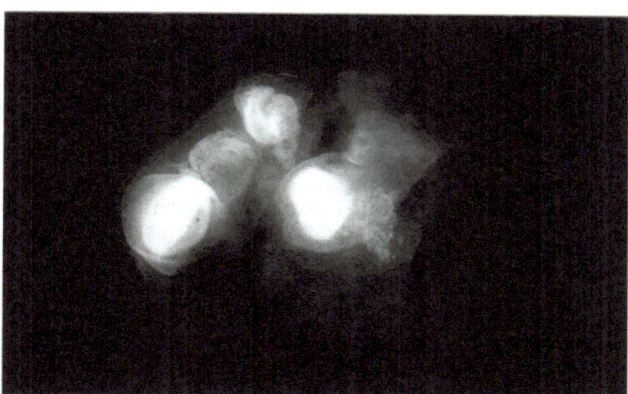

Fig. 9.26 X-ray of the nodule shown in preceding figure reveals partially formed teeth

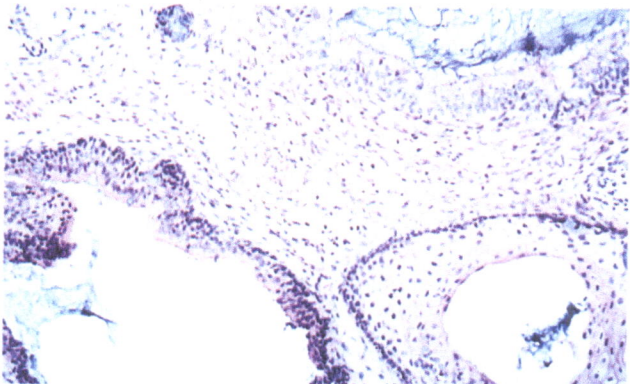

Fig. 9.27 Different types of epithelia line mature glandular structures in this example of a benign ovarian teratoma. H&E × 120

should identify immature tissues and overtly malignant elements (yolk sac tumour, embryonal carcinoma, dysgerminoma and choriocarcinoma).

A correlation seems to exist between the degree of immaturity and metastatic potential. This is the basis of a histological grading system proposed by Norris et al.[34] which takes account of the degree of immaturity, presence of neuroepithelium and its quantity. Their study, however, involved mostly adults; as immature ovarian teratomas of children are not so extensively studied, these criteria are not necessarily relevant[10]. Other good prognostic signals are low stage tumours, a young age and small-sized lesions[34].

Neuroepithelium (neuroectoderm) is the most common type of immature tissue found in ovarian teratoma, usually comprising medullary canals (embryonic neural tubes), or 'neuroblastomatous' growth. Other immature elements, whose malignant potential remains questionable, include fetal cartilage, kidney and primitive mesenchyme. Neuroepithelium may be the dominant or sole component of some ovarian tumours[35].

Implants on the pelvic or abdominal peritoneum composed entirely or mainly of mature glial tissue are referred to as gliomatosis peritonei, and does not as such imply malignancy. Intraperitoneal dispersal of the mature glial tissue through a defect in the tumour capsule is the usual explanation for their occurrence[36]. While gliomatosis peritonei is usually associated with ovarian teratoma, it has been reported in a newborn with a gastric teratoma[37]. Mature or relatively mature glial tissue may also be located in the subcapsular sinuses of lymph nodes within the drainage area of ovarian teratomas. This is referred to as nodal gliomatosis and is also not thought to have ominous significance[13]. The latter condition may coexist with gliomatosis peritonei.

TESTICULAR TERATOMAS

Testicular tumours are rare in children and the usual clinical presentation is a painless testicular mass[38]. In children aged 18 years and less, about 70% are germ cell tumours[39], the majority comprising yolk sac tumours or embryonal carcinoma. A review of 556 tumours in prepubertal testes showed 76% to be germ cell neoplasms[40]. Yolk sac tumour tends to predominate in infancy while embryonal carcinoma tends to affect adolescents and young adults. Yolk sac tumour and embryonal carcinoma may occur in isolation or in combination, or as part of a mixed (malignant) teratoma. Seminoma is virtually confined to the postpubertal testis and a pure testicular choriocarcinoma is the least common gonadal germ cell tumour[1].

Benign teratomas of the testis show the usual diversity of structures, as seen in other benign teratomas. The survival rate in testicular yolk sac tumour is in excess of 90%[14].

MEDIASTINAL TERATOMAS

Germ cell tumours account for about 20% of tumours arising in the anterior mediastinum[41]. About 7% of all germ cell/teratomas in children involve the anterior mediastinum[1]. Clinical presentation is generally related to the compression or invasion of important adjacent structures. Thus chest pain, dyspnoea and dysphagia are frequent. As many as 50% of children with mediastinal teratomas are asymptomatic and, in such cases, a mass is incidentally discovered on a chest X-ray. Germ cell tumours of the mediastinum may be:

(a)   Mature teratomas,
(b)   Immature teratomas,
(c)   'Pure' germ cell neoplasms,
(d)   Mixed germ cell neoplasms, and
(e)   Mixed (malignant) teratomas.

About half to three-quarters of the teratomas arising at this site are histologically mature[42]. Grossly, they are multicystic and encapsulated and smooth-surfaced, free from the contiguous structures. Immature teratomas are the least common, accounting for only 1% of mediastinal tumours. Their behaviour tends to be age related in that affected children under 15 years of age generally follow a benign course, while metastases are likely in older patients.

Despite reports to the contrary, mediastinal 'pure' yolk sac tumours are occasionally encountered in girls[43,44]. The polyvesicular vitelline microscopic pattern is unusual at this site; Schiller–Duval bodies are commonly seen[11].

Several reports have indicated an association between mediastinal (non-dysgerminomatous) germ cell tumour and Klinefelter syndrome. Haematological malignancies have been linked with mediastinal germ cell tumours but may be therapy related[45].

A small number of the tumours are situated within the pericardium near the base of the heart[1]. A picture in the neonatal period of congenital heart disease, cardiomegaly or hydrops fetalis is the usual mode of clinical presentation. No instance of histologically malignant pericardial teratoma has been reported[1]. Intracardiac teratomas are documented rarely[46].

ABDOMINAL TERATOMAS

Because of variation in clinical presentation and implications for differential diagnosis, abdominal teratomas are usefully separated into those that affect the retroperitoneum and others[3]. A wide age spectrum is involved but a significant proportion of these tumours occur in children. The neoplasms are often encapsulated and, as in other teratomas, naked eye examination discloses a combination of cystic and solid areas[3].

Microscopically, the constituent tissues are no different from those found in teratomas at other sites, apart from a seemingly greater incidence of somatic immaturity[1]. The rate of malignancy is however not especially high, and is apparently less than that found in sacrococcygeal tumours. Tissue indistinguishable from Wilms' tumour has been described in retroperitoneal teratomas[47,48].

Retroperitoneal teratomas should also be separated from sacrococcygeal tumours that have a large intrapelvic extension. Another potential source of confusion is a metastasis from an occult testicular primary growing in a retroperitoneal lymph node[3].

TERATOMAS OF THE STOMACH

Teratomas at this site are distinctly rare and males are chiefly affected[1,3]. The tumours may be predominantly intragastric or extragastric and often are located on the posterior wall or lesser curvature. The neoplasms may attain an enormous size[3]. The microscopic appearance is usually that of a mature teratoma although immature elements, such as neuroectoderm, have been described[3]. There is no reported instance of an invasive or metastasizing gastric teratoma in a child and frankly malignant elements are yet to be described[1].

TERATOMAS OF THE LIVER

Teratomas arising in the liver are also rare[49]. Mature and immature somatic structures are derived from all three germ layers. Liver tissue is often well-represented in hepatic teratomas and, in such cases, the distinction from hepatoblastoma may be difficult. This is especially so in certain cases of mixed hepatoblastomas referred to as teratoid hepatoblastomas[50]. In addition to the usual mesenchymal and epithelial components of a mixed hepatoblastoma, they include combinations of mature cartilage, skeletal muscle, intestinal-type and keratinized squamous epithelium, and melanin pigment. The problem is compounded by the finding of a raised serum level of alpha-fetoprotein in cases of hepatic teratoma[49].

Children with hepatic teratomas generally have a favourable outcome. So far, only one case has been reported to be malignant[51]. This tumour, however, displayed a large hepatic component and whether it was a true teratoma or a complex hepatoblastoma is questionable[52]. The liver is rarely the primary seat of a pure yolk sac tumour[53].

TERATOMAS OF THE KIDNEY

Teratomas of renal origin have been reported rarely in children[54]. Confusion may arise with Wilms' tumour expressing diverse tissue differentiation (see Chapter 2). The presence of microscopic features resembling Wilms' tumour excludes a true teratoma of the kidney. Beckwith[55] proposed strict criteria for the identification of renal teratoma. These were: (a) an unequivocal intrarenal origin and (b) attempts to form organs other than the kidney.

INTRACRANIAL TERATOMAS

Central nervous system teratomas are a special category of intracranial neoplasm. Most commonly they present as a midline supratentorial mass in the pineal or hypothalamic region. There is a predilection for the first two decades of life. Those presenting in the newborn are regarded as a special subgroup, as the patients are generally females and the tumours tend to be massive[3]. Hydrocephalus is a common complication and surgical removal may be impossible as the brain is often extensively involved.

Grossly, these teratomas display a variegate appearance with solid and cystic areas, contrasting with germinomas (or areas of germinoma) which tend to be soft, white and homogeneous[3].

There is microscopic similarity to other teratomas with mature and immature structures derived from all three germ cell layers, in varying combination. Germinoma, yolk sac tumour and choriocarcinoma have all been described in this location, either in pure form or as part of a mixed teratoma. The histological appearance of intracranial germinoma is no different from that seen elsewhere.

The differential diagnosis includes intracranial epidermoid cysts[3] and cerebral metastases from an extracranial primary teratoma[22]. Pineal or parapineal germinomas should also be distinguished from a true pinealoma.

TERATOMAS INVOLVING UNUSUAL SITES

The heart, lung, intestine, spleen and placenta have all been reported as primary sites of origin of teratomas[3]. A dermoid cyst in the pancreas has been reported[56].

REFERENCES

1. Dehner LP. Gonadal and extragonadal germ cell neoplasms-teratomas in childhood. In: Finegold, editor. Pathology of neoplasia in childhood and adolescents. Vol. 18 in the series Monographs of Problems in Pathology. Philadelphia: WB Saunders Co. 1986:282–312.
2. Malogolowkin MH, Mahour GH, Krailo M, Ortega JA. Germ cell tumors in infancy and childhood: a 45-year experience. Pediatr Pathol. 1990;10:231–41.
3. Gonzalez-Crussi F. Extragonadal teratomas. In: Atlas of tumor pathology (Series 2, fascicle 118). Washington, DC: Armed Forces Institute of Pathology; 1982:
4. Alpers CE, Harrison MR. Fetus in fetu associated with an undescended testis. Pediatr Pathol. 1985;4:37–46.
5. Marsden HB, Birch JM, Swindell R. Germ cell tumours of childhood: a review of 137 cases. J Clin Pathol. 1981;34:879–83.
6. Grosfeld JL, Ballantine, Lowe D, Baehner RL. Benign and malignant teratomas in children: analysis of 85 patients. Surgery. 1976;80:297–305.
7. Dehner LP. Gonadal and extragonadal germ cell neoplasia of childhood. Hum Pathol. 1983;14:493–511.
8. Harms D, Jänig U. Germ cell tumours of childhood. Virchows Arch (Pathol Anat). 1986;409:223–39.
9. Brodeur GM, Howarth CB, Pratt CB, Caces J, Hustu HO. Malignant germ cell tumors in 57 children and adolescents. Cancer. 1981;48:1890–8.
10. Kooijman CD. Immature teratomas in children. Histopathology. 1988;12:491–502.
11. Truong LD, Harris L, Mattioli C et al. Endodermal sinus tumor of the mediastinum. A report of seven cases and review of the literature. Cancer. 1986;58:730–9.
12. Tallerman A. Endodermal sinus (yolk sac) tumor elements in testicular germ-cell tumors in adults. Comparison of prospective and retrospective studies. Cancer. 1980;46:1213–17.
13. Perrone T, Steiner M, Dehner LP. Nodal gliomatosis and alpha-fetoprotein production. Two unusual facets of grade I ovarian teratoma. Arch Pathol Lab Med. 1986;110:975–7.
14. Hawkins EP, Finegold MJ, Hawkins HK, Krischner JP, Starling KA, Weinberg A. Nongerminomatous malignant germ cell tumors in children. A review of 89 cases from the Pediatric Oncology Group, 1971–1984. Cancer. 1986;58:2579–84.
15. Tapper D, Lack EE. Teratomas in infancy and childhood. A 54-year experience at the Children's Hospital Medical Center. Ann Surg. 1983;198:398–410.
16. Malogolowkin MH, Ortega JA, Krailo M et al. Immature teratomas: identification of patients at risk for malignant recurrence. J Natl Can Inst. 1989;81:870–4.
17. Dehner LP. Yet another face of the yolk sac tumor. Arch Pathol Lab Med. 1989;113:1113–14.
18. Manivel JC, Jessurun J, Wick MR, Dehner LP. Placental alkaline phosphatase immunoreactivity in testicular germ-cell neoplasms. Am J Surg Pathol. 1987;11:21–9.
19. Pallesen G, Hamilton-Dutoit SJ. Ki-1 (CD30) antigen is regularly expressed by tumor cells of embryonal carcinoma. Am J Pathol. 1988;133:446–50.
20. Scully RE. Tumors of the ovary and maldeveloped gonads. In: Scully RE, editor. Atlas of tumor pathology (Series 2. fascicle 16). Washington, DC: Armed Forces Institute of Pathology; 1982: 226–45.
21. Uchida T, Shimoda T, Miyata H et al. Immunoperoxidase study of alkaline phosphatase in testicular tumor. Cancer. 1981;48:1455–62.
22. Chandra SA, Gilbert EF, Viseskul C, Strother CM, Haning RV, Javid MJ. Neonatal intracranial choriocarcinoma. Arch Pathol Lab Med. 1990;114:1079–82.
23. Kurman RJ, Norris HJ. Embryonal carcinoma of the ovary. A clinicopathologic entity distinct from endodermal sinus tumor resembling embryonal carcinoma of the adult testis. Cancer. 1976;38:2420–33.
24. Lack EE. Extragonadal germ cell tumors of the head and neck region. Review of 16 cases. Hum Pathol. 1985;16:56–64.
25. Bale PM. Sacrococcygeal developmental abnormalities and tumors in children. Perspect Pediatr Pathol. 1984;1:9–56.
26. Fraumeni F, Li FP, Dalager N. Teratomas in children: epidemiological features. J Natl Can Inst. 1973;51:1425–9.
27. Altman RP, Randolph JG, Lilley JR. Sacrococcygeal teratoma: American Academy of Pediatrics Surgical Section Survey – 1973. J Pediatr Surg. 1974;9:389–98.
28. Valdiserri RO, Yunis EJ. Sacrococcygeal teratomas: a review of 68 cases. Cancer. 1981;48:217–21.
29. Tebbi K, Ragab AH, Ternberg JL, Vietti TJ. An extrarenal Wilms' tumor arising from a sacrococcygeal teratoma. Clin Pediatr. 1974;13:1019–21.
30. Ward SP, Dehner LP. Sacrococcygeal teratoma with nephroblastoma (Wilms' tumor): a variant of extragonadal teratoma in childhood. A histologic and ultrastructural study. Cancer. 1974;33:1355–63.
31. Gonzalez-Crussi F. Case 6. Retroperitoneal tumor. Pediatr Pathol. 1985;4:181–5.
32. Gonzalez-Crussi F, Winkler RF, Mirkin DL. Sacrococcygeal teratomas in infants and children. Relationship of histology and prognosis in 40 cases. Arch Pathol Lab Med. 1978;102:420–5.
33. Dehner LP, Mills A, Talerman A, Billman GF, Krous HF, Platz CE. Germ cell tumors of the head and neck soft tissues: a pathologic

spectrum of teratomatous and endodermal sinus tumors. Hum Pathol. 1990;21:309–18.

34. Norris HJ, Zirkin HJ, Benson WL. Immature (malignant) teratoma of the ovary. A clinical and pathologic study of 58 cases. Cancer. 1976;37:2359–72.

35. Aquirre P, Scully RE. Malignant neuroectodermal tumor of the ovary, a distinctive form of monodermal teratoma. Report of five cases. Am J Surg Pathol. 1982;6:283–92.

36. Robboy SJ, Scully RE. Ovarian teratoma with glial implants on the peritoneum. An analysis of 12 cases. Hum Pathol. 1970;1:643–53.

37. Coulson WF. Peritoneal gliomatosis from a gastric teratoma. Am J Clin Pathol. 1990;94:87–9.

38. Fernandes ET, Etcubanas E, Rao BN, Kumar APM, Thompson EI, Jenkins JJ. Two decades of experience with testicular tumors in children at St Jude Children's Research Hospital. J Pediatr Surg. 1989;24:677–82.

39. Leonard MP, Jeffs RD, Leventhal B, Gearhart JP. Pediatric testicular tumors: the Johns Hopkins Experience. Urology. 1991;37:253–6.

40. Brosman SA. Testicular tumors in prepubertal children. Urology. 1979;6:581–8.

41. Canty TG, Siemens R. Malignant mediastinal teratoma in a 15-year-old girl. Cancer. 1978;41:1623–6.

42. Carter D, Bibro MC, Touloukian RJ. Benign clinical behaviour of immature mediastinal teratoma in infancy and childhood: report of two cases and review of the literature. Cancer. 1982;49:398–402.

43. Hijiya N, Horikawa R, Matsushita T, Yamaguchi M, Noda E. Malignant mediastinal germ cell-tumors in childhood: a report of two cases achieving long-term disease-free survival. Am J Pediatr Hematol Oncol. 1989;11:437–40.

44. Gooneratne S, Keh P, Sreekanth S, Recant W, Talerman A. Anterior mediastinal endodermal sinus (yolk sac) tumor in a female infant. Cancer. 1985;56:1430–3.

45. deMent S. Association between mediastinal germ cell tumors and hematologic malignancies. Hum Pathol. 1990;21:699–703.

46. Cox JN, Friedli B, Mechmeche R, Ismail MB, Oberhaensli I, Faidutti B. Teratoma of the heart. A case report and review of the literature. Virchows Arch (Pathol Anat). 1983;402:163–74.

47. Malik TK, Malik GB, Diesh G. Retroperitoneal teratoma with nephroblastic tissue as the main component. Intern. Surg. 1967;47:246–9.

48. Carney JA. Wilms' tumor and renal cell carcinoma in retroperitoneal teratoma. Cancer. 1975;35:1179–83.

49. Witte DP, Kissane JM, Askin FB. Hepatic teratomas in childhood. Pediatr Pathol. 1983;1:81–92.

50. Conran RM, Hitchcock CL, Waclawiw MA, Stocker JT, Ishak KG. Hepatoblastoma; the prognostic significance of histological type. Pediatr Pathol. 1992;12:167–83.

51. Misugi K, Reiner CB. A malignant true teratoma of the liver in childhood. Arch Pathol. 1965;80:409–12.

52. Dehner LP. Hepatic tumors in the pediatric age group: a distinctive clinicopathologic spectrum. Perspect Pediatr Pathol. 1978;4:217–68.

53. Hart WR. Primary endodermal sinus (yolk sac) tumor of the liver. First reported case. Cancer. 1975;35:1453–8.

54. Dehner LP. Intrarenal teratoma occurring in infancy: report of a case with discussion of extragonadal germ cell tumors in infancy. J Pediatr Surg. 1973;8:369–78.

55. Beckwith JB. Wilms' tumor and other renal tumors of childhood. In: Finegold, editor. Pathology of neoplasia in childhood and adolescents. Vol. 18 in the series Monographs of Problems in Pathology. Philadelphia: WB Saunders Co; 1986:313–32.

56. DeCourcy JL. Dermoid cyst of the pancreas: case report. Ann Surg. 1943;75:394–5.

Vascular tumours

10

HAEMANGIOMAS

Haemangiomas are the most commonly encountered tumours in paediatric practice[1,2]. Whether they are true neoplasms or hamartomas is still an outstanding issue[2]. The skin and/or subcutaneous tissue are the sites usually involved, although any part of the body may be affected, including deeper structures. Despite not being seen for days or weeks, the majority of haemangiomas are present at birth. The lesions are divided into capillary, cavernous, intracutaneous capillary haemangioma (port-wine stain) and haemangiomatous varicosities; the latter may be associated localized haemangiomatous gigantism or local organ overgrowth[1]. It is well known that a child with one haemangioma often has another at a more distant site. Several syndromes are recognized to be associated with multiple haemangiomas affecting the skin or deeper structures[1,2].

CAPILLARY HAEMANGIOMA (STRAWBERRY NAEVUS)

Capillary haemangiomas are the single largest group of haemangiomas[3]. The most common sites are the head and the neck, and the lesion is usually located in the skin and subcutaneous tissue. Lesions are present at birth or are noted soon after. An initial period of rapid growth may continue for weeks or months. At this time, the growth often doubles in size over a few days or weeks[2]. The maximal size is generally achieved at around 6 months of age. This is followed by a stationary period, and then, over several years, a period of slow regression. More than 70% of these lesions show complete involution by 7 years of age, leaving little trace of the original lesion[2].

Naked eye examination shows the tumours to be flat, raised or even pedunculated; capillary haemangioma may occur as a 'pure' lesion or combined with a cavernous haemangioma.

The histology depends largely on the stage of the lesion[1]. The initial growth is characterized by a lobular pattern (Figure 10.1) with solid areas of marked cellularity and moderate numbers of mitoses (Figure 10.2). Inconspicuous vascular spaces lined by plump endothelial cells, together with infiltration of the adjacent normal tissues, may mimic a sarcoma[4]. However, the characteristic lobulation and distinct vascular spaces generally allow a correct diagnosis in the majority of cases. Various terminologies have been applied to this form of capillary haemangioma; 'cellular haemangioma of infancy' seems preferable to the older term 'haemangioendothelioma' as the latter may be confused with a variety of other conditions, sometimes with malignant connotation[4].

Maturation usually commences at the periphery of the lobules and is accompanied by enlargement of the vascular spaces and flattening of the endothelium (Figure 10.3). Ultimately, the lesion resembles a capillary haemangioma (Figure 10.4) or cavernous haemangioma. Interstitial fibrosis marks the stage of regression (Figure 10.5), and excision (or biopsy) at this period reveals a picture called 'sclerosing haemangioma'.

'Cellular haemangioma of infancy' is the most common benign tumour of the parotid in infancy[5]. The lesions may be accompanied by haemangioma of the overlying skin.

The differential diagnosis lies predominantly with infantile haemangiopericytoma although, ultrastructur-ally, endothelium is identified in both conditions[4,6]. A reticulin stain may be useful in separating the two histologically; the cells of cellular haemangioma of infancy are contained within the vascular sheath (Figure 10.6), while those of the haemangiopericytoma lie outside the vascular sheath; additionally, the pericytes of haemangiopericytoma are individually encompassed by reticulin (Figure 10.15).

CAVERNOUS HAEMANGIOMA

These growths are less often seen than capillary haemangiomas, and are composed of large dilated blood-filled vascular spaces lined by well-differentiated innocuous endothelium (Figure 10.7)[3]. The age and anatomical distribution are similar to that of capillary haemangioma, being usually present at birth or appearing shortly thereafter[2]. They differ from capillary haemangioma by their larger size and lack of circumscription. Spontaneous involution is also very common in these lesions, although it is usually less complete than in capillary lesions[2]. They may be combined with capillary haemangioma[1,2].

PORT-WINE STAINS

The port-wine stain (or haemangioma simplex) is an intradermal type of capillary lesion that is present at birth[1]. The skin has a purplish hue and the face is most commonly affected. These stains persist for life and show no tendency to regress. A cavernous haemangioma may be present elsewhere[2].

HAEMANGIOMATOUS VARICOSITIES

These lesions generally involve the extremities but may extend onto the trunk. The skin surface is often discoloured, and, when the lesion is extensive, overgrowth of the extremity or even hemihypertrophy may occur. The latter condition is referred to as the Klippel–Trenaunay–Weber syndrome[7].

HAEMANGIOMA OF SKELETAL MUSCLE

Allen and Enzinger[8] reported this lesion as a distinct entity. In two relatively large series, 12 out of 89 cases[8], and 20 out of 61 cases[9] involved children younger than 10 years old. The lower extremity is usually affected. Three histological types are recognized[8]: small vessel type (Figure 10.8), large vessel type and mixed type. The small vessel type is the most common and occurs in adults and children. These lesions resemble the capillary haemangiomas of skin. Adipose tissue is a component in all three types. The small vessel type, as might be expected, causes more diagnostic confusion than the other types. The lesion is locally aggressive and has a high rate of recurrence, most often in association with incomplete surgical resection. Haemangioma of skeletal muscle is probably related to the lesion previously referred to as infiltrating angiolipoma[10].

LYMPHANGIOMA

This is the principal lesion of lymphatics in childhood. Any part of the body served by lymphatics may be

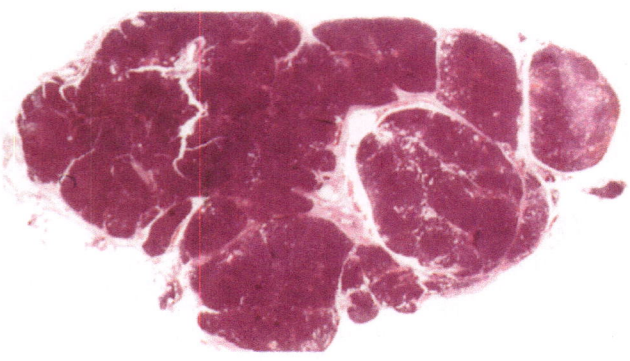

Fig. 10.1 A cellular haemangioma of infancy viewed at low magnification to demonstrate the lobular pattern that is characteristic of the lesion (actual size)

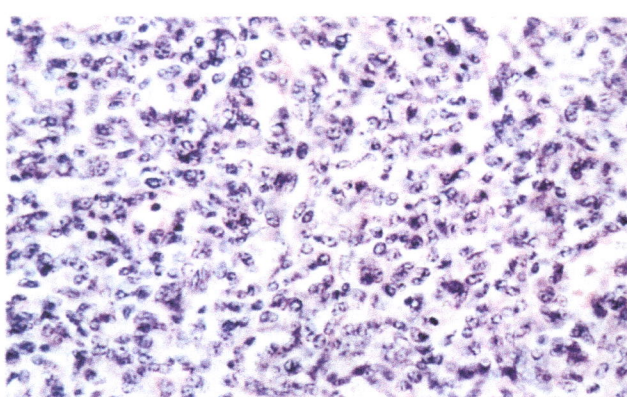

Fig. 10.2 The same lesion as in Figure 10.1 viewed at higher magnification; it is composed of sheets of closely apposed small round cells with an interposed (hardly discernible) fine vascular network. H&E × 300

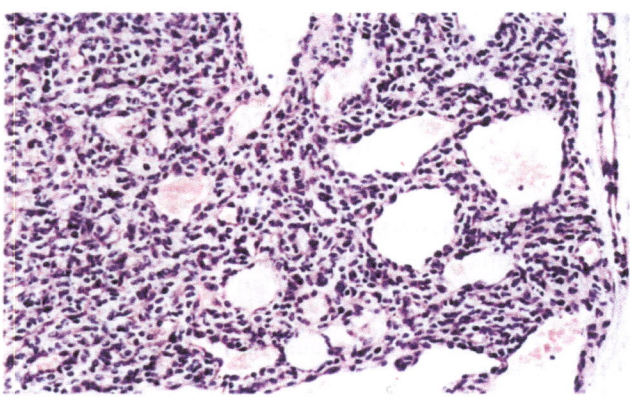

Fig. 10.3 Maturation in a cellular haemangioma of infancy usually commences at the periphery of the lobules, characterized by enlarging vascular spaces and flattening of the endothelium. H&E × 185

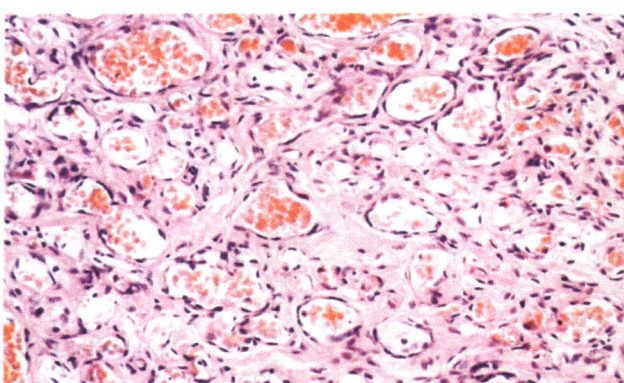

Fig. 10.4 A leash of variable-sized but generally small blood-filled channels lined by flattened endothelial cells characterizes a mature capillary haemangioma. H&E × 75

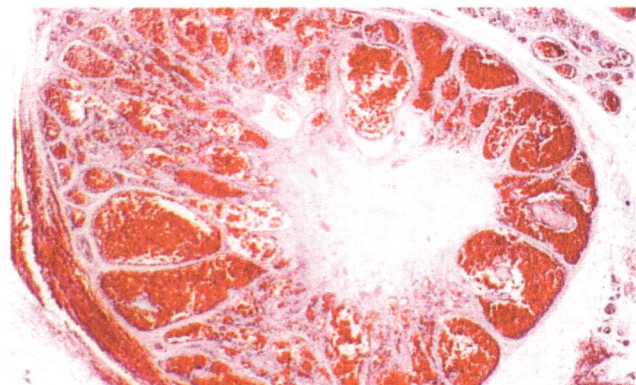

Fig. 10.5 A lobule of capillary haemangioma showing central sclerosis of the lesion during the early stage of involution. H&E × 30

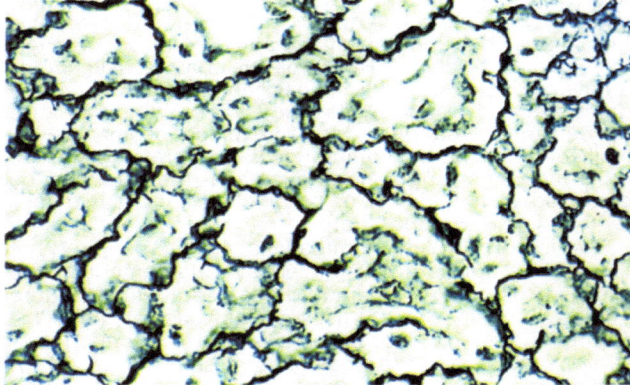

Fig. 10.6 A Gomori reticulin preparation of a cellular haemangioma of infancy shows reticulin fibres outlining individual vascular channels encompassing the endothelial cells. × 600

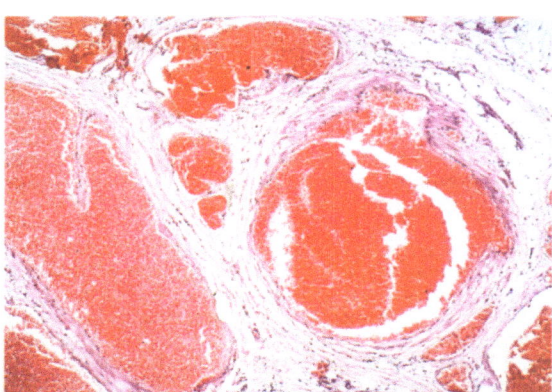

Fig. 10.7 A cavernous haemangioma with large irregular vascular channels lined by flattened endothelium and filled with red blood cells. H&E × 48

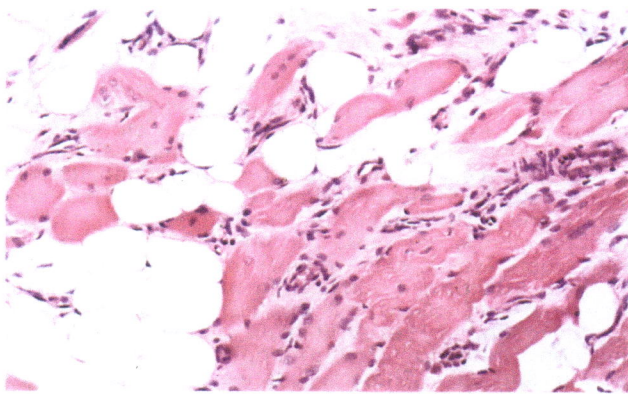

Fig. 10.8 Haemangioma of skeletal muscle of small vessel type reveals several capillary-sized channels infiltrating between muscle fibres and adipose tissue. H&E × 185

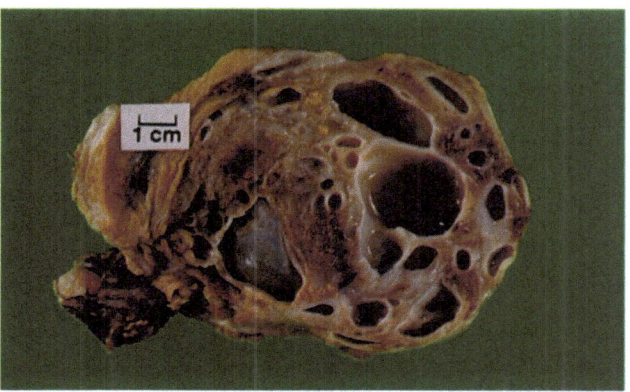

Fig. 10.9 Cystic lymphangioma. The patient was a 12-year-old boy who presented with abdominal pain. Laparotomy showed a large retroperitoneal cystic mass that was enucleated. The mass is well circumscribed and the cut surface shows several variable-sized cysts, some of which contain gelatinous material. The surgical specimen measured 15 cm in maximal extent

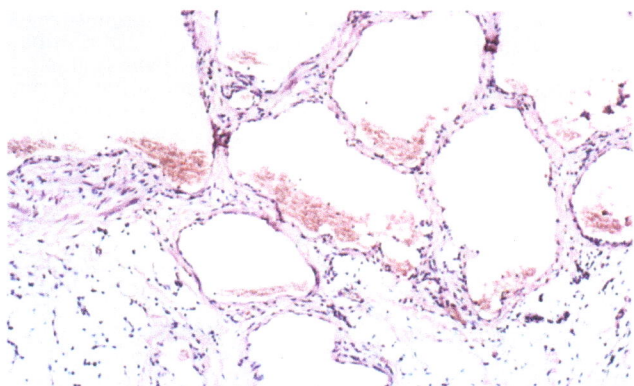

Fig. 10.10 Lymphangioma shows irregular vascular channels largely filled with lymph, but also containing a small amount of blood probably resulting from surgical trauma. H&E × 75

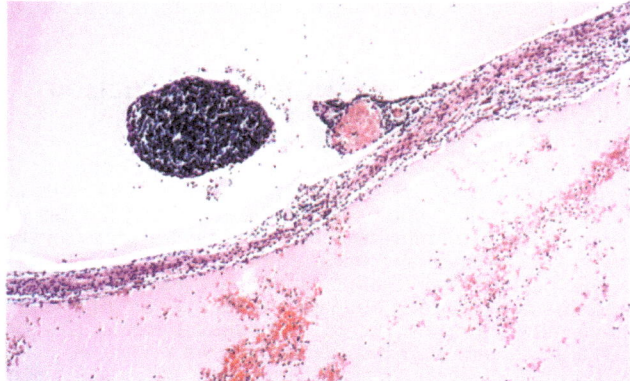

Fig. 10.11 Two lymph-filled spaces are separated by a thin fibrous wall containing lymphocytes. A nodule of lymphoid tissue projects into the upper part of the cavity. Some red blood cells are present in the lower cavity. H&E × 60

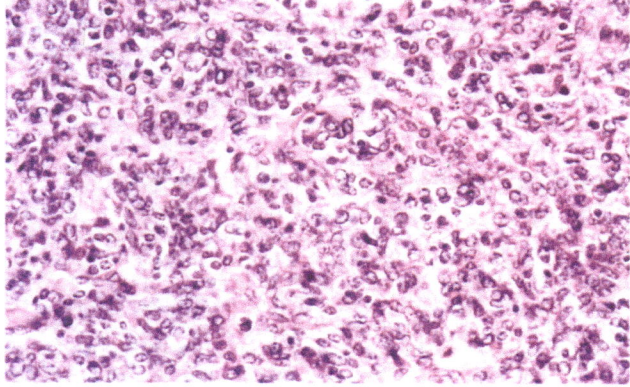

Fig. 10.12 Infantile haemangiopericytoma in which the dominant pattern is one of solid sheets of small cells with little evidence of vasoformation, similar in appearance to that seen in Figure 10.2. The patient was born with a large non-tender swelling above the right ankle. H&E × 300

affected. The head, neck and axilla account for a half to three-quarters of all cases. Many lymphangiomas (50–60%) are already present at birth, and, by the end of the second year, about 90% are present[11]. The lesions are regarded as developmental abnormalities (hamartomas, rather than true neoplasms). The masses are clinically poorly defined, usually soft and often compressible.

Morphological variants include simple lymphangioma (cutaneous lymphangioma simplex), cavernous lymphangioma and cystic lymphangioma (Figure 10.9)[12]. When lymphangiomas are large, the term 'cystic hygroma' is often used. Most cystic hygromas involve the neck, and, of these, 10% have a significant mediastinal component. The lung, liver, spleen, bone and gastrointestinal tract are other recognized sites. Within the abdomen, the usual location is the mesentery; the retroperitoneum is relatively seldom affected[12]. These lesions may become inflamed and a clinical diagnosis of appendicitis may be suggested.

The origin of cystic lymphangioma is unknown, but early developmental sequestration of lymphatic vessels is a widely held view, the sequestered channels becoming distended secondary to accumulation of lymph[13]. However, this theory fails to explain the often invasive character of the lesions. Generalized involvement by lymphangioma has been reported[14].

The vascular spaces of some lymphangiomas may contain blood, presumably the result of surgical trauma, and, in such instances, distinction from haemangiomas may be difficult (Figure 10.10). At least some of the spaces of true lymphangiomas are filled exclusively with lymph, however, and intraluminal projections of subendothelial lymphoid follicles are also helpful in their identification (Figure 10.11).

HAEMANGIOLYMPHANGIOMAS

Some children have tumours in which both lymph-filled and blood-filled spaces are admixed[2]. Clinically, these lesions generally behave as lymphangiomas, with only occasional evidence of regression. Mediastinal[15] and diffuse visceral[16] involvement have been reported.

SPINDLE CELL HAEMANGIOENDOTHELIOMA

This is an uncommon vascular tumour that affects both sexes over a wide age range[17]. Clinical presentation is often in childhood and there is a predilection for the distal extremity. Fifty per cent of patients have multiple lesions.

Microscopically, there is an admixture of dilated thin-walled vascular spaces and solid spindle cell areas, the latter containing red blood cells in slit-like spaces. Clusters of smooth muscle cells are also admixed, as are small numbers of round cells with intracytoplasmic vacuolation, reminiscent of histiocytoid haemangioma (see below). The lesion has been variously interpreted as non-neoplastic and also as a low-grade malignancy[18].

INFANTILE HAEMANGIOPERICYTOMA

Congenital or infantile haemangiopericytomas require separate consideration from the 'adult type' because their clinical behaviour is invariably benign[19]. They are present at birth or are recognized during infancy, involving the subcutis almost exclusively. Boys are more commonly affected than girls. Multiple tumours are rarely reported[20].

A partially or completely encapsulated multilobulated growth is the usual gross appearance[19]. Consistency varies from soft to firm and the size of the lesions varies from 0.3 to 6 cm.

Histologically, the neoplasm is composed of lobules of closely packed cells which are arranged around a rich fine vascular network (Figure 10.12), the latter often

forming spaces which may be small and inconspicuous (Figure 10.13) or, less often, large and sinusoidal (Figure 10.14). Cellular areas may alternate with areas that are collagenized. The tumour cells may be round, oval or spindled, and numerous mitoses are often seen. Haemorrhage and necrosis may be present. Unlike the 'adult-type' of haemangiopericytoma, these features do not indicate malignancy. The ramifying vascular structures typical of the 'adult-type' are less often seen in the infant variant[21].

Infantile haemangiopericytoma bears a close microscopic resemblance to cellular haemangioma of infancy. Endovascular endothelial proliferation may occur as a feature of both conditions[6], and a reticulin stain is useful in their distinction: in infantile haemangiopericytoma the pericytes lie outside the vascular sheath and are individually encircled by reticulin fibres (Figure 10.15)[22]. The constituent cells of cellular haemangioma of infancy, by comparison, are encompassed by the vascular sheath. The cells of infantile haemangiopericytoma also mark positively for smooth muscle actin, and may be diagnostically helpful[4].

Due to the lack of specific cytological features, the tumour may be difficult to distinguish from many other mesenchymal tumours. Haemangiopericytoma-like areas are seen in infantile myofibromatosis, mesenchymal chrondrosarcoma, fibrous histiocytoma, and synovial sarcoma. Tumours of smooth muscle, fibroblasts and the glomus tumour should also be considered in the differential diagnosis. Infantile haemangiopericytoma may be difficult to segregate from infantile myofibromatosis and congenital-infantile fibrosarcoma as these entities may all exhibit cellular spindle-cell areas (Figure 10.16)[21]. Haemangiopericytoma may also form a component of benign mesenchymomas[23] (see Chapter 13).

The 'adult-type' of haemangiopericytoma carries a more uncertain outlook and patients may include older children[19]. In the latter series of 106 cases of the 'adult-type', one case affected a child less than 9 years of age; 4% of cases were aged between 10 and 19 years.

GLOMUS TUMOUR (GLOMANGIOMA)

This tumour also has its origin in the pericyte. Children are rarely affected[24]. Three histological types are encountered[24]: mucoid–hyaline, angiomatous–glomangioma and the solid type. The angiomatous–glomangioma is the most common histological type found in children (Figure 10.17). The glomus cell is a cuboidal cell with a round nucleus and faint-staining cytoplasm. Most lesions are single. Multiple lesions may be inherited as an autosomal dominant trait[24].

HISTIOCYTOID HAEMANGIOMA (EPITHELIOID HAEMANGIOMA; ANGIOLYMPHOID HYPERPLASIA WITH EOSINOPHILIA)

This is a benign condition presenting clinically as a cutaneous reddish or blue nodular lesion[25]. Growth is generally indolent and, while the lesion predominates in women in early or mid-adult life, children are occasionally affected. The head and neck region is usually involved.

Microscopically[25], there is an exuberant proliferation of endothelial cells coupled with a conspicuous inflammatory infiltrate (Figure 10.18). The cells are round, oval or cuboidal, resembling histiocytes or even epithelial cells. The nuclei are vesicular and frequently folded, and the cytoplasm is abundant and eosinophilic. The cells are usually arranged in compact masses separated by fibrous tissue, or they occur singly. Mitoses are uncommon. Intracytoplasmic vacuolation of the endothelial cells is a distinctive microscopic feature (Figure 10.19). The vacuoles in the cytoplasm increase in size by enlargement and progressive fusion. Vascular channels of varying diameter are present. Red blood cells are plentiful and haemosiderin-laden macrophages are common. The degree and composition of the inflammatory infiltrate is variable, but lymphoid tissue and eosinophils predominate. Surgical excision is the treatment of choice but recurrence often follows incomplete removal. The question has been raised whether histiocytoid haemangioma represents a specific entity[26].

PAPILLARY ENDOTHELIAL HYPERPLASIA (MASSON'S VEGETANT INTRAVASCULAR HAEMANGIOENDOTHELIOMA)

There is no age predilection for this entity and about one third of cases occur in children[27]. The head and neck regions are most often involved and the dermis or subcutis is usually affected. The lesion may occur de novo or arise in a pre-existing lesion, such as a pyogenic granuloma or haemangioma.

Microscopically, tufts and fronds, either lying apparently free or attached to the wall by a stalk, project into vascular lumina (Figure 10.20). The papillae may or may not contain stroma, and are covered by a monolayer of hyperplastic endothelium. The endothelial cells are neither clustered nor layered; yet their nuclei may show mild-to-moderate atypia (Figure 10.21). There is no cellular anaplasia. Thrombotic material, an important diagnostic feature, is often present[27]. The histogenesis is not entirely clear, but the lesion probably represents atypical organization of thrombus by endothelial cells. Because of the complex papillary infoldings, the lesion may be mistaken for angiosarcoma. Features that assist in making the distinction are solid areas, necrosis, piling up of endothelium and frequent mitotic figures in angiosarcoma[28]. Simple excision of papillary endothelial hyperplasia is usually curative and recurrences are uncommon, unless the pre-existing lesion is an intramuscular haemangioma or infantile haemangiomatosis[3].

ENDOVASCULAR PAPILLARY ANGIOENDOTHELIOMA (DABSKA TUMOUR)

In 1969, Dabska[29] described six cases of an unusual vascular neoplasm of the skin and subcutaneous tissue of infants and young children. Their ages ranged from 4 months to 15 years. The growths tended to be locally invasive and, in two of the cases, metastasized to regional lymph nodes. Despite these features, all the cases survived after surgical excision, although two patients received radiotherapy.

Microscopically, the neoplasm shows intercommunicating vascular channels lined by endothelial cells which are flattened, cuboidal or tall cylindrical[31]. Mitoses are rare. The cells are clustered to form papillary structures that project into the vascular lumina. The vascular spaces also contain apparent free-floating cells, singly or in groups. Intervening stroma may be fibrotic and display solid nests of endothelium. The stroma may contain lymphoid aggregates.

The endothelial cells exhibit immunoreactivity for factor VIII-related antigen, Ulex europaeus, blood group iso-antigens and vimentin, and histochemical data suggest that the underlying basis of the lesion is one of high endothelial differentiation[30], an idea previously proposed by Manivel et al.[31]. A similar lesion involving the spleen of a child has been reported[30].

The differential diagnosis includes low-grade angiosarcoma and papillary endothelial hyperplasia. Angiosarcomas are exceedingly rare in children and are usually characterized by cellular pleomorphism. The presence of thrombotic material aids in the diagnosis of papillary endothelial hyperplasia.

ANGIOSARCOMA (MALIGNANT HAEMANGIOENDOTHELIOMA)

Kauffman and Stout[32] reported nine cases of angiosarcoma in children, and a further nine cases were identified from the literature. Of 101 tumours on the files of the Armed Forces Institute of Pathology in the United States of America, 11% involved patients under 11 years of age[33].

The soft tissues are most commonly affected and the tumour is rarely present at birth. The presence of anastomosing vascular channels lined by neoplastic endothelium is the usual microscopic picture[33] (Figure 10.22). The endothelium may form a single layer or may be heaped up to form papillae, or the neoplastic cells may occlude the entire lumen. Tumour cells are large and hyperchromatic. Mitotic activity is variable and may be sparse in well-differentiated tumours. Necrosis may be present.

KAPOSI'S SARCOMA

Children outside Africa are rarely affected. Contrasting with adults, the condition is extremely rare in children in association with acquired immune deficiency syndrome. Between 1982 and 1985, 4% of children with acquired immune deficiency syndrome developed Kaposi's sarcoma according to the Centers for Disease Control in the United States of America[34]. In children with acquired immune deficiency syndrome, both the lymphadenopathic[35] and the cutaneous form of Kaposi's sarcoma occur[36]; the former is more common and should be distinguished from other vascular lesions of the lymph node, including the entity referred to as intranodal haemorrhagic spindle cell tumour[37]. In the cutaneous form of Kaposi's sarcoma, the skin shows a variable number of tender and non-tender purplish nodular lesions.

The microscopic pattern is no different from that seen in adults, and includes the presence of spindle cells, vascular slits and extravasated red blood cells and haemosiderin. The cells lining the clefts and the intervening spindle cells are positive for factor VIII-related antigen[38].

Although indolent cutaneous lesions may occur, children in Africa usually present with a rapidly proliferative lymphadenopathic form of disease. Dutz and Stout[39], who extensively reviewed the literature on Kaposi's sarcoma in children, found that a fulminating course tended to parallel an age less than 6 years.

KAPOSI-LIKE INFANTILE HAEMANGIOENDOTHELIOMA

A retroperitoneal tumour with a distinctive microscopic pattern affecting an infant was reported by Tsang and Chan[40]. From the literature, the authors identified seven other cases. The patients were less than 1 year old and they often presented with an abdominal mass and jaundice, sometimes with bleeding. There was a high mortality, with only three of eight babies surviving.

Microscopically, the index case showed an infiltrative growth composed of lobules of spindle cells and vascular channels separated by fibrous septa. The nuclei of the spindle cells were elongated and regular and the chromatin was fine. The mitotic count was less than one per 20 high-power fields. The cytoplasm was moderate in amount, lightly eosinophilic or even clear. No eosinophilic globules were identified. The spindle cells express determinants for factor VIII-related antigen, Ulex europaeus, and blood group A and H isoantigens.

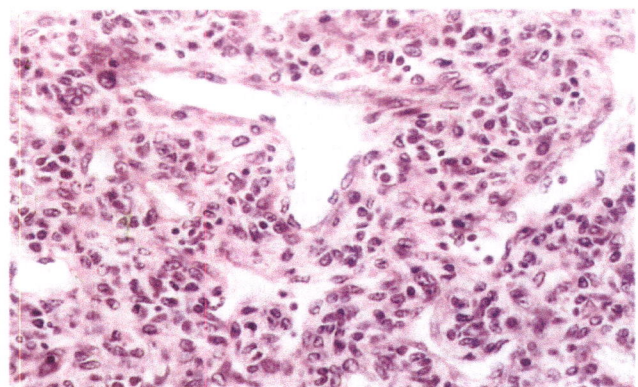

Fig. 10.13 Different microscopic field of the lesion depicted in Figure 10.12 provides a clue to its vascular nature; there are several irregular vascular channels. H&E × 300

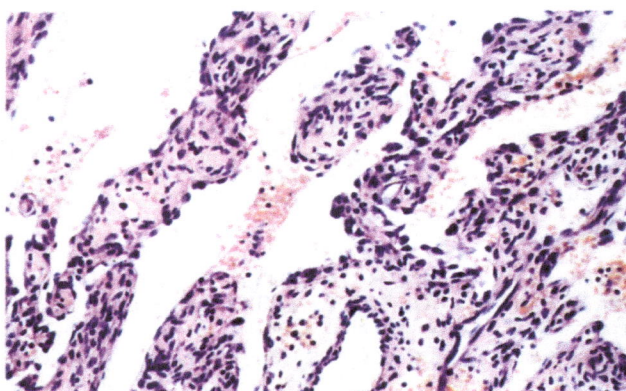

Fig. 10.14 Large irregular vascular spaces lined by prominent endothelium are shown in this infantile haemangiopericytoma; intervening areas are cellular. Necrosis was fairly extensive. A vascular lesion on the lower leg was present at birth. H&E × 185

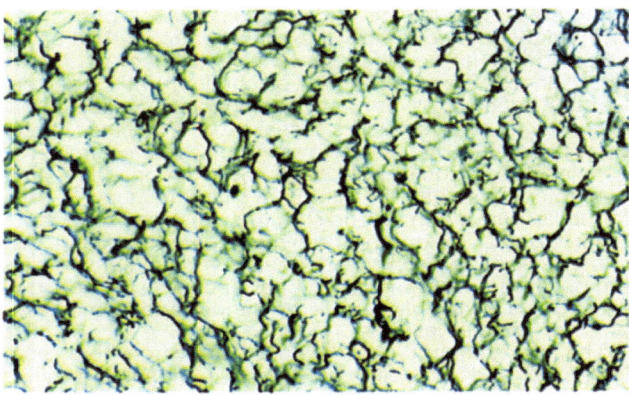

Fig. 10.15 Infantile haemangiopericytoma shows individual cells to be encompassed by reticulin fibres. Compare with Figure 10.6. Gomori reticulin × 600

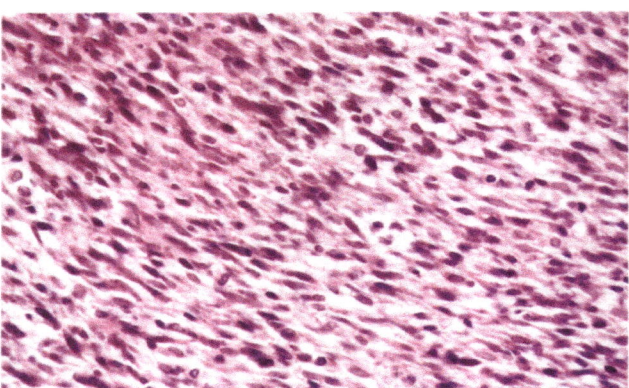

Fig. 10.16 This area of infantile haemangiopericytoma is composed of spindle cells that may be difficult to distinguish from congenital–infantile fibrosarcoma. H&E × 300

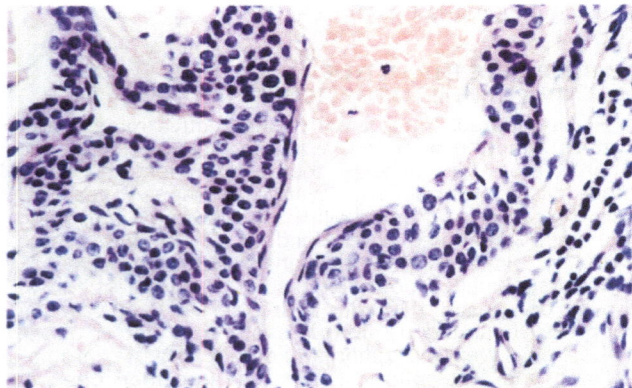

Fig. 10.17 A large vessel in a glomus tumour is outlined by a stratified layer of cells with eosinophilic cytoplasm and a central vesicular nuclei characteristic of the glomus cell. H&E × 300

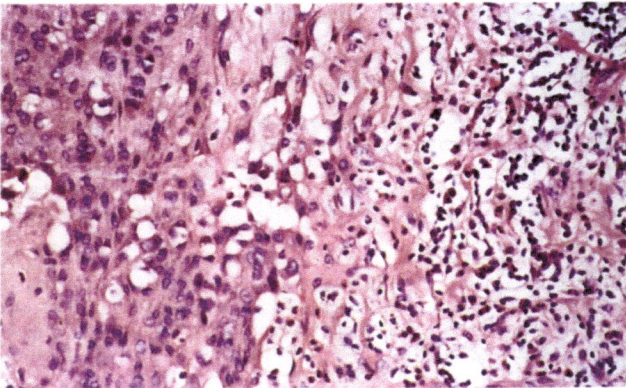

Fig. 10.18 Histiocytoid haemangioma shows a swathe of syncytial epithelioid cells composed of copious pink cytoplasm and prominent cytoplasmic vacuolation to the left of the field; a cellular infiltrate is present on the right, partially masking the lesion. H&E × 185

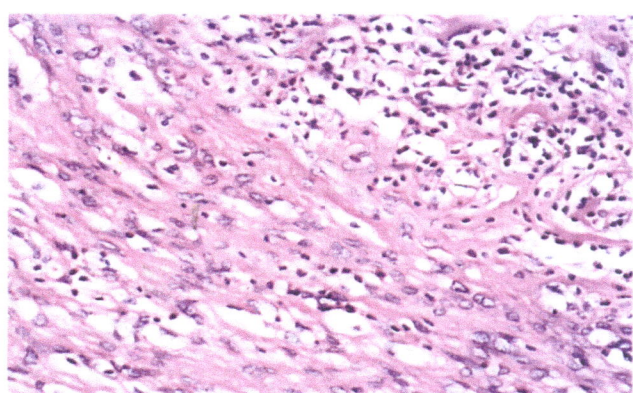

Fig. 10.19 A different view of the lesion shown in the preceding figure demonstrates conspicuous cytoplasmic vacuolation. An inflammatory component is seen to the right in the upper part of the field. H&E × 185

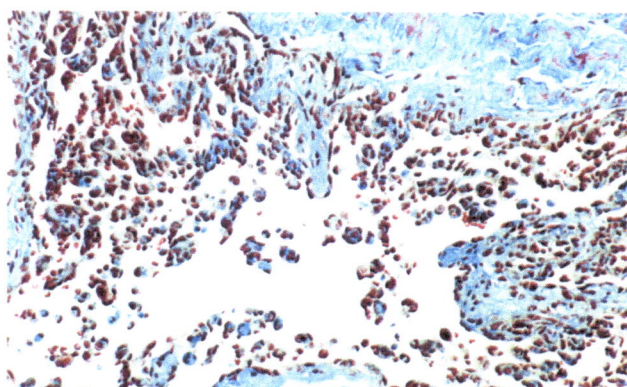

Fig. 10.20 Papillary endothelial hyperplasia shows fibrous cores of the papillary processes covered by a single layer of prominent endothelium. Masson's trichrome × 185

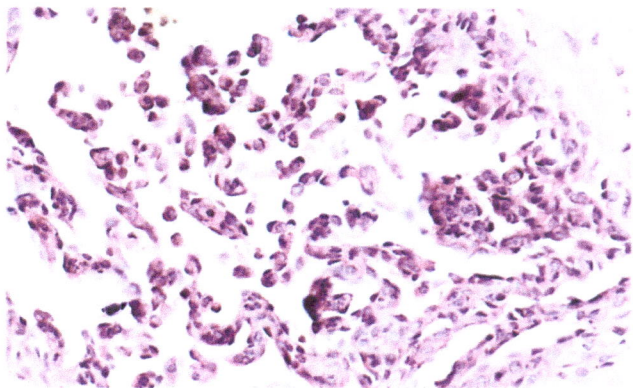

Fig. 10.21 Papillary endothelial hyperplasia demonstrates numerous papillary processes covered by endothelium in which the nuclei are often slightly atypical. The lesion was excised from the forehead of a 2½-year-old boy. H&E × 300

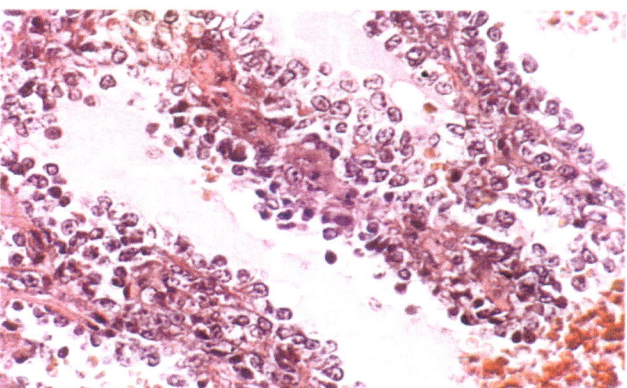

Fig. 10.22 Postmortem histology of a hepatic angiosarcoma that was part of a widely disseminated tumour in a 3½-month-old girl. The lesion is composed of large vascular spaces lined by plump endothelial cells that are often layered. Nuclear pleomorphism is of moderate degree. H&E × 300

Kaposi's sarcoma may be distinguished on several counts[36]:

(a)   It is exceptionally rare under 1 year of age;
(b)   It is typically multicentric and grows in a diffuse or multinodular pattern;
(c)   It lacks reticulin fibres and basal lamina material;
(d)   It contains PAS-positive hyaline globules and shows an insignificant number of pericytes.

REFERENCES

1. Martin LW, MacCollum DW. Hemangiomas in infants and children. Am J Surg. 1961;101:571–80.
2. Williams HB. Hemangiomas and lymphangiomas. Adv Surg. 1981;15:317–49.
3. Enzinger FM, Weiss SW. Benign tumors and tumorlike lesions of blood vessels. In: Enzinger FM, Weiss SW, editors. Soft tissue tumors. St Louis, Toronto, London, C.V. Mosby, 1983:379–421.
4. Gonzalez-Crussi F, Reyes-Mugica M. Cellular hemangiomas ('hemangioendotheliomas') in infants. Light microscopic, immunohistochemical, and ultrastructural observations. Am J Surg Pathol. 1991;15:769–78.
5. Nagoa K, Matsuzaki O, Shigematsu O, Kaneko T, Katoh T, Kitamura T. Histopathologic studies of benign infantile hemangioendothelioma of the parotid gland. Cancer. 1980;46:2250–6.
6. Alpers CE, Rosenau W, Finkbeiner WE, de Lorimier AA, Kronish D. Congenital (infantile) hemangiopericytoma of the tongue and sublingual region. Am J Clin Pathol. 1984;81:377–82.
7. Matsubara O, Tanaka M, Ida T, Okeda R. Hemimegalencephaly with hemihypertrophy (Klippel–Trenaunay–Weber syndrome). Virchows Arch (Pathol Anat). 1983;400:155–62.
8. Allen PW, Enzinger FM. Hemangioma of skeletal muscle. An analysis of 89 cases. Cancer 1972;29:8–22.
9. Beham A, Fletcher CDM. Intramuscular angioma: a clinicopathological analysis of 74 cases. Histopathology. 1991;18:53–9.
10. Lin JJ, Lin F. Two entities in angiolipoma. A study of 459 cases of lipoma with review of literature on infiltrating angiolipoma. Cancer. 1974;34:720–7.
11. Hilliard RI, McKendry JBJ, Phillips MJ. Congenital abnormalities of the lymphatic system: a new clinical classification. Pediatrics, 1990;86:988–94.
12. Leonidas JC, Brill PW, Bhan I, Smith TH. Cystic retroperitoneal lymphangioma in infants and children. Radiology. 1978;127:203–8.
13. Godart S. Embryological significance of lymphangioma. Arch Dis Childh. 1966;41:204–6.
14. Morphis LG, Arcinue EL, Krause MD. Generalized lymphangioma in infancy with chylothorax. Pediatrics. 1970;46:566–75.
15. Toye R, Armstrong P, Dacie JE. Lymphangiohaemangioma of the mediastinum. Br J Radiol. 1991;64:62–4.
16. Koblenzer PJ, Bukowski MJ. Angiomatosis (hamartomatous hemlymphangiomatosis). Report of a case with diffuse involvement. Pediatrics. 1961;28:65–76.
17. Fletcher CDM, Beham A, Schmid C. Spindle cell haemangioendothelioma: a clinicopathological and immunohistochemical study indicative of a non-neoplastic lesion. Histopathology. 1991;18:291–301.
18. Weiss SW, Enzinger FM. Spindle cell hemangioendothelioma. A low-grade angiosarcoma resembling a cavernous haemangioma and Kaposi's sarcoma. Am J Surg Pathol. 1986;10:521–30.
19. Enzinger FM, Smith BH. Hemangiopericytoma, an analysis of 106 cases. Hum Pathol. 1976;7:61–82.
20. Seibert JJ, Seibert RW, Weisenburger DS, Allsbrook W. Multiple congenital hemangiopericytomas of the head and neck. The Laryngoscope. 1978;88:1006–11.
21. Chung EB. Pitfalls in diagnosing benign soft tissue tumors in infancy and childhood. Pathol Annu. 1985;20:323–86.
22. Kauffman SL, Stout AP. Hemangiopericytoma in children. Cancer. 1960;13:695–710.
23. Le Ber MS, Stout AP. Benign mesenchymomas in children. Cancer. 1962;15:598–605.
24. Dehner LP. Soft tissue, peritoneum, and retroperitoneum. In: Dehner LP, editor. Pediatric surgical pathology, 2nd edn. Baltimore: Williams & Wilkins; 1987:882.
25. Rosai J, Gold J, Landy R. The histiocytoid hemangiomas. Hum Pathol. 1979;10:707–30.
26. Cooper PH. Is histiocytoid hemangioma a specific pathological entity? Am J Surg Pathol. 1988;12:815–7.
27. Clearkin KP, Enzinger FM. Intramuscular papillary endothelial hyperplasia. Arch Pathol Lab Med. 1976;100:441–4.
28. Kuo T, Sayers CP, Rosai J. Masson's 'vegetant intravascular hemangioendothelioma': a lesion often mistaken for angiosarcoma. Cancer. 1976;38:1227–36.
29. Dabska M. Malignant endovascular papillary angioendothelioma of the skin in childhood. Clinicopathological study of 6 cases. Cancer. 1969;24:503–10.
30. Katz JA, Mahoney DH, Shukla LW, Smith CW, Gresik MV, Hawkins HK. Endovascular papillary angioendothelioma in the spleen. Pediatr Pathol. 1988;8:185–93.
31. Manivel JC, Wick MR, Swanson PE, Patterson K, Dehner LP. Endovascular papillary angioendothelioma of childhood: a vascular lesion possibly characterized by 'high' endothelial cell differentiation. Hum Pathol. 1986;17:1240–4.
32. Kauffman SL, Stout AP. Malignant hemangioendothelioma in infants and children. Cancer. 1961;14:1186–96.
33. Enzinger FM, Weiss SW. Malignant vascular tumors. In: Enzinger FM, Weiss SW, editors. Soft tissue tumours. St Louis, Toronto, London: CV Mosby; 1983:422–49.
34. Rodgers M, Thomas P, Starcher E, Noa M, Bush T, Jaffe H. Acquired immune deficiency syndrome in children: report of the Centers for Disease Control National Surveillance, 1982–1985. Pediatrics. 1987;79:1008–14.
35. Buck BE, Scott GB, Valdes-Dapena M, Parks WP. Kaposi sarcoma in two infants with acquired immune deficiency syndrome. J Pediatr. 1983;103:911–13.
36. Connor E, Boccon-Gibod L, Joshi V et al. Cutaneous acquired immunodeficiency syndrome-associated Kaposi's sarcoma in pediatric patients. Arch Dermatol. 1990;126:791–3.
37. Bisceglia M, Amini M, Bosman C. Primary Kaposi's sarcoma of the lymph node in children. Cancer. 1988;61:1715–18.
38. Nadji M, Morales AR, Ziegles-Weissman J, Penneys NS. Kaposi's sarcoma. Immunohistologic evidence for an endothelial origin. Arch Pathol Lab Med. 1981;105:274–5.
39. Dutz W, Stout AP. Kaposi's sarcoma in infants and children. Cancer. 1960;13:684–94.
40. Tsang WYW, Chan JKC. Kaposi-like hemangioendothelioma. A distinctive vascular neoplasm of the retroperitoneum. Am J Surg Pathol. 1991;15:982–9.

The fibromatoses

11

These are predominantly non-metastasizing tumours whose precise definition is still a matter of debate (Table 11.1). Terminology is complex and little agreement exists as to the most suitable classification. The microscopic picture varies considerably but there is a common tendency towards a high degree of cellularity, local invasiveness and a high rate of recurrence after surgery[1]. The cellularity, mitotic activity and infiltrative nature of the growth often give an impression of biological aggression. Many of these lesions (infantile myofibromatosis, desmoid, fibrous hamartoma of infancy, recurrent digital fibromatosis) demonstrate an origin from the myofibroblast. As a group, the neoplasms tend to occur more commonly in boys. A study of 900 soft-tissue tumours in children found that 12% belonged to the category of fibromatoses[2].

Table 11.1 The fibromatoses

Infantile myofibromatosis
Fibrous hamartoma of infancy
Infantile digital fibromatosis
Palmar and plantar fibromatosis
Sternomastoid tumour
Juvenile aponeurotic fibromatosis
Hyaline fibromatosis
Infantile (desmoid-type) fibromatosis
Congenital–infantile fibrosarcoma
Nasopharyngeal angiofibroma

INFANTILE MYOFIBROMATOSIS (CONGENITAL GENERALIZED FIBROMATOSIS; GENERALIZED HAMARTOMATOSIS; MULTIPLE CONGENITAL MESENCHYMAL TUMOURS; DIFFUSE CONGENITAL FIBROMATOSIS; MULTIPLE VASCULAR LEIOMYOMAS OF THE NEWBORN)

Infantile myofibromatosis is a rare proliferative disorder of mesenchyme[3]. Terminological confusion has resulted from the previous application of a wide variety of labels. Infantile myofibromatosis is, currently, the preferred term because of the histological resemblance to smooth muscle and its frequent occurrence in newborns and infants[4]. Of all the different types of fibromatoses, it is the one most likely to be encountered by the pathologist[2].

The majority of patients present before the age of 2 years and, of these, more than half are present at birth. Older children and adults are rarely affected[4]. Many of the tumours regress in the postnatal period, although initially after birth, there may be an increase in size and number. New growths may continue to develop later in childhood[5].

The aetiology of infantile myofibromatosis is unknown[6], although some evidence suggests an effect of exposure *in utero* to oestrogenic hormones[7]. Familial occurrence has been described, however[5], but the precise mode of inheritance is still in doubt. Congenital malformation is rarely associated[8].

The number of lesions varies from one to several, and, in some individuals, may reach a hundred. Chung and Enzinger[4] reported solitary lesions to be three times more common than multiple tumours. About 20% of solitary lesions appear in older individuals and are found most often in the skin, muscle or subcutaneous tissue. Solitary lesions predominate in the head/neck region; the skeletal muscle is involved in about 65% of cases[9].

Thirty-seven per cent of infants presenting with multiple lesions have visceral involvement[6]; they usually manifest palpable tumours at birth[6]. Both forms of the disease may affect the skin, subcutis, muscle and bone. Boys are more often involved in the solitary form, whereas in the multiple type girls are mainly affected[4]. Any organ may be affected in the visceral form. A firm, hard to rubbery nodule or nodules in the skin or underlying tissue is the usual clinical expression. They tend to be easily mobile while deeply located nodules are usually fixed.

Of the parenchymal organs, the lung is the most commonly affected, while involvement of the central nervous system appears exceptional[10]. Two patterns of pulmonary involvement are reported; the first shows nodules associated with bronchioles or pulmonary vessels; in the second pattern, parenchymal nodules are unrelated to these structures and the appearance is similar to that of lesions found elsewhere[7].

Bone lesions, which may be solitary or multiple, are found in 55% of patients[3]. In the multiple form, the lesions arise most commonly in the skull and the metaphyses of long bones. Radiologically, the osseous lesions are central and lytic, but a sclerotic rim is not uncommon in the calvarium[11]. The cortex of bones may be expanded and may easily fracture. Solitary lesions most commonly affect the craniofacial region and should be distinguished microscopically from other fibrous tumours, such as fibrous dysplasia and desmoplastic fibroma[11]; other entities that should be considered in the differential diagnosis include metaphyseal fibrous defect, neurofibroma and fibrosarcoma.

Individual nodules of infantile myofibromatosis are discrete and are generally well-delineated; they measure some 0.5–7 cm in diameter and are firm to rubbery in consistency[4]. The cut surface often reveals a central, necrotic or cystic area. On account of their prominent vascularity, lesions located near the skin surface may be mistaken clinically for haemangiomas[4,10].

Microscopically, a distinct zoning phenomenon is present; cellularity tends to predominate in the centre, where characteristic angular gaping vascular channels (reminiscent of haemangiopericytoma) are often encountered (Figure 11.1)[4]. In this part of the lesion, the cells are closely packed and have an immature appearance. Plump or elongated cells with pale-staining or slightly eosinophilic cytoplasm, reminiscent of smooth muscle fibres, are distributed more peripherally (Figure 11.2); these cells are often arranged in compact intertwining bundles or whorls.

The overall cellularity varies between lesions and between areas within the same lesion. The number of mitoses is variable but usually sparse; abnormal forms are not encountered. Collagen production tends to be minimal. Hyalinization, necrosis and calcification (Figure 11.3) are frequent, although these features are generally lacking in visceral lesions. Nodular growth into vascular spaces has been described[4].

A tumour capsule is poorly defined and there is often extension into the adjacent tissues, but this is not as marked as in other types of fibromatoses. Solitary and multiple lesions show a similar histology, but those found

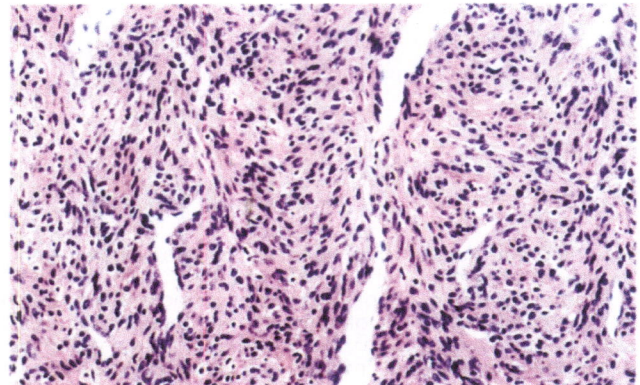

Fig. 11.1 Infantile myofibromatosis. Angular gaping vascular channels, a feature commonly found in infantile myofibromatosis, are prominent in this field. The lesion was resected from the soft tissue of the left leg of a 5-day-old boy. H&E × 185

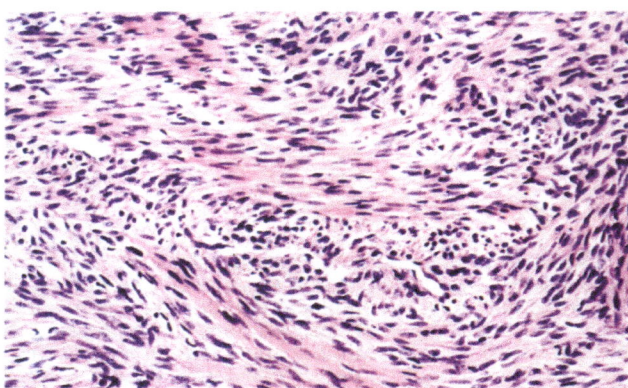

Fig. 11.2 Infantile myofibromatosis. Same tumour as depicted in Figure 11.1. Spindle-shaped tumour cells arranged in compact intertwining bundles are better defined at the edge of the tumour. H&E × 185

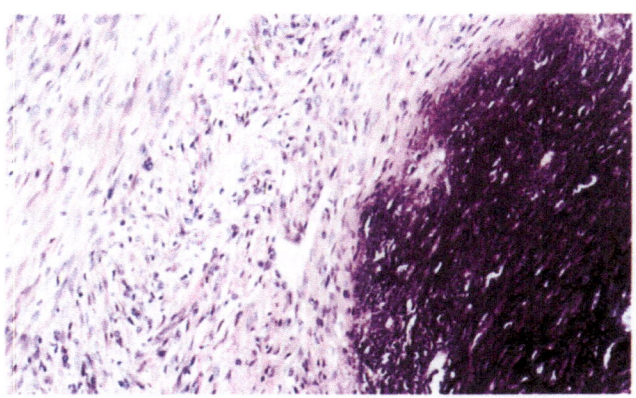

Fig. 11.3 Infantile myofibromatosis. Part of the lesion is calcified. The tumour was removed from the scalp of the same patient at the age of 2 years. H&E × 75

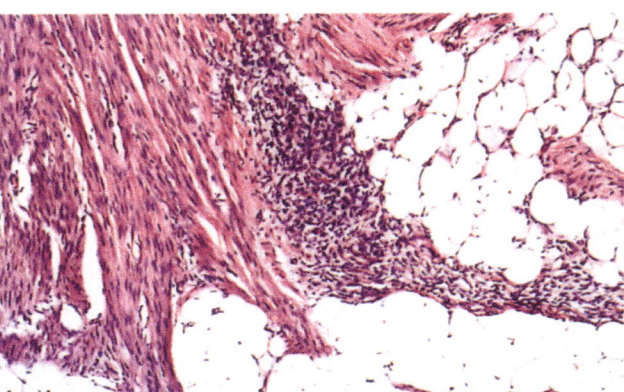

Fig. 11.4 Fibrous hamartoma of infancy shows three major components: fibrocollagenous trabeculae, primitive mesenchymal stroma and adipose tissue. H&E × 75

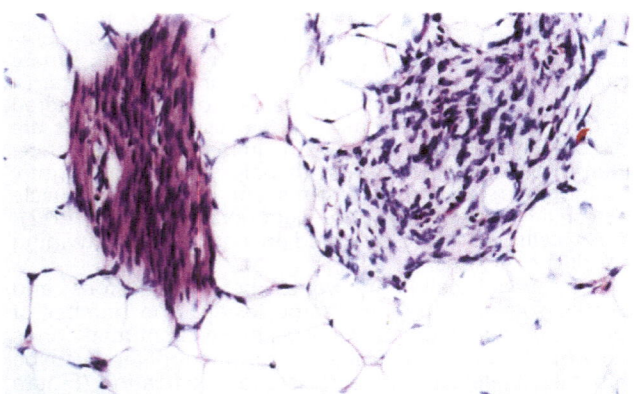

Fig. 11.5 The three histological components of fibrous hamartoma of infancy are demonstrated at higher magnification. The primitive mesenchymal stroma is arranged as a ball-like structure. The lesion arose in the left hip of a 12-month-old boy. H&E × 185

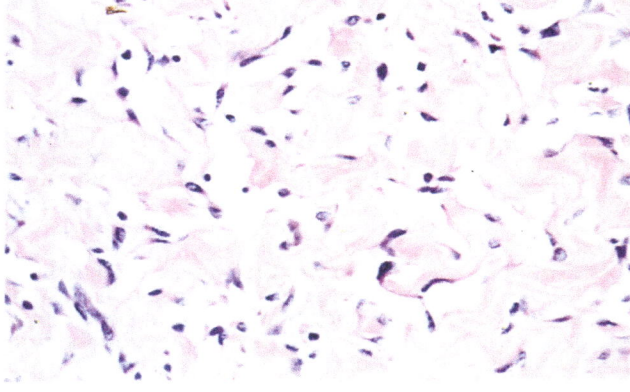

Fig. 11.6 This fibrous hamartoma of infancy shows an unusual microscopic pattern composed of thick wavy bundles of mature collagen, superficially resembling neurofibroma. Although this was the predominant microscopic picture of the lesion, foci of more typical features were identified peripherally. H&E × 300

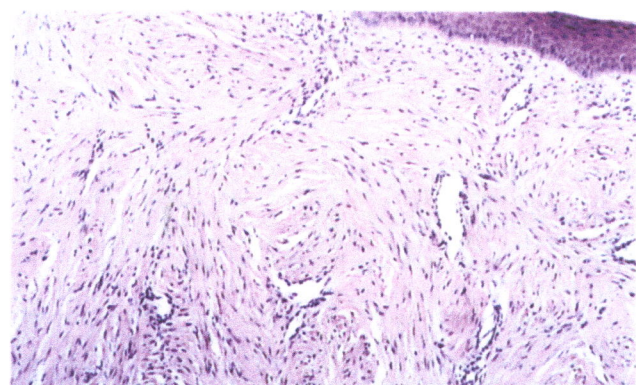

Fig. 11.7 Infantile digital fibromatosis. Low-magnification view shows a pattern of fibromatosis in which vascular channels are particularly prominent. The lesion was resected from the second right toe of a 9-month-old girl. H&E × 75

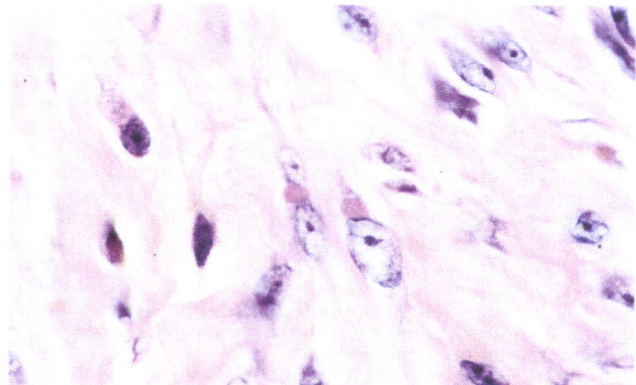

Fig. 11.8 Infantile digital fibromatosis. Same lesion as in Figure 11.7. Characteristic eosinophilic inclusions are seen in the cytoplasm of several spindle cells. H&E × 750

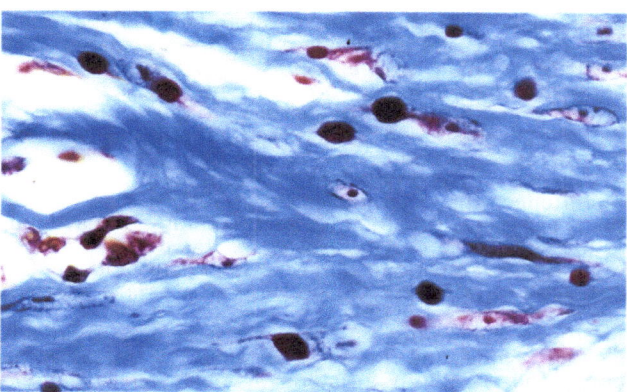

Fig. 11.9 Infantile digital fibromatosis. The cytoplasmic inclusions stain magenta with Masson's trichrome. × 750

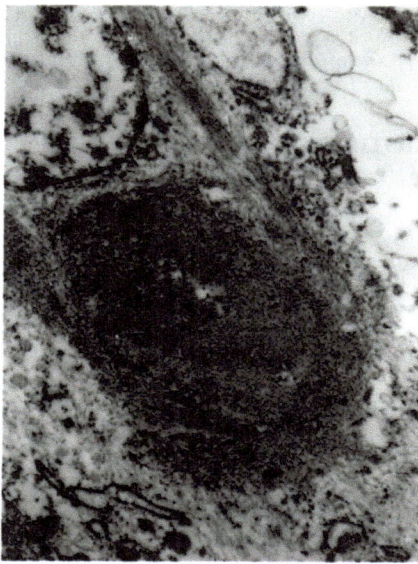

Fig. 11.10 Ultrastructural view of infantile digital fibromatosis shows a detailed strucfure of an intracytoplasmic inclusion. This is sharply outlined, occupies a juxtanuclear position, and is composed of closely packed electron dense finely granular and fibrillary material. × 11 250

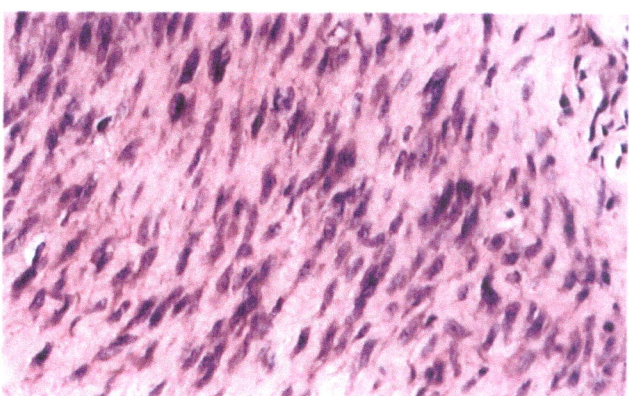

Fig. 11.11 Closely packed fibroblasts with minimal intervening collagen characterize the proliferative stage of plantar fibromatosis. The lesion was resected from the sole of the right foot of an 11-year-old girl. H&E × 300

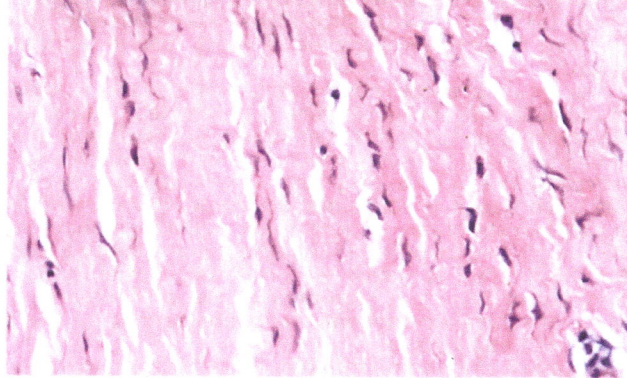

Fig. 11.12 A lesser degree of cellularity with correspondingly more collagen characterize plantar fibromatosis in a more quiescent phase. H&E × 300

in bone and viscera tend to be less differentiated[9]. PAS staining is usually negative[12], a feature that may assist in distinguishing such lesions from a true smooth muscle tumour[9]. However, a recent study has invoked true smooth muscle differentiation in the histogenesis of infantile myofibromatosis[12].

The microscopic differential diagnosis includes all other forms of fibromatoses, as well as mesenchymal neoplasms exhibiting a spindle-cell pattern. An important diagnostic pointer to infantile myofibromatosis is the presence of haemangiopericytoma-like areas[4,5]. With the exception of congenital fibrosarcoma-like fibromatosis (see below), other types of fibromatosis do not seem to exhibit this feature. (NB: Haemangiopericytoma-like foci may be found also in synovial sarcoma, fibrous histiocytoma and mesenchymal chondrosarcoma.)

Solitary intestinal fibromatosis is rarely reported; they are generally poorly demarcated congenital growths that most often affect the small and large bowel[13]. The outlook for solitary intestinal tumours is considerably better compared with intestinal tumours associated with multicentric/visceral disease. Lesions limited to the skin and superficial soft tissue, with or without osseous involvement, are generally associated with a benign clinical course. Most infants with multiple lesions die soon after birth[1], especially when the cardiorespiratory or gastrointestinal systems are involved. The outcome is especially poor when the lungs are affected[7,14]. The recurrence rate after excision of solitary lesions is less than 10%[4,5].

FIBROUS HAMARTOMA OF INFANCY (FHI)

FHI is an uncommon benign soft-tissue lesion of unknown histogenesis[15,16]. Children in their first year are usually affected and the tumour may present at birth. Lesions are occasionally discovered in later childhood. They are three times more likely to occur in boys than in girls.

A solitary firm freely movable mass in the subcutaneous tissue is the usual clinical finding. Ninety per cent of tumours are located in the upper part of the body. Thirty-seven per cent occur in the axillary region[15]. Less commonly, the forearm, chest and groin are affected but FHI never seem to involve the hands and feet.

The lesions are generally poorly circumscribed and unencapsulated; a few are well circumscribed[15] or, rarely, encapsulated[16]. The majority measure 2.5–5 cm in greatest diameter. Sometimes the lesion is attached to the underlying fascia, and extension into the subepidermal zone may occur.

The microscopic picture is usually distinctive[3,15]. Three components in variable proportions are found (Figure 11.4): (a) well-defined fibrocollagenous trabeculae; (b) primitive mesenchymal stroma; and (c) mature adipose tissue.

The various tissue components are usually sharply delineated, but transition may be detected[17]. Cellular pleomorphism, nuclear hyperchromatism, mitoses and calcification are not seen. Blood vessels are conspicuous especially in relation to the primitive mesenchymal stroma; this often shows a concentric arrangement with whorls or ball-like structures (Figure 11.5). A mild lymphocytic infiltration may be present. The amount of adipose tissue may be difficult to gauge as the lesion is often poorly demarcated from the surrounding tissue. Tumours in which the fatty component predominates may be misdiagnosed as a lipoma.

An unusual pattern, thought to be related to older lesions, is composed of short wavy thick bundles of mature collagen and superficially resembles a neurofibroma (Figure 11.6)[15]. It is usually confined to the central part of the tumour, blending peripherally with the more typical histological elements. Diagnostic difficulties

occasionally arise when this pattern dominates the histological picture.

The natural history of fibrous hamartoma of infancy is unknown. Simple excision is usually curative; recurrences are unusual[15,18].

INFANTILE DIGITAL FIBROMATOSIS (RECURRING DIGITAL FIBROMATOSIS OF CHILDHOOD; RECURRING DIGITAL FIBROMA; INFANTILE DIGITAL MYOFIBROBLASTOMA; INCLUSION BODY FIBROMATOSIS; REYE TUMOUR)

Reye[19] first called attention to this lesion in 1965. The age distribution, topography and morphology are distinctive. The exact incidence is difficult to gauge because of the widely varying terms previously used, but there is general agreement as to its rarity. The great majority of cases arise during the first year after birth and some lesions have been congenital[3,9,17]. The sex incidence is approximately equal. No known genetic predisposition is recognized. There may be functional impairment and the joint may be deformed[9,17].

Most lesions are multiple[3], involving several fingers or toes; they are sessile and generally measure 1.0 cm or less in diameter. Fingers are more often affected than toes and, curiously, the thumbs and big toes are spared. One digit may contain several lesions. The fingers and toes are occasionally affected together. The tumours are sited on the dorsum or sides of the distal digits; they elevate and stretch the overlying skin, and superficial ulceration may be encountered.

One survey recorded recurrences in 75% of cases[3]. Recurrences may continue throughout the first decade but are unusual after the fifth year. The tumour may recur at the site of the previous lesion or involve an adjacent digit. Regression and resolution often occur[9] and metastases are not observed. Observation after simple excision is the treatment of choice.

Grossly, the tumour is rubbery in consistency, unencapsulated, white and homogeneous[1,9]. The microscopic appearance is fairly consistent[3], revealing an ill-defined lesion composed of interlacing bundles or whorls of closely apposed spindle-shaped fibroblasts (Figure 11.7). Nuclei are plump, oval and vesicular. Pleomorphism is non-existent and mitoses are rare. Multinucleated cells are occasionally found. The lesion often extends into the underlying connective tissue and encircles skin adnexae. The papillary dermis is frequently involved but the overlying epidermis is generally spared.

The presence of inclusions in the cytoplasm of the spindle cell represents the most remarkable feature of the lesion (Figure 11.8)[1,3,9]. The inclusions are eosinophilic and range in size from 6 to 24 μm. They are located adjacent to the nuclei which are often indented, but may also be found in the extracellular matrix. Their number varies from case to case, and from area to area in the same tumour, but, in some instances, they may be difficult to find. Allen[1] referred to two cases in which the lesions conformed clinically and morphologically to this entity but, despite extensive searching, inclusions could not be demonstrated. Similar inclusions have not yet been reported in the other types of fibromatoses.

The cytoplasmic inclusions are usually obvious on haematoxylin and eosin staining. They also display a range of tinctorial qualities, including a bright red reaction to Masson's trichrome (Figure 11.9) and purple with phosphotungstic acid haematoxylin (PTAH)[3]; PAS and alcian blue staining are negative. Viral stains, such as phloxine tartrazine, feulgen and methyl green pyronine, are negative.

Ultrastructure supports an origin from the myofibroblast[20,21]. The cells are elongated with irregular nuclei. The cytoplasm contains bundles of longitudinally aligned microfilaments interspersed with dense bodies, reminiscent of the contractile unit of smooth muscle. The inclusions consist of rounded non-membrane-bound electron-dense bodies composed of closely packed finely granular and fibrillary material (Figure 11.10). The intracytoplasmic microfilaments and the electron-dense bodies are often intimately connected or continuous. Apart from supporting a myofibroblastic derivation, these appearances also suggest that the cytoplasmic inclusions are derived from a contractile protein, possibly the Z line. Particles resembling viruses are not seen.

A morphologically similar tumour is reported to occur rarely in adults in an extradigital location; recurrence in such cases appears to be unusual[22].

PALMAR AND PLANTAR FIBROMATOSIS

Plantar fibromatosis affects all age groups while palmar fibrosis rarely occurs in children[3,23]. Patients with plantar fibrosis usually complain of a burning sensation on the sole of the foot. A nodule projecting from the plantar fascia towards the dermis is the usual clinical finding[3].

The age of the lesion determines the microscopic picture[3,24]. Thus, in the proliferative stage, the pattern is one of dense cellularity and abundant mitoses, and little collagen (Figure 11.11). The involutional stage is characterized by the presence of more collagen and correspondingly less cellularity. A dense collagenized pattern with a few compressed fibroblasts characterizes the residual stage (Figure 11.12). The residual stage is associated with contractions.

About 10% of plantar lesions are bilateral[3]. Both palmar and plantar lesions rarely arise in the same patient. A recurrence rate of 57% is reported for plantar fibromatosis after simple excision[3]. Wide excision is necessary to safeguard against recurrence.

STERNOMASTOID TUMOUR (FIBROMATOSIS COLLI; CONGENITAL TORTICOLLIS)

This is a fibroproliferative lesion that usually arises in the distal third of the sternomastoid muscle. Its incidence is variably estimated to be 4 per 1000 (in Minnesota) and 5 per 10 000 births (in Singapore)[25]. It is the most common cause of a mass in the neck in the perinatal period[25].

A firm spindle-shaped swelling measuring 0.5 to 3 cm in diameter appears usually within the first 2–6 weeks after birth. For the first 2–3 months, the tumour remains stable in size; it then gradually decreases in size. The lesion is limited to the sternomastoid muscle[9]. Most cases can be diagnosed confidently on clinical grounds and a biopsy is generally not necessary; it should be reserved for where the diagnosis is uncertain[25]. Bilateral tumours are rarely reported.

The histology varies with the age of the patient[3,9]. Fibrous proliferation with variable amounts of collagen invading the adjacent muscle characterizes the early stage of the lesion (Figure 11.13). Muscle fibres that have become entrapped and separated frequently undergo degeneration[17]. The proliferating cells are uniform and bland, and mitoses are rarely encountered. Focal infiltration of lymphocytes may be present. Haemosiderin is usually absent. Later, acellular collagen replaces the fibroblastic tissue which may extend through the entire muscle, leading to cicatrization and torticollis[3].

However, torticollis may develop without evidence of a preceding tumour[3]; conversely, not all patients with a sternomastoid tumour develop torticollis. The cause of the condition is still debatable, and while birth trauma and intramuscular haematoma are appealing as explanations, they are difficult to reconcile with an absence of significant haemosiderin deposition, and also its reported occurrence after Caesarean section[1,9].

JUVENILE APONEUROTIC FIBROMATOSIS (JAF) (CARTILAGE ANALOGUE OF FIBROMATOSIS; CALCIFYING APONEUROTIC FIBROMA)

This is a slow-growing painless mass that usually involves the volar aspects of the hands and feet of children and young adults[17,26]. The hand is more commonly affected than the foot; most lesions arise in the palm or fingers. Less often, they involve the soft tissue of the extremities more proximally[3,9]. Most lesions are encountered in the first 10 years of life (56%). Occasionally they are present at birth[3,9].

Grossly, the lesions are ill-defined or poorly circumscribed, firm to rubbery and grey–white in colour. Those arising in the hands and feet are usually the size of a small pea, rarely exceeding 2 cm in diameter[9,17]. They may be larger when the soft tissues of the extremities are involved[3].

The microscopy is quite distinct. There is marked cellularity comprising plump fibroblasts with round-to-oval nuclei and ill-defined cytoplasm (Figure 11.14)[3,9,17]. Despite the degree of cellularity, mitoses are difficult to find. In areas, the cells appear to 'stream' in one direction, or they are arranged haphazardly; elsewhere, they interdigitate to form bundles or even a storiform pattern. This cellular pattern differs from the usual interdigitating arrangement seen in other types of fibromatoses[3]. Multiple processes of tumour characteristically extend into the surrounding adipose tissue and muscle (Figure 11.15), encircling blood vessels and nerves[3,9].

Linear or granular flecks of calcification are common, as are foci of chondroid differentiation. However, these features are more often seen in the tumours from older children and adolescents[17]. Their presence has given rise to such terms as 'calcifying aponeurotic fibroma' and 'cartilage analogue of fibromatosis'. Cells pallisaded around foci of calcification is a common feature and may mimic a granuloma[3]. Giant cells resembling osteoclasts are seen occasionally.

The lesion is locally invasive and the recurrence rate following surgery is about 50%[3,9]. Lesions are more likely to recur in infants and young children under 5 years old[3]. There are no reliable histological criteria to indicate the likelihood of recurrence. Surgery should aim at conservative resection of recurrences, rather than involving complex mutilating procedures[1,3].

Palmar and plantar fibromatoses may give rise to problems in the differential diagnosis[1,9]. When the lesion occurs more proximally, the differential diagnosis should include infantile (desmoid) fibromatosis and fibrous hamartoma of infancy[9]. The high degree of cellularity may suggest fibrosarcoma[17].

HYALINE FIBROMATOSIS (FIBROMATOSIS HYALINICA MULTIPLEX JUVENALIS)

This is a rare hereditary disorder with an onset between 3 months and 4 years[9,27]. Subcutaneous tumour nodules and gingival hyperplasia are characteristic features. The nodules vary in size from 0.5 to 5 cm[9]. The scalp is frequently involved. New nodules continue to appear up to the age of about 12 years. Joint contractures develop frequently and bone lesions, in the form of erosions or punched-out osteolytic areas, may be seen radiologically.

Histologically[17,27], streaks of spindle cells with oval-to-round nuclei and pale-to-clear cytoplasm are embedded in copious amorphous hyaline eosinophilic ground sub-

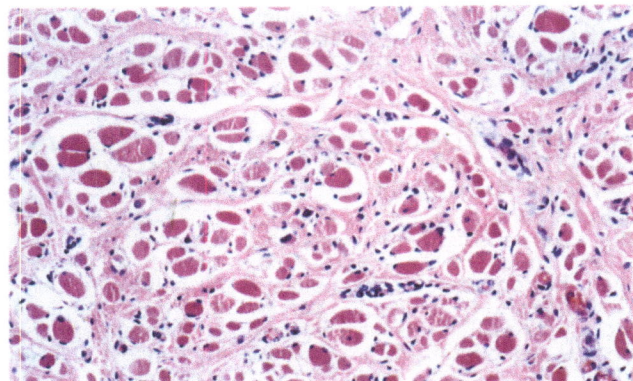

Fig. 11.13 Sternomastoid tumour in a 3-month-old female infant reveals muscle fibres separated by fibrocollagenous tissue. This was an incidental discovery at autopsy in an infant who died as SIDS. H&E × 185

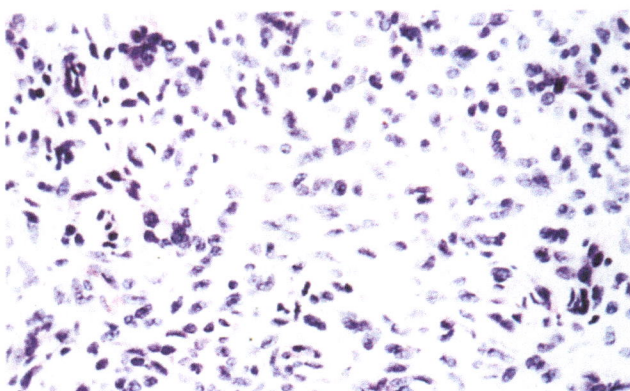

Fig. 11.14 Plump fibroblasts with haphazard arrangement are typical of a juvenile aponeurotic fibroma. H&E × 300

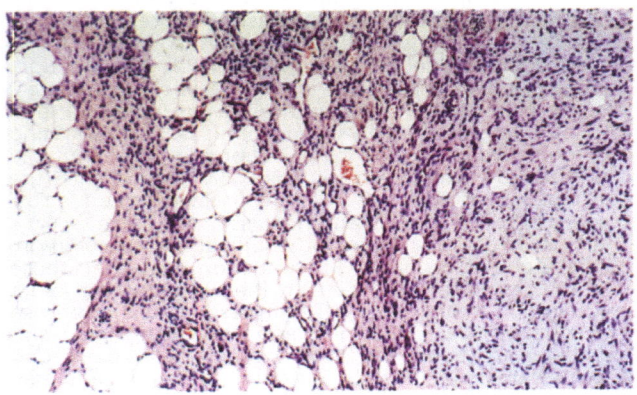

Fig. 11.15 A marked degree of cellularity and diffuse infiltration of adjacent adipose tissue are other features of juvenile aponeurotic fibroma. H&E × 75

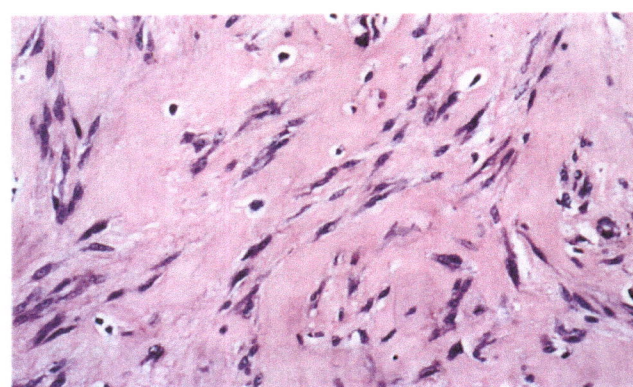

Fig. 11.16 Hyaline fibromatosis. This 12-year-old girl presented with multiple generalized subcutaneous nodules. Histology shows cords of fibroblasts amidst large amounts of hyalinized collagen-like material. H&E × 185

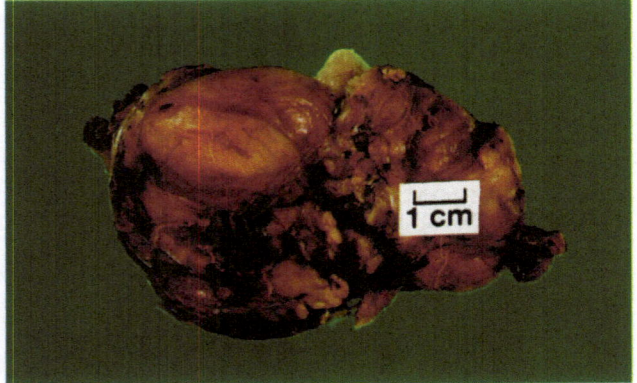

Fig. 11.17 Naked-eye appearance of infantile (diffuse-type) fibromatosis resected from the soft tissue at the back of the right thigh of a young boy. The tumour is lobulated and well-circumscribed; it measured 7 cm in maximal extent and weighed 99 g

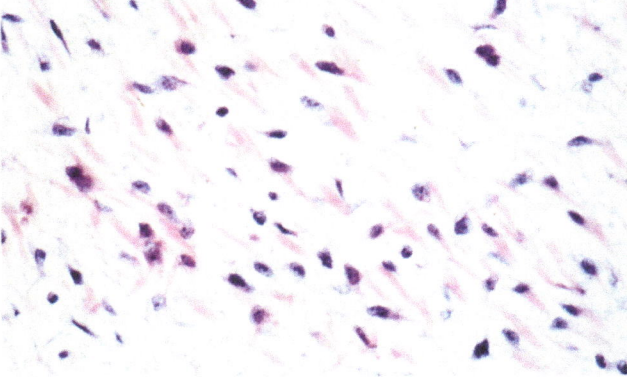

Fig. 11.18 Infantile (diffuse-type) fibromatosis. Histology shows haphazardly arranged primitive mesenchymal cells set in abundant mucoid matrix. H&E × 300

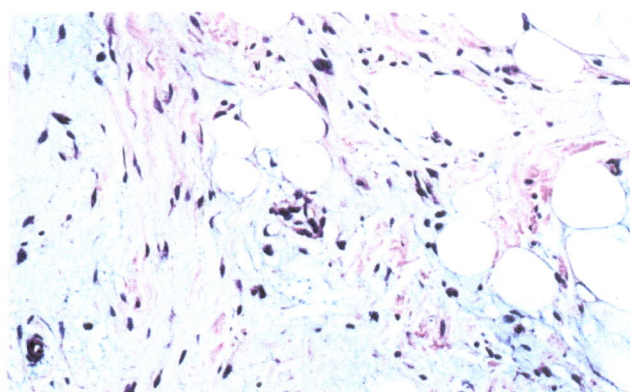

Fig. 11.19 Contiguous adipose tissue is diffusely infiltrated by infantile 'diffuse-type' fibromatosis at the periphery of the tumour. H&E × 185

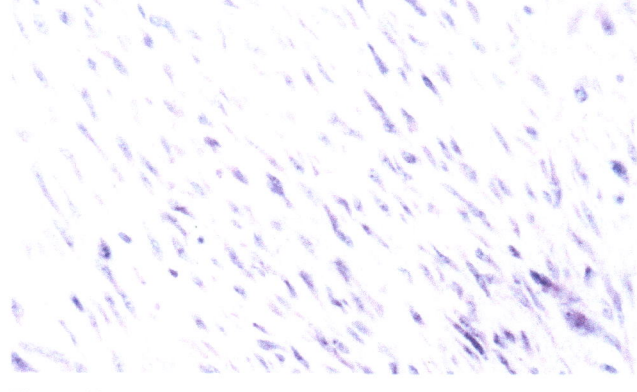

Fig. 11.20 Infantile (desmoid-type) fibromatosis demonstrates a relatively cellular tumour composed of spindle cells. The degree of cellularity is typically variable and another area of the same lesion with a lesser degree of cellularity is depicted in Figure 11.21. The patient was a 4-year-old boy who had a tumour in the middle of the left sternomastoid muscle. H&E × 300

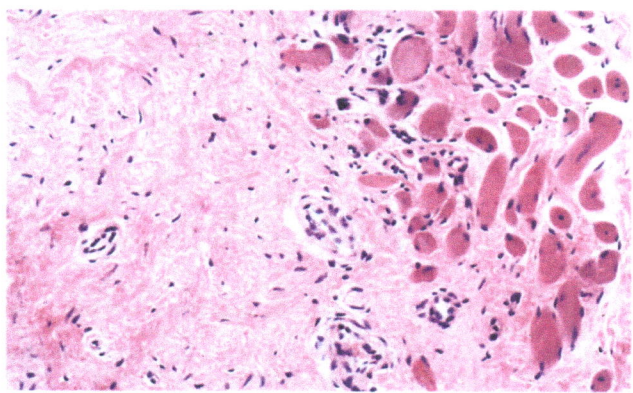

Fig. 11.21 A less cellular area of the lesion depicted in Figure 11.20 demonstrates infiltration of the neighbouring skeletal muscle. H&E × 185

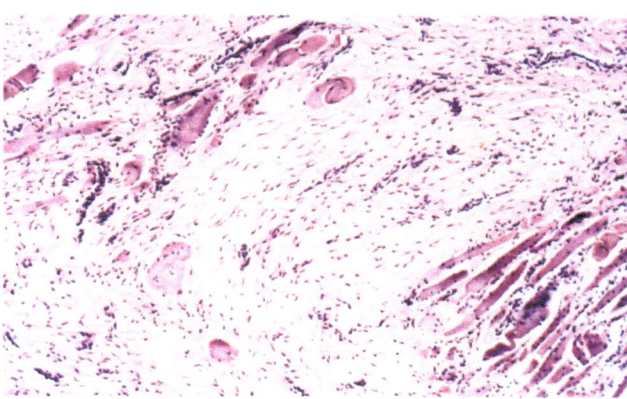

Fig. 11.22 The tumour was removed from the soft tissue over the right scapula of a 22-year-old male. Microscopy shows poorly cellular fibrous tissue with corresponding increase in collagen infiltrating neighbouring skeletal muscle; the age and microscopic picture is typical of musculo-aponeurotic fibromatosis which is regarded as the adult version of desmoid-type fibromatosis. H&E × 75

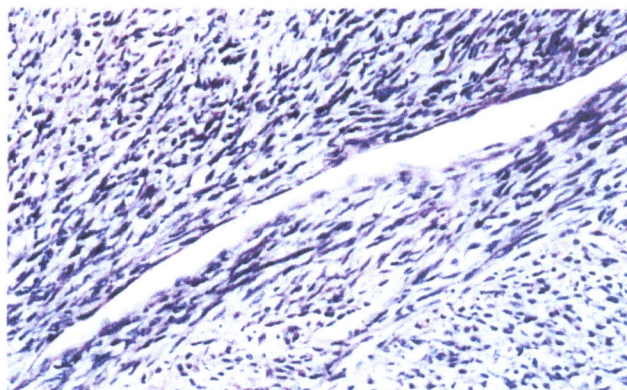

Fig. 11.23 Congenital–infantile fibrosarcoma shows a highly cellular spindle cell tumour around a distorted vascular channel. The tumour was resected from the chest wall of a 6-week-old boy; there was no recurrence during a 10-year period of follow-up. H&E × 185

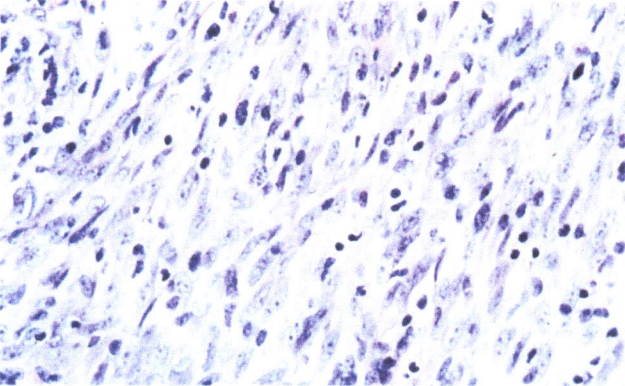

Fig. 11.24 Microscopic view of congenital–infantile fibrosarcoma shows a spindle-cell tumour with a marked degree of cellularity and an admixture of lymphocytes. The patient was a neonate who presented with a large retroperitoneal mass. H&E × 300

stance (Figure 11.16). The tumour cells are arranged singly or in groups. The ground substance is PAS positive, diastase-resistant.

The only effective treatment is surgical excision but the lesions may recur[9]. This condition is distinct from infantile systemic hyalinosis, a condition in which the deposits of hyaline material are far more widespread, and which includes involvement of the internal organs[28].

INFANTILE (DESMOID-TYPE) FIBROMATOSIS (DESMOID TUMOUR; MUSCULOAPONEUROTIC FIBROMATOSIS; AGGRESSIVE FIBROMATOSIS; DESMOPLASTIC FIBROMA)

This is a relatively uncommon fibrous tissue proliferation known for its ability to infiltrate and spread locally[29]. A painless solitary mass arising in skeletal muscle or adjacent fascia, aponeurosis or periosteum is the usual presentation[9,23]. While the lesion occurs most commonly in the muscles of the head and neck, any anatomical site may be involved[30]. In the head and neck region, the tongue is commonly affected, followed in frequency by the mandibular region and mastoid area[9]. The shoulder, upper arm and thigh are other common sites. Some reports have noted a female predominance[31], albeit slight; others have documented a male predominance[2,29].

Desmoid-type fibromatosis covers a wide age range and has a peak age incidence in the third decade; 15–30% of cases are diagnosed in patients less than 20 years old[2]. Some of the lesions may be multifocal and others may arise at the sites of previous surgery. Familial examples have been described, and instances associated with Gardner's syndrome are reported[2,30]. Rarely is there an association with other congenital abnormalities[29]. Trauma and hormonal factors have been implicated in the histogenesis[31], but the situation remains unclear.

Tumour size varies from 2 to 15 cm in diameter[29]. The lesions are relatively well circumscribed, although never encapsulated (Figure 11.17). Consistency is usually rubbery, and the cut surface is greyish-white to yellowish-tan with a whorled or lobulated appearance; focal haemorrhages are occasionally noted[29].

The microscopic picture is variable and generally corresponds to the patient's age[9,23]. The pattern usually found during the early months of life is a haphazard arrangement of primitive mesenchymal cells set in a diffuse myxoid matrix (Figure 11.18)[23], scattered lymphoid cells are often noted, as are large amounts of adipose tissue (Figure 11.19). This pattern is referred to as the 'diffuse type' and is least common[23].

The second pattern, usually referred to as the desmoid type, predominates in the older child[23]. It exhibits moderately cellular fibrous tissue with an intertwining fascicular pattern. Those lesions with more mature-appearing spindle-shaped fibroblasts are accompanied by variable amounts of collagen (Figure 11.20). The cytoplasmic borders of the fibroblasts are ill-defined; mitoses are variable, though never brisk, and nuclear pleomorphism is absent. Mononuclear cells, including mast cells, are often scattered within the stroma of the tumour. There is a strong propensity for the tumour to infiltrate adjoining skeletal muscle and adipose tissue; atrophic muscle is often entrapped at the periphery (Figure 11.21).

Some examples of desmoid-type fibromatosis display unusually high degrees of cellularity, and the term 'aggressive fibromatosis' is usually reserved for such variants[9].

Less cellular examples of the tumour associated with larger amounts of collagen are encountered in older subjects (Figure 11.22), and are usually referred to as musculoaponeurotic fibromatosis[31]. The microscopic cut-off point between the two patterns is ill-defined, and the two terms are sometimes used interchangeably. A combination of the 'diffuse type' and the more mature pattern may be found in the same tumour[23].

The differential diagnosis in the 'diffuse type' includes lipoblastomatosis, myxoid liposarcoma and embryonal (myxoid) rhabdomyosarcoma[23]. The differential diagnosis of the more mature pattern includes other types of fibromatoses. Aggressive fibromatosis (cellular examples of infantile desmoid) may be difficult to distinguish from congenital–infantile fibrosarcoma in the young, and from fibrosarcoma in older patients. As a rule, aggressive fibromatosis reveals residual muscle fibres and adipocytes at the tumour edge; it also often includes a variable growth pattern characterized histologically by alternating hypercellular and collagenous areas[9].

Local resection with wide surgical margins is the treatment of choice. Because of their location, the management of tumours of the head and neck is especially problematic. Preoperative chemotherapy has been advocated for some cases[29]; radiotherapy and endocrine therapy appear to have little or no benefit[30]. Recurrence after surgery is well recognized, and recurrence rates of 68%[30] and 60%[32] have been documented. Tumour recurrences as late as 5 and 10 years after initial surgery have been reported[9]. In the young, tumours are more likely to recur, probably correlating with greater mitotic activity of the tumour at this age[29]. Disagreement exists over whether tumour size affects the rate of recurrence[30,31]. The histologies of the primary and recurrent tumour are always identical[33]. Metastases have not been documented.

Desmoplastic fibroma of bone is considered the osseous counterpart of the soft-tissue desmoid tumour[29]. The differential diagnosis of this entity includes fibrous dysplasia of bone, osteogenic fibroma and infantile myofibromatosis. Desmoplastic tumour of bone is exceedingly rare; Dahlin could identify only four such tumours out of a total of 6221 bone tumours[34].

Intra-abdominal fibromatosis probably belongs to this category of tumours[23]. They may occupy the mesentery of the small intestine, omentum, mesocolon or retroperitoneum[3]. A wide age range is affected and the entity is especially associated with Gardner's syndrome.

CONGENITAL–INFANTILE FIBROSARCOMA (CONGENITAL, INFANTILE OR JUVENILE FIBROSARCOMA; CONGENITAL FIBROSARCOMA-LIKE FIBROMATOSIS; AGGRESSIVE FIBROMATOSIS)

This is a rare category of fibromatosis in which the clinical behaviour is notoriously unpredictable and correlates poorly with histological pattern[35]. The lesion comprised 13% of 108 fibroblastic–myofibroblastic tumours recorded by Coffin and Dehner[2]. In one large series, the average age at diagnosis was found to be 8.6 months[35]. Fifty per cent of cases were diagnosed in the first 3 months and of these, a large proportion was already present at birth. A review of 52 cases of congenital tumours[36] (i.e. those present at birth or within the first 3 months) found an equal sex distribution. The large majority of the tumours arose in the extremity; none regressed spontaneously and there was no familial or inherited tendency. The lesion may involve virtually any anatomical site, apart from the central nervous system.

A painless non-tender swelling or mass is the usual clinical presentation, and there is a tendency for rapid growth[35]. The presence of dilated blood vessels in the superficial part of the growth may impart a bluish or violaceous hue to the overlying skin[1].

Grossly, the tumour is poorly circumscribed and often deeply infiltrative. Consistency varies from soft to firm; the cut surfaces are variably pale pink, grey–white or tan.

The lesion may be small or large enough to encompass an entire limb. The size ranges from 1.2 to 13.5 cm in diameter[35].

Microscopically, the neoplasm exhibits fibroblastic differentiation marked by a high degree of cellularity (Figure 11.23). The cells are often arranged in interlacing bundles or irregularly coursing fascicles. Mitoses are common but vary in number between tumours and between fields within the same tumour. There is little nuclear pleomorphism. Cytoplasm is ill-defined and collagen production is variable. The prominence of reticulin fibres generally parallels the degree of cellularity, cells being individually encompassed by reticulin. Irregular cleft-like or cavernous vascular channels are often found, and sometimes scattered chronic inflammatory cells are present (lymphocytes and plasma cells) (Figure 11.24)[35]. Cystic areas, haemorrhage and necrosis are noted occasionally, and are especially seen in large and deep-seated neoplasms. The cellularity, mitotic activity and local invasiveness of the lesion is reminiscent of adult-type fibrosarcoma.

The microscopic differential diagnosis includes many spindle-cell tumours that are known to occur in childhood[35,38] (see Table 12.1). Congenital fibrosarcoma is generally more cellular than desmoid fibromatosis[37], but may be difficult to segregate from 'aggressive fibromatosis'[38]. The microscopic picture overlaps with congenital infantile haemangiopericytoma as both tumours may show cellular areas composed of immature spindle cells with irregular vascular channels[9] (see Chapter 10)[1].

Wide local excision is recommended and the majority of patients have an excellent outlook. A 5-year survival rate of 84% has been reported for 48 patients[35]. In a retrospective review of 110 infants and children with 'fibrosarcoma', those 10 years of age and above had a metastatic rate of 50%; patients less than 5 years old had a 7.3% chance of developing metastases[39].

A local recurrence rate, reported by Chung and Enzinger[35] and Soule and Pritchard[39], was 17% and 43%, respectively. For 52 congenital tumours, the overall local recurrence rate was reported as 32%[36], and was similar for axial and extremity tumours. Recurrences usually occur within 12 months of initial surgery[35]. More recent reports[2,38,40] suggest that the recurrence rate may not be as high as previously recorded[36,40], even when the surgical margins are positive. Late recurrence and metastases have been described and long-term follow-up of patients is necessary[35].

Chung and Enzinger[35] reported metastatic disease in four of 53 cases (8.3%). In a review of 52 cases (47 from the literature)[36], seven (13.5%) developed metastatic disease. Rosenberg et al.[3] identified 13 cases in the literature in which 'aggressive fibromatosis' was reported to have metastasized; some patients were in their first year. By these authors' criteria, metastases invalidate the diagnosis which should be altered to one of 'true' fibrosarcoma; others question the inclusion of such lesions within the category of fibromatoses[41].

NASOPHARYNGEAL ANGIOFIBROMA

This is a benign highly vascular tumour virtually confined to adolescent males[42]. The median age of onset is 13 years and the age spread is 8–27 years[3]. Common symptoms are nasal obstruction, epistaxis and nasal discharge, although bulging of the cheek or palate and exophthalmos occur occasionally. The tumour may regress at puberty, suggesting an endocrine role in its pathogenesis. The growth is always unilateral but neighbouring bones may be extensively involved.

Grossly, the tumour is firm, white and polypoid with a spongy cut surface. The size of the lesion varies[3] from 2–5 cm. Microscopically, abundant loose or collagenous stroma separates variable-sized thin-walled vascular channels. When the stroma is loose, the component cells are plump or stellate; when the stroma is collagenous, the cells are elongated and compressed. Mitoses are uncommon. Inflammatory cells are usually concentrated at the surface. Adjacent tissues are often invaded. Surgical excision, even if incomplete, is the treatment of choice. Recurrence may follow.

REFERENCES

1. Allen PW. The fibromatoses: a clinicopathologic classification based on 140 cases (Part 2). Am J Surg Pathol. 1977;2:305–21.
2. Coffin CM, Dehner LP. Fibroblastic–myofibroblastic tumors in children and adolescents: a clinicopathological study of 108 examples in 103 patients. Pediatr Pathol. 1991;11:569–87.
3. Rosenberg HS, Stenback WA, Spjut HS. The fibromatosis of infancy and childhood. Perspect Pediatr Pathol. 1978;4:269–348.
4. Chung EB, Enzinger FM. Infantile myofibromatosis. Cancer. 1981;48:1807–18.
5. Bračko M, Cindro L, Golouh R. Familial occurrence of infantile myofibromatosis. Cancer. 1992;69:1294–9.
6. Wiswell TE, Davis J, Cunningham BE, Solenberger R, Thomas PJ. Infantile myofibromatosis: The most common fibrous tumour of infancy. J Pediatr Surg. 1988;23:314–18.
7. Roggli VL, Kim H-S, Hawkins E. Congenital generalized fibromatosis with visceral involvement. A case report. Cancer. 1980;45:954–60.
8. Michel M, Ninane J, Claus D, Gosseye S, Wese FX, Moulin D. Major malformations in a case of infantile myofibromatosis. Eur J Pediatr. 1990;149:251–2.
9. Chung EB. Pitfalls in diagnosing benign soft tissue tumors in infancy and childhood. Pathol Annu. 1985;20:323–86.
10. Adickes ED, Goodrich P, AuchMoedy J et al. Central nervous system involvement in congenital visceral fibromatosis. Pediatr Pathol. 1985;3:329–40.
11. Inwards CY, Unni KK, Beabout JW, Shives TC. Solitary congenital fibromatosis (infantile myofibromatosis) of bone. Am J Surg Pathol. 1991;15:935–41.
12. Fletcher CDM, Achu P, van Noorden S, McKee PH. Infantile myofibromatosis: a light microscopic, histochemical and immuno-histochemical study suggesting true smooth muscle differentiation. Histopathology. 1987;11:245–58.
13. Srigley JR, Mancer K. Solitary intestinal fibromatosis with perinatal bowel obstruction. Pediatr Pathol. 1984;2:249–58.
14. Wiswell TE, Sakas EL, Stephenson SR, Lesica JL, Reddoch SR. Infantile myofibromatosis. Pediatrics. 1985;76:981–4.
15. Enzinger FM. Fibrous hamartoma of infancy. Cancer. 1965;18:241–8.
16. Paller AS, Gonzalez-Crussi F, Sherman JO. Fibrous hamartoma of infancy. Eight additional cases and a review of the literature. Arch Dermatol. 1989;125:88–91.
17. Enzinger FM, Weiss SW. Fibrous proliferations of infancy and childhood. In: Enzinger, FM, Weiss SW, editors. Soft tissue tumors. St Louis, Toronto, London: CV Mosby; 1983:71–102.
18. Lee JT, Girvan DP, Armstrong RF. Fibrous hamartoma of infancy. J Pediatr Surg. 1988;23:759–61.
19. Reye RDK. Recurring digital fibrous tumors of childhood. Arch Pathol. 1965;80:228–31.
20. Bhawan J, Bacchetta C, Joris I, Majno G. A myofibroblastic tumour. Infantile digital fibroma (recurrent digital fibrous tumor of childhood). Am J Pathol. 1979;94:19–36.
21. Yun K. Infantile digital fibromatosis. Immunohistochemical and ultrastructural observations of cytoplasmic inclusions. Cancer. 1988;61:500–7.
22. Viale G, Doglioni C, Iuzzolino P et al. Infantile digital fibromatosis-like tumour (inclusion body fibromatosis) of adulthood: report of two cases with ultrastructural and immunocytochemical findings. Histopathology. 1988;12:415–24.
23. Enzinger FM, Weiss SW. Fibromatoses. In: Enzinger FM, Weiss SW, editors. Soft tissue tumors. St Louis, Toronto, London: CV Mosby; 1983:45–70.
24. MacKenzie DH. The fibromatoses. In MacKenzie DH, editor. The differential diagnosis of fibroblastic disorders. Oxford: Blackwell Scientific Publications; 1970:67–102.
25. Thompsen JR, Koltai RJ. Sternomastoid tumor of infancy. Ann Otol Rhinol Laryngol. 1989;98:955–9.
26. McKenzie DH. The fibromatoses. In McKenzie DH, editor. The differential diagnosis of fibroblastic disorders. Oxford and Edinburgh. Blackwell Scientific Publications; 1970:78–81.

27. Kitano Y. Juvenile hyalin fibromatosis. Arch Dermatol. 1976; 112:86–8.
28. Landing BH, Nadorra R. Infantile systemic hyalinosis. Report of four cases of a disease, fatal in infancy, apparently different from juvenile systemic hyalinosis. Pediatr Pathol. 1986;6:55–79.
29. Ayala AG, Ro JY, Goepfert H, Cangir A, Khorsand J, Flake G. Desmoid fibromatosis: a clinicopathological study of 25 children. Semin Diagnost Pathol. 1986;3:138–50.
30. Rock MG, Pritchard DJ, Reiman HM, Soule EH, Brewster RC. Extra-abdominal desmoid tumours. J Bone Jt Surg. 1984;66:1369–74.
31. Enzinger FM, Shiraki M. Musculo-aponeurotic fibromatosis of the shoulder girdle (extra-abdominal desmoid). Analysis of thirty cases followed up for ten or more years. Cancer. 1967;20:1131–40.
32. Kofoed H, Kamby C, Anagnostaki L. Aggressive fibromatosis. Surg Gynecol Obstet. 1985;160:124–7.
33. Lagace R, Bouchard H-Ls, Delage C, Seemayer TA. Desmoplastic fibroma of bone. An ultrastructural study. Am J Surg Pathol. 1979;3:423–30.
34. Dahlin DC. Bone tumours. General aspects and data on 6,211 cases,

3rd edn. Springfield: Charles C. Thomas; 1978:325–8.
35. Chung EB, Enzinger FM. Infantile fibrosacroma. Cancer. 1976;38:729–39.
36. Blocker S, Koenig J, Ternberg J. Congenital fibrosacroma. J Pediatr Surg. 1987;22:665–70.
37. Balsaver AM, Butler JJ, Martin RG. Congenital fibrosarcoma. Cancer. 1967;20:1607–16.
38. Wee E, Pho RWH. Infantile fibrosarcoma. Report of cases. Arch Pathol Lab Med. 1979;103:236–8.
39. Soule EH, Pritchard DJ. Fibrosarcoma in infants and children. A review of 110 cases. Cancer. 1977;40:1711–21.
40. Wilson MB, Stanley W, Sens D, Garvin AJ. Infantile fibrosarcoma – a misnomer. Pediatr Pathol. 1990;10:901–7.
41. Ninane J, Gosseye S, Panteon E, Claus D, Rombouts JJ, Cornu G. Congenital fibromatosis. Preoperative chemotherapy and conservative surgery. Cancer. 1986;58:1400–6.
42. Sinha PP, Aziz HI. Juvenile nasopharyngeal angiofibroma. A report of seven cases. Radiology. 1978;127:501–5.

Rhabdomyosarcoma (RMS) 12

RMS is the most common soft tissue sarcoma in children[1]. It comprises about two thirds of all soft tissue sarcomas in children and represents 5% of all paediatric malignancies[2]. Because of its origin within the soft tissues, almost any part of the body may be affected. The more common soft tissue sarcomas of adults (synovial sarcoma, liposarcoma, fibrosarcoma, leiomyosarcoma and irradiation-associated sarcomas) are diagnosed about one third as often as RMS in children[3].

Diagnosis of RMS depends on the histological recognition of rhabdomyoblasts that are generally easily recognized by the presence of variable amounts of intensely acidophilic cytoplasm (Figure 12.1). They assume a variety of shapes, being round, oval, spindled, strapped, racquet and tadpole shaped, with or without cytoplasmic cross-striations. Cytoplasmic cross-striations are reported to be present in less than half of the tumours[4,5].

The cytoplasm stains deep blue with Phosphotungstic acid haematoxylin (PTAH) and deep red with Masson's trichrome[6] (Figure 12.2). PTAH staining is often useful in augmenting cytoplasmic cross-striations, usually already evident on conventional staining. (Cytoplasmic cross-striations have assumed a lesser diagnostic importance since the introduction of immunohistochemistry.) The more differentiated rhabdomyoblasts are rich in cytoplasmic glycogen, showing an *en-bloc* positivity (Figure 12.3), readily demonstrated on the PAS/diastase reaction. The likelihood of a positive PAS reaction decreases in the less differentiated rhabdomyoblasts. The yield of positive PAS reactions is appreciably increased with prior fixation in absolute alcohol, or in frozen sections. Tumour cells may exhibit phagocytosis[7].

A substantial proportion of tumours are poorly differentiated, lacking rhabdomyoblastic differentiation, and are consequently difficult to separate from other small-cell tumours, especially neuroblastoma, non-Hodgkin's lymphoma, Ewing's sarcoma and neuroepithelioma. Immunohistochemistry and electron microscopy are useful in identifying cell lineage. The stage of disease is determined by the extent of the tumour and degree of resectability[8]. The histological subtypes of RMS include embryonal, alveolar and pleomorphic patterns[9].

EMBRYONAL RMS

The embryonal subtype is more commonly encountered than other subtypes. It has a modal age distribution of 3–5 years. While the tumour predominates in the head, neck and genitourinary tract (including the epididymis), the thorax, biliary tree, retroperitoneum and perineum are other recognized primary sites. Tumours that affect the nasopharynx, paranasal sinuses and middle ear are associated with a poor survival because of their parameningeal location and the propensity for early invasion of the neural axis[10]. Boys are affected more commonly than girls. Congenital tumours are described occasionally[11,12].

Botryoid RMS is a special variant of embryonal RMS and is characterized by a grape-like structure which grows beneath the mucous membrane of hollow viscera (Figure 12.4). This subtype predominates in the genitourinary tract where it involves the trigone of the bladder, the anterior wall of the vagina and the prostate, but may also arise in the middle ear, paranasal and maxillary sinuses, nasopharynx and soft palate.

Embryonal tumours show a predominantly myxoid or spindled pattern. Stellate and spindle cells arranged in a loose syncytium set in a mucoid stroma (Figure 12.5) is the usual microscopic pattern associated with the myxoid pattern. Nuclei are hyperchromatic but mitoses are generally scant; pleomorphism and anaplasia are unusual. Cytological preparations reveal cells with pale nuclei, prominent nucleoli and slender tapering cytoplasm (Figure 12.6).

In the botryoid variant, the submucosal layer is cellular ('cambium' layer), while the underlying tissue is hypocellular and myxoid[13] (Figure 12.7). The cells in the 'cambium' layer range from large and eosinophilic to small and undifferentiated (Figure 12.8). Myxoid liposarcoma, lipoblastomatosis, neurothekeoma, 'diffuse type' of infantile fibromatosis and extraskeletal myxoid chondrosarcoma should be considered in the differential diagnosis when the myxoid pattern prevails.

The spindle-cell pattern of embryonal RMS (Figure 12.9) may be confused with a wide range of spindle-cell tumours (Table 12.1). In such cases, the diagnosis of RMS rests on the identification of rhabdomyoblastic differentiation, either in conventional sections (Figure 12.10) or with the aid of ancillary methods. Cytogenetically, trisomy 2 has been identified in eight out of nine cases of embryonal RMS studied by Wang-Wuu *et al.*[14].

Table 12.1 Tumours with a spindle-cell pattern that may mimic RMS

Fibromatoses
Synovial sarcoma (monophasic variant)
Fibrosarcoma
Haemangiopericytoma
Malignant fibrous histiocytoma
Malignant peripheral nerve sheath tumour

ALVEOLAR RMS

Alveolar RMS accounted for some 20% of cases of RMS in the Intergroup Rhabdomyosarcoma Study (IRS) experience[15]. Compared with the embryonal subgroup, alveolar RMS tends to affect an older age group, and there is a notable predilection for the soft tissues of the extremities. The tumours predominate in males (as they do in non-botryoid embryonal RMS). Compared with embryonal RMS, alveolar RMS is generally associated with more aggressive behaviour and an adverse clinical outcome[15,16].

This subgroup is recognized by the microscopic pattern of irregular and variable-sized spaces or 'alveoles' separated by connective tissue septa of variable thickness (Figure 12.11)[6,12,17]. 'Alveoles' vary substantially in size, ranging from small spaces with a smooth outline (Figure 12.12) to spaces that are large and irregular (Figure 12.13). The spaces or 'alveoles' often contain dehiscent or 'floating' cells that are karyorrhectic and pyknotic (Figure 12.13); occasionally they display rhabdomyoblastic differentiation (Figure 12.14). The 'alveoles' are lined by tumour cells that are seemingly attached to the connective tissue septa and frequently have an epithelioid appearance. Mitoses are generally inconspicuous. Multi-

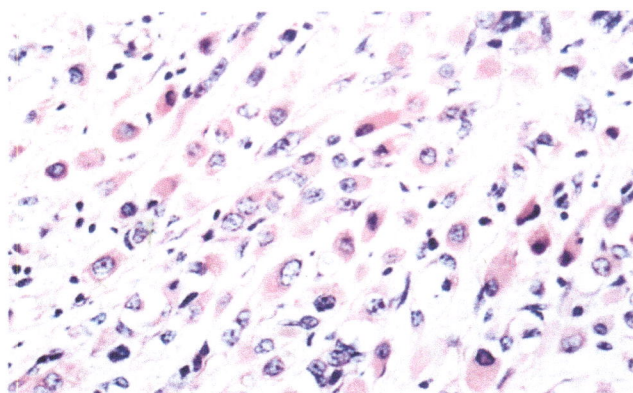

Fig. 12.1 Microscopy of embryonal rhabdomyosarcoma reveals well-differentiated rhabdomyoblasts. H&E × 300

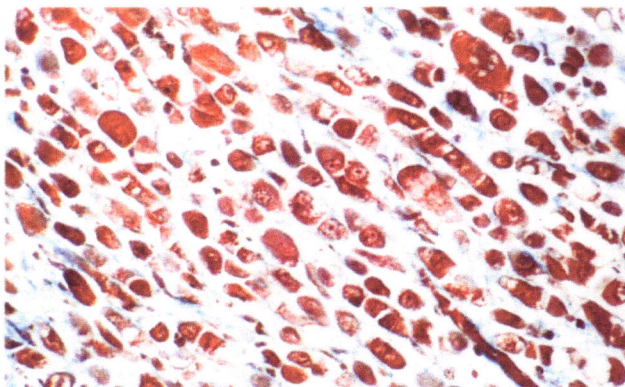

Fig. 12.2 The cytoplasm of the rhabdomyoblasts from the same tumour depicted in Figure 12.1 stains reddish-brown with Masson's trichrome. Masson's trichrome × 300

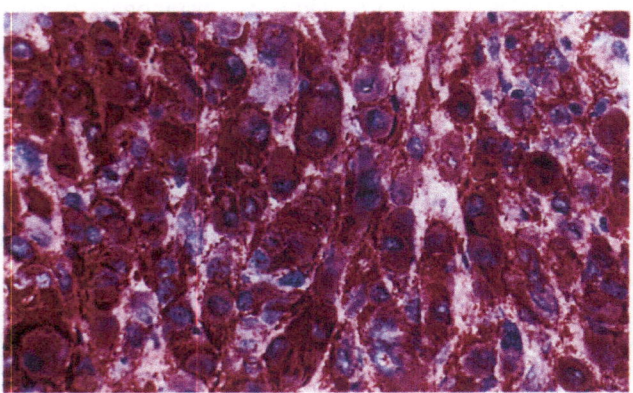

Fig. 12.3 There is strong PAS-positivity, reflecting abundant cytoplasmic glycogen, a feature of the well-differentiated rhabdomyoblast. Same tumour as in Figure 12.2. PAS × 300

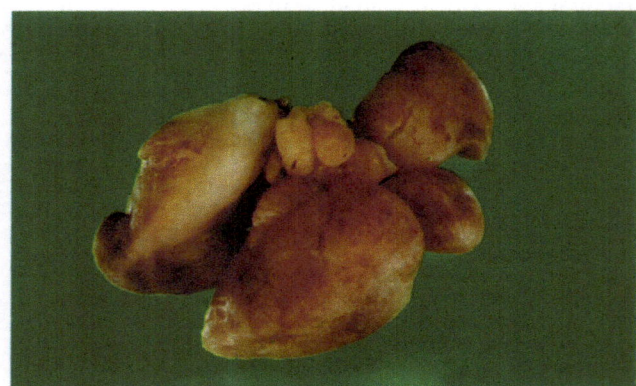

Fig. 12.4 Mucosa-covered polypoid growth is characteristic of botryoid embryonal rhabdomyosarcoma. This tumour arose in the middle ear of a 2-year-old boy. 3.5 × original size

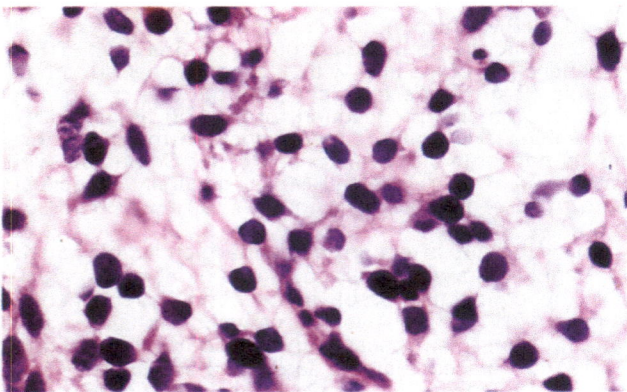

Fig. 12.5 Myxoid pattern of embryonal rhabdomyosarcoma shows spindle and stellate cells suspended in a myxoid stroma. Evidence of rhabdomyoblastic differentiation was difficult to find. The tumour arose in the right buttock of a 1-month-old girl. H&E × 750

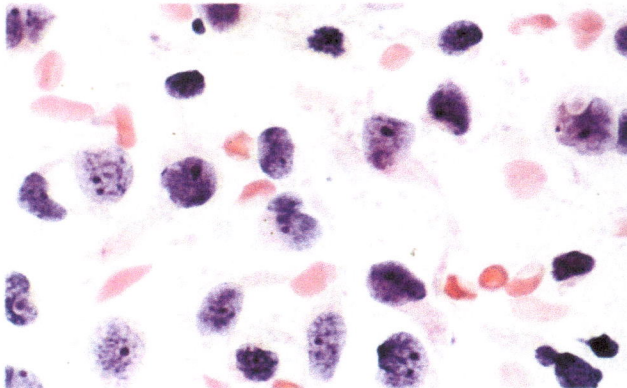

Fig. 12.6 Cytological preparation of a myxoid embryonal rhabdomyosarcoma (same tumour as above) shows slightly irregular nuclei and prominent nucleoli. Cytoplasm is scant and often forms elongated processes. H&E × 750

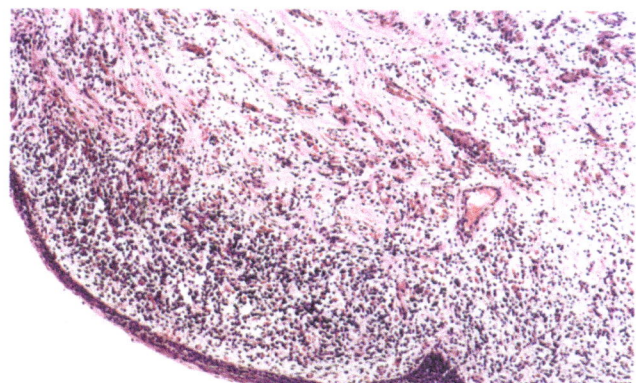

Fig. 12.7 Poorly differentiated tumour cells are clustered beneath the epithelium producing the so-called cambium layer that is typical of botryoid embryonal rhabdomyosarcoma. The tumour arose in the vagina of a 3-month-old girl. H&E × 75

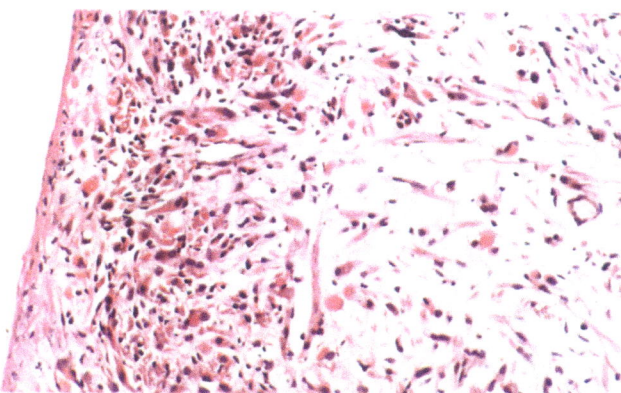

Fig. 12.8 The rhabdomyoblasts of a botryoid embryonal rhabdomyosarcoma show relatively advanced differentiation. The microscopy is from a biopsy of bladder wall tumour in a 2-month-old boy. H&E × 185

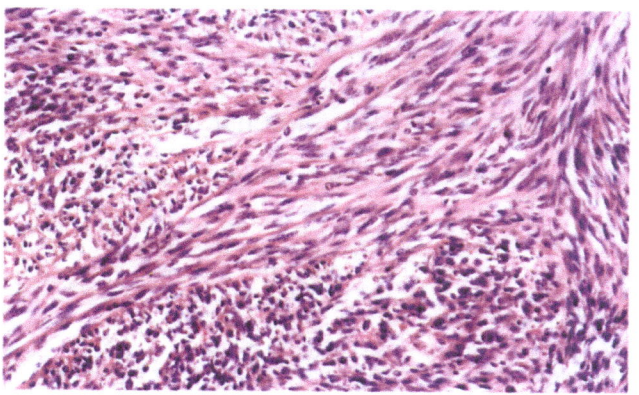

Fig. 12.9 Embryonal rhabdomyosarcoma with a predominant spindle-cell pattern mimics other types of spindle-cell tumour. H&E × 185

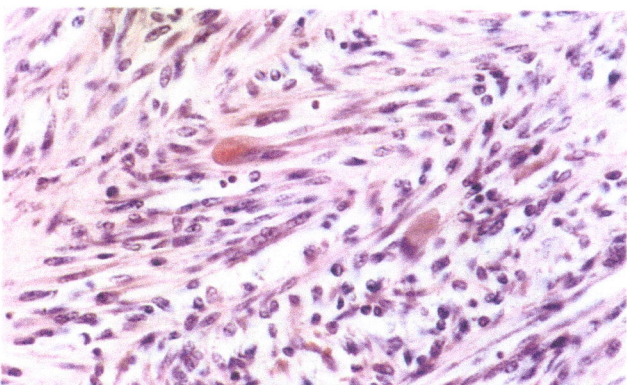

Fig. 12.10 Occasional foci of rhabdomyoblastic differentiation of a spindle-cell lesion (see Figure 12.9) reveal its true lineage. H&E × 300

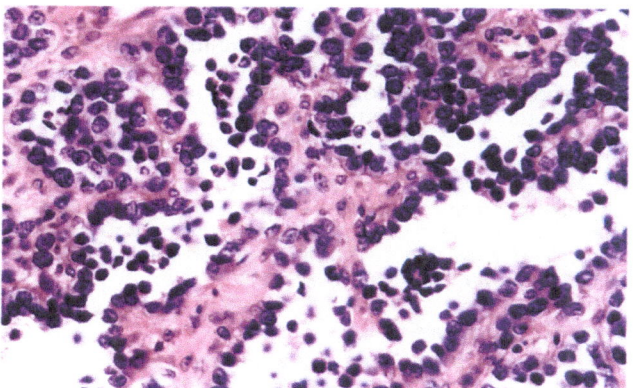

Fig. 12.11 Alveolar rhabdomyosarcoma shows irregular 'alveoles' lined by tumour cells and separated by bands of fibrous tissue. Dehiscent or 'free-floating' cells lie within the spaces. The tumour was removed from the neck of a 15-year-old girl; the primary site was not identified. H&E × 300

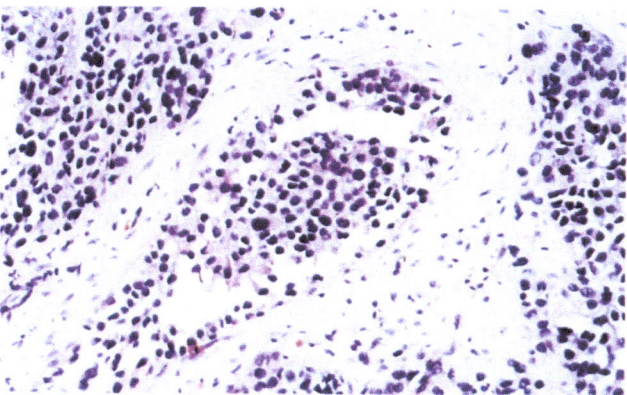

Fig. 12.12 Alveolar rhabdomyosarcoma removed from the buttock of a 12-year-old boy shows an occasional island of tumour undergoing 'disintegration' to form an early 'alveole'. H&E × 185

nucleated tumour giant cells with a wreath of peripherally placed nuclei are fairly common (Figure 12.15); these cells surprisingly do not exhibit cross-striations despite having generous amounts of cytoplasm. They are fairly common in the alveolar subtype and represent an important diagnostic clue[6,9].

The alveolar pattern may coexist with areas of tumour lacking 'alveoles'. Hence, the examination of multiple sections may be necessary for their identification. The alveolar spaces are thought to represent a degenerative phenomenon and, consequently, are more likely to be found centrally where the vascularization is expected to be minimal. A form of alveolar RMS has been described in which alveolar spaces are deficient or absent, a pattern referred to as the monomorphous round cell or 'solid variant' of alveolar RMS (Figure 12.16)[18]. These tumours are cytologically similar to conventional alveolar RMS and share a similar, if not identical, prognosis.

Alveolar RMS tends to metastasize to lymph nodes, lung, pleura, pancreas and bone[6]. (RMS is one of the few sarcomas that are metastatic to lymph nodes.) Twenty-nine per cent of cases of RMS are reported to have bone marrow metastases at diagnosis[19]. Patients with disseminated disease, including lymph nodal and bone marrow involvement, may have a leukoerythroblastic blood picture, simulating a haemopoietic malignancy[20]. Lymphadenopathic or systemic form are terms that have been used for this clinical presentation. Undifferentiated blast cells have been described in the peripheral blood of such patients[7]. The primary tumour may be difficult to detect, even after exhaustive clinical study or at post-mortem examination[20].

Aveolar RMS appears to arise in pre-existent skeletal muscle while embryonal tumours seem to originate in uncommitted primitive mesenchyme. However, the anatomical distribution of alveolar RMS is not limited to skeletal muscle as they also overlap with sites usually associated with the embryonal histology[21]. Thus, the periorbital, perianal and perineal soft tissues are other recognized primary sites for alveolar RMS.

Coexistence within the same tumour of the embryonal and alveolar pattern is well documented[4,11,22]. These tumours are sometimes referred to as mixed RMS[12]; their behaviour usually conforms to that associated with the alveolar subtype[18].

A balanced translocation t(2;13) (q37;q14) has been found repeatedly in association with alveolar RMS[23,24], and promises to be an important tool in diagnosis and providing greater insight into tumour biology.

OTHER VARIANTS OF RMS

Large series of cases of RMS in children occasionally include pleomorphic RMS. The reported variable prevalence of 0.7–5%[11] attests to the probable application of different histological criteria. Therapy may induce a microscopic picture that resembles the pleomorphic pattern[16]. For all practical purposes, according to Dehner, pleomorphic RMS do not affect children[25].

RMS with intermediate filament cytoplasmic inclusions have been described recently[26]. Tumours with embryonal or alveolar histology are affected and, on immunohistochemistry, the inclusions express vimentin and desmin. These tumours form a small but important group as they may be mistaken for extrarenal rhabdoid tumour, a neoplasm with a greater potential for aggressive behaviour.

RMS therapy may induce maturation of tumour cells, the formation of chondroid areas, ballooning of cells and cellular anaplasia[5,27].

PRIMITIVE RMS

Various terminologies have been used for soft-tissue tumours that lack differentiation at light microscopy. These include 'sarcoma of undetermined histogenesis', 'undifferentiated mesenchymal sarcoma', 'mesenchymal sarcoma, probably RMS' and 'embryonal sarcoma'[6,11,12]. Their numbers have understandably declined since the advent of immunohistochemical markers. The main differential diagnosis lies with the soft-tissue variant of Ewing's sarcoma[28], as other small round-cell tumours are unlikely contenders at this site. The demonstration of intracellular glycogen by PAS/diastase reaction may assist in making this distinction[10]: the small cells of extraosseous Ewing's sarcoma often reveal punctate intracytoplasmic glycogen; by contrast, the small cells of the primitive RMS are generally negative. When neither glycogen nor myogenic differentiation is found, the tumour is reasonably relegated to the category 'sarcoma, not otherwise specified (NOS)'[10,28].

Ultrastructural investigation is also recommended as a means of separation of primitive RMS from extraskeletal Ewing's sarcoma[28]. As both entities show similar behaviour and response to therapy, it may be argued that a distinction is merely academic. It should be noted, however, that some soft-tissue Ewing's tumours may exhibit a neural phenotype[29], placing it within the category of PNETS, a group currently known for its aggressive behaviour.

TUMOURS INVOLVING SPECIFIC PRIMARY SITES

Head and neck tumours (excluding orbital tumours)

The head and neck are the sites most frequently affected by RMS[15], and the embryonal pattern is the predominant subtype. Specific sites include the nasopharynx, palate, tongue, maxillary sinus, external and middle ear[30]. The poor prognosis of RMS at this site is related to:

(a) A high rate of unresectability[15], and
(b) Frequent direct extension into the adjacent central nervous system because of the parameningeal location of many of the tumours[10,16].

Orbital tumours

In childhood, RMS is the most common malignant tumour of the orbit[31]. In the latter study, the ages of the six cases ranged from newborn to 19 years. The most common presenting sign was a rapid onset of proptosis. Extension of the tumour into one of the eyelids is common, and botryoid pattern, presenting as a multinodular subconjunctival mass, is sometimes seen. In this location, embryonal and alveolar histological subtypes are both described but the embryonal pattern is far more common, accounting for almost three quarters of cases. The embryonal tumours usually arise in the superior nasal part of the orbit, displacing the eye downwards and outwards while alveolar tumours tend to occur in the lower part of the orbit. In the IRS experience, orbital tumours were associated with one of the best survival rates, compared with tumours at other primary sites[32].

Hepatic tumours

The botyroid variant is the usual pattern seen in tumours of the liver[2,33]. They may arise in the intrahepatic or extrahepatic biliary tree and obstructive jaundice is the major clinical feature. The common bile duct is frequently involved[33] and a choledochal cyst is the most common clinical impression[19]. The precise site of origin of the tumour may be difficult to localize at operation[19].

Genitourinary and pelvic tumours

In children, approximately 20–40% of RMS affect the genitourinary tract and pelvis[5,15]. The tumours may involve the bladder, prostate (or both), paratesticular structures or the female reproductive organs[34]. Of these sites, the most favourable outcome occurs in association with paratesticular involvement. Loughlin et al.[34] found the event-free survival in such cases to be 88%. Paratesticular tumours are thus best considered separately from a prognostic standpoint. One study showed the embryonal pattern to be present in 97% of paratesticular tumours[35].

Perianal/perineal tumours

This is an uncommon primary location for RMS[15]. Of 36 patients with perineal tumours, 56% showed an alveolar pattern and 30% showed an embryonal pattern; 14% showed other types of sarcoma[36]. In the IRS series referred to by Hays et al.[15], 69% were of the alveolar type and 23% were of the embryonal type. Patients with perineal involvement have a particularly poor outlook, probably due to the high incidence of an alveolar subtype and a location that is related to late-onset symptomatology[36].

Tumours of the extremities

This is a fairly common location for RMS[15] and involves embryonal and alveolar subtypes; the alveolar histology is more prevalent[15]. The lower extremity seems to be more commonly involved than the upper extremity[37]. Extremity tumours are associated with a poor prognosis[15].

Retroperitoneal tumours

These tumours are exclusive of those arising in the genitourinary and hepatobiliary systems. In the IRS series, retroperitoneal RMS were uncommon, accounting for only 11% of tumours. They were associated with a poor survival mainly because of their large size at presentation, advanced clinical stage and the poor surgical resectability[32,38].

Histologically, 58% of the tumours were of embryonal or botryoid pattern and 8% showed an alveolar pattern[38]; other sarcomas encountered in this location included extraosseous Ewing's sarcoma, undifferentiated sarcoma and unspecified sarcoma.

Tumours of the trunk

RMS of the trunk may be separated into those affecting the chest, paraspinal region and abdominal wall[39]; most of the tumours arise in the chest wall. As a group, the prognosis is intermediate between the more favourable genitourinary tumours and the less favourable extremity tumours.

Paraspinal tumours show the most favourable outcome, while the outlook is least favourable when the chest wall is affected. The poor outcome with chest wall tumours may be attributable to the high incidence of distant metastases at the time of presentation, and the relatively high proportion of alveolar tumours at this site[39].

Intrathoracic tumours

By 1982, 2.6% of patients registered with the IRS had intrathoracic soft tissue sarcomas[38]. These were mainly located in the mediastinum; other sites included the pleura and lung.

Tumour subtype was predominantly embryonal. This site was associated with advanced disease at presentation, a high rate of unresectability and high mortality. The children tended to be older compared with RMS at other sites[38].

Renal tumours

The kidney is rarely a primary site for RMS, and when it occurs, presents a diagnostic dilemma[40]. Most paediatric renal tumours with skeletal muscle are examples of Wilms' tumour (see Chapter 2). Malignant rhabdoid tumour of the kidney may be mistaken for renal RMS, particularly as the former may express muscle-related antigens[40].

IMMUNOHISTOCHEMISTRY OF RMS

A number of antisera are available against muscle-related antigens for use in immunohistochemical study. These antigens include desmin, myoglobin, isoenzymes of creatine kinase, myosin (fast and slow), muscle specific actin (MSA) and Z-band protein[41]. Desmin and myoglobin are currently used most widely. Myoglobin, though specific for skeletal muscle, lacks sensitivity, and, compared with desmin, it is expressed later in embryonic myogenesis. Myoglobin readily marks differentiated rhabdomyoblasts whose nature is usually already apparent in conventional sections[42].

Desmin is the intermediate filament found in smooth muscle and skeletal muscle[43,44] and its demonstration is thus non-specific for RMS. Smooth muscle tumours are, however, unusual in children and, hence, in practice, positivity for desmin in soft-tissue tumours is usually accepted to indicate skeletal muscle lineage. Several studies have alluded to the greater sensitivity of desmin, compared with myoglobin, in delineating the less differentiated cellular component in alveolar and embryonal RMS[43,44].

Desmin is also expressed in other neoplasms and thus caution is required in interpretation; e.g. tumours in which skeletal muscle is part of a complex morphology (such as teratomas, Wilms' tumours, mesenchymomas and ectomesenchymomas), and those with diverse immunophenotype (such as peripheral primitive neuroectodermal tumour, extraosseous Ewing's sarcoma, fibromatous lesions, embryonal sarcoma of the liver[42] and malignant rhabdoid tumours[45]).

Suboptimal fixation and lack of adequate differentiation of the tumour cells are some factors that may result in the tumour cells of RMS failing to react to antisera[46]. Alcohol fixation appears to enhance the sensitivity of markers such as desmin[42]. Caution is necessary in the evaluation of undifferentiated tumours in or near normal skeletal muscle (Figure 12.17) as deeply entrapped non-neoplastic fibres are likely to immunoreact to muscle-related antisera. Tumour metastatic to skeletal muscle may sufficiently damage the muscle to cause leakage of antigen which is then ingested by reactive macrophages[47]. The macrophages may express the antigen and could lead to diagnostic error.

A small proportion of RMS react positively for neuron-specific enolase, cytokeratin and S-100 protein[48,49] and such results should not be overinterpreted. Most RMS express vimentin (in common with Ewing's sarcoma, non-Hodgkin's lymphoma and some cases of neuroblastoma) but expression may be weak or absent in well-differentiated RMS[50].

ELECTRON MICROSCOPY

At the light microscopic level, rhabdomyoblasts are likely to be confused with cells from a number of other conditions, such as rhabdoid tumour, epithelioid sarcoma, alveolar soft part sarcoma and malignant melanoma. The value of electron microscopy lies mainly in its potential to

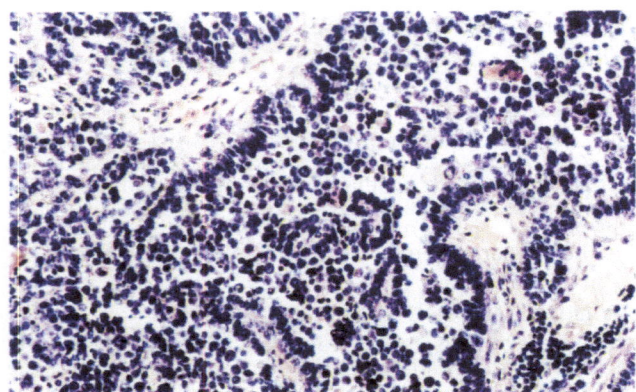

Fig. 12.13 The spaces or 'alveoles' in this alveolar tumour are larger than those seen in the preceding figure. The spaces are filled with dehiscent or 'free floating' tumour cells and rows of tumour cells are seen attached along the connective tissue bands. The tumour arose in the triceps muscle of a 1¹/₂-year-old girl and was metastatic to an axillary lymph node on the same side. H&E × 185

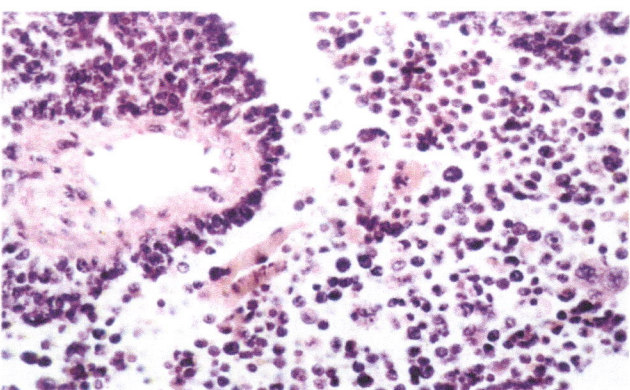

Fig. 12.14 Another example of alveolar rhabdomyosarcoma demonstrates large 'alveoles' with many 'free-floating' cells, some of which show rhabdomyoblastic differentiation. H&E × 300

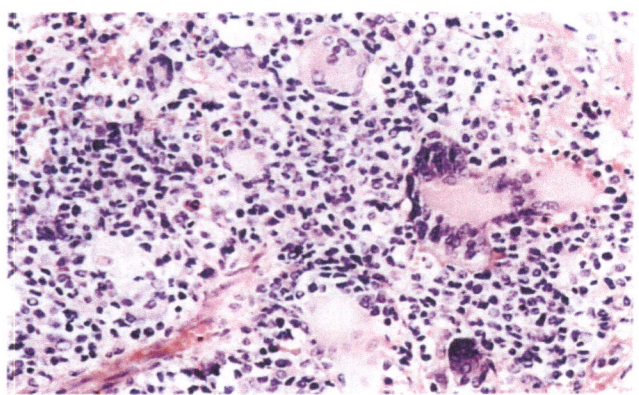

Fig. 12.15 'Alveoles' were difficult to identify in this neoplasm. Several tumour giant cells with peripherally arranged nuclei are evident, a common feature of alveolar rhabdomyosarcoma. H&E × 185

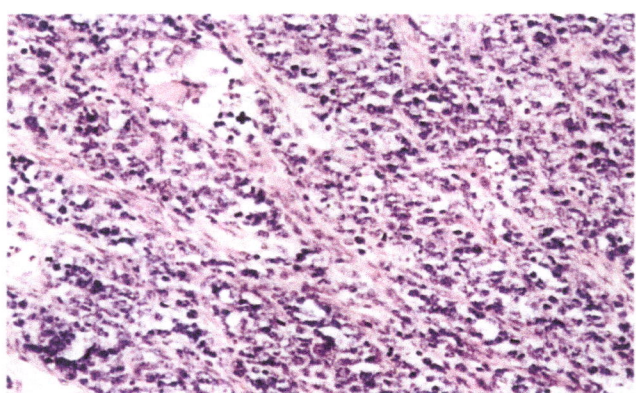

Fig. 12.16 A 'solid variant' of alveolar rhabdomyosarcoma shows sheets of tumour cells with some intervening fibrous stroma. Occasional rhabdomyoblasts and the immunohistochemical expression of desmin revealed a myogenic lineage. The patient was 12 years of age and presented with bilateral groin masses, a large left gluteal and a perirectal mass. H&E × 185

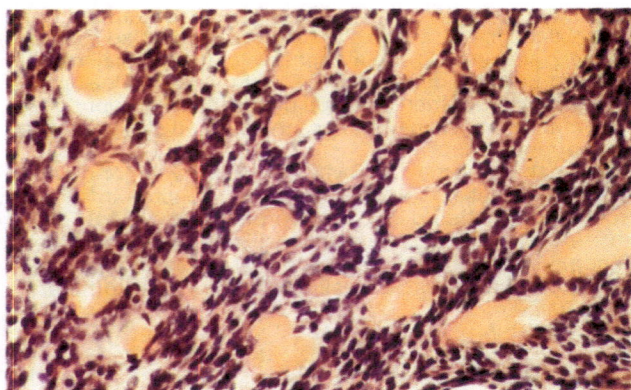

Fig. 12.17 The skeletal muscle is infiltrated by poorly differentiated rhabdomyosarcoma. The presence of indigenous skeletal muscle within a tumour may lead to erroneous diagnosis, but the degree of differentiation of the infiltrated muscle is too advanced. The neoplasm was resected from the back of the tongue of a 4-month-old boy. H&E × 300

Fig. 12.18 Ultrastructure of embryonal rhabdomyosarcoma of the urinary bladder shows a cluster of intracytoplasmic alternating thick (myosin) and thin (actin) filaments, the minimal criteria advocated for confirmation of rhabdomyosarcoma

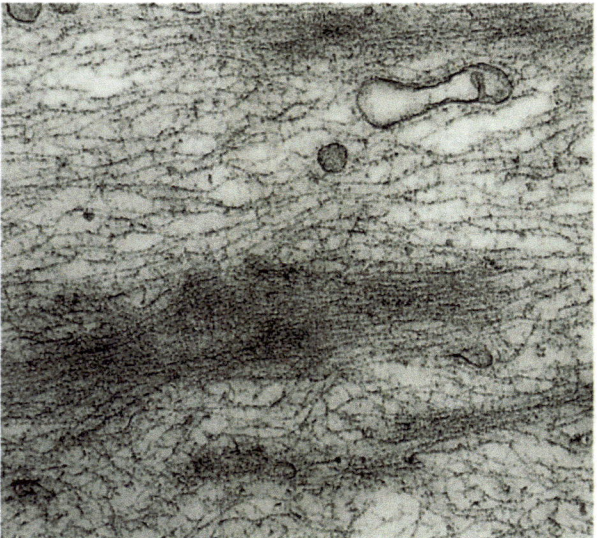

Fig. 12.18

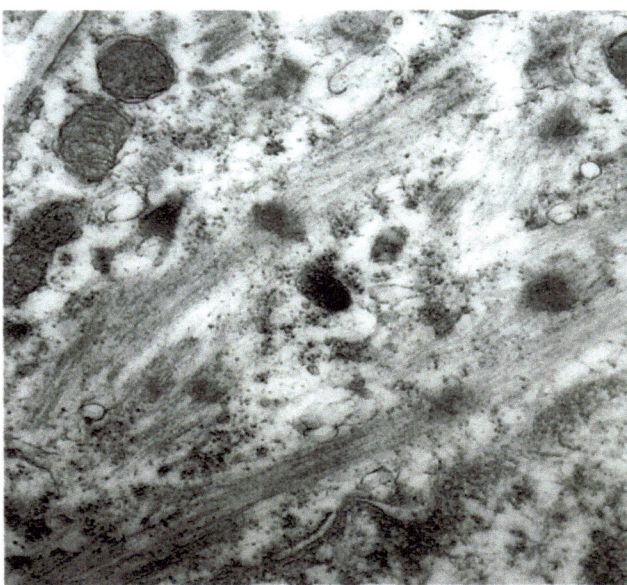

Fig. 12.19 Ultrastructure of embryonal rhabdomyosarcoma shows diagnostic intracytoplasmic sheaves of thick and thin filaments interrupted by rectangular densities. It is the same tumour as seen in Figure 12.17. × 39 000

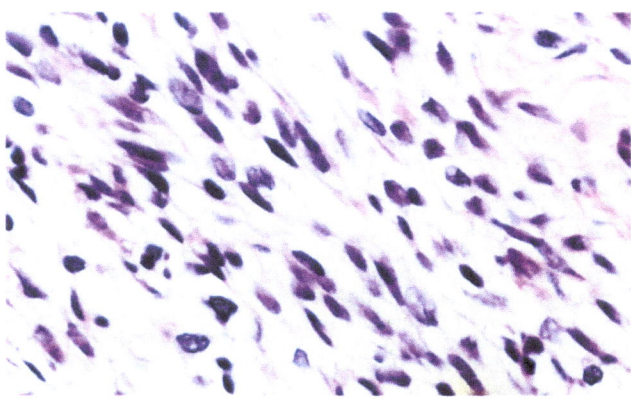

Fig. 12.20 Microscopy of rhabdomyoma removed from the right post-auricular area of a 2-month-old boy shows haphazardly arranged primitive mesenchymal cells. Tumour cell nuclei are only mildly irregular, and mitoses are rare. The gross specimen was a circumscribed and partially encapsulated nodule that measured 1.5 × 1.2 × 1.0 cm. H&E × 750

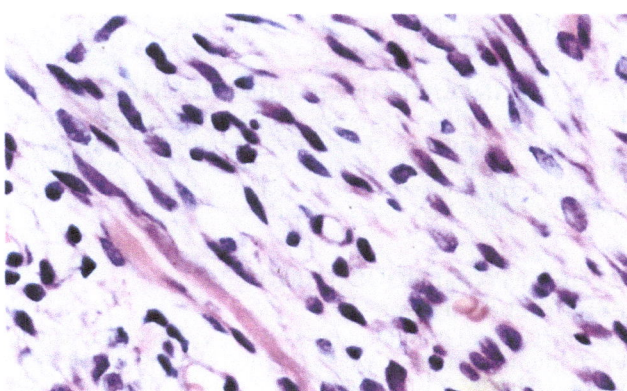

Fig. 12.21 Same tumour as above (fetal rhabdomyoma). Immature skeletal muscle fibres are especially conspicuous along the edge of the tumour. H&E × 750

delineate sarcomeric organization that is the fundamental contractile unit of normal skeletal muscle[51-54]. The minimal ultrastructural criteria advocated for the diagnosis of RMS are the presence of alternating thick (myosin) and thin (actin) filaments arranged in bundles (Figure 12.18)[54,55]. The intermittent occurrence of Z-band material at rectangular densities, with the long axis at right angles to the alignment of the filaments, is an additional diagnostic feature (Figure 12.19)[55].

These ultrastructural parameters are, however, less readily discerned in the small primitive-cell type of RMS in which the features are expected to lack specificity. Nonspecific features include monoparticulate cytoplasmic glycogen, intermediate filaments lacking structural organization, pinocytotic vesicles, primitive cell attachments and basement membrane-like material around cells. In the better-differentiated tumours, these features may, of course, accompany sarcomeric organization.

Tumour cell junctions are more common and myofilament formation less advanced in alveolar RMS compared with embryonal RMS[52]. When RMS infiltrate normal skeletal muscle, caution is required to separate these entrapped fibres from those integral to the tumour. This can usually be resolved by finding an advanced degree of myofilament organization in the entrapped fibres paralleling that seen in normal skeletal muscle.

IN VITRO INDUCTION OF DIFFERENTIATION

Poorly differentiated growth of RMS in culture can be induced to undergo differentiation using a variety of agents[56]. Diagnosis is supplemented by the application of immunohistochemistry, ultrastructure or even cytogenetics to the harvested growth.

OTHER MYOGENOUS TUMOURS

Fetal rhabdomyoma

The fetal type of rhabdomyoma occurs virtually exclusively in children less than 3 years old, and the tumour is often present shortly after birth[57,58]. The great majority of the lesions are solitary and there is a marked male preponderance. The lesion is benign and the usual location is in the dermis and subcutaneous tissues of the head and neck. There is a notable predilection for the posterior auricular region.

The tumour appears to be a hamartoma rather than a neoplasm, although the precise histogenesis remains obscure. Unlike the cardiac rhabdomyoma, it is not associated with tuberous sclerosis. Fetal rhabdomyoma is less common than the adult type of rhabdomyoma.

Grossly, the lesions are well-circumscribed but unencapsulated, with an average size of 2–5 cm; the cut surface has a homogeneous glistening mucoid appearance. Histologically, there is a mixture of undifferentiated mesenchymal cells with indistinct cytoplasm and haphazardly arranged immature skeletal muscle fibres. The cells vary in stage of differentiation and are set in a mucoid stroma (Figure 12.20). The differentiated larger muscle fibres are generally located at the periphery of the lesion (Figure 12.21). Nuclear atypicality and nuclear hyperchromatism are absent and mitoses are extremely rare. Electron microscopy reveals myotubular differentiation and, immunohistochemically, the immature muscle fibres express desmin.

Embryonal RMS is the main differential diagnosis[58]. RMS occupies a deeper location, is less well-circumscribed and exhibits a more irregular cellular pattern. RMS also shows a greater degree of mitotic activity, nuclear pleomorphism and hyperchromasia, and focal necrosis is more frequent. However, the histology of fetal rhabdomyoma may occasionally evoke sufficient concern to warrant a reasonable period of post-excision follow-up[57].

NON-MYOGENOUS TUMOURS WHICH MAY BE CONFUSED WITH RMS

Pseudosarcomatous myofibroblastic proliferation of the urinary bladder refers to a benign polypoid growth[59]. The cause is unknown and the lesions appear unrelated to trauma. Painless haematuria is a common symptom. Histology shows interlacing fascicles of spindle cells interspersed with oedematous and myxoid areas. The overlying urothelium is commonly ulcerated. The postoperative course, so far, has been benign and without recurrence.

Vaginal polyps with features similar to the botryoid pattern of rhabdomyosarcoma have been reported[60]. While this is predominantly a condition of adults, infants are occasionally affected.

HISTOLOGICALLY COMPLEX TUMOURS THAT MAY INCLUDE SKELETAL MUSCLE OR RMS AS A COMPONENT

Ectomesenchymoma, mesenchymoma, pulmonary blastoma, nephroblastoma, teratoma, neuromuscular hamartoma and malignant peripheral nerve sheath tumour ('Triton tumour') may exhibit microscopic evidence of skeletal muscle, usually as a component of a more complex morphology. The term rhabdomyomatous mesenchymal hamartoma has been applied to a dermal lesion composed of mature skeletal muscle and adipose tissue[61].

REFERENCES

1. Soule EH, Mahour GH, Mills SD, Lynn HB. Soft tissue sarcomas of infants and children: a clinicopathological study of 135 cases. Mayo Clin Proc. 1968;43:313–26.
2. IRAC. International incidence of childhood cancer. Lyon: IRAC Scientific Publications. No. 87;1988.
3. Pratt CB. Some aspects of childhood cancer epidemiology. Pediatr Clin N Am. 1985;32:541–56.
4. Weichert KA, Bove KC, Aron BS, Lampkin B. Rhabdomyosarcoma in children. A clinicopathological study of 35 patients. Am J Clin Pathol. 1976;66:692–701.
5. Bale PM, Parsons RE, Stevens MM. Diagnosis and behaviour of juvenile rhabdomyosarcoma. Hum Pathol. 1983;14:596–611.
6. Enzinger FM, Shiraki M. Alveolar rhabdomyosarcoma. An analysis of 110 cases. Cancer. 1969;24:18–31.
7. Fitzmaurice RJ, Johnson PRE, Liu Yin JA, Freemont AJ. Rhabdomyosarcoma presenting as 'acute leukaemia'. Histopathology. 1991;18:173–5.
8. Maurer HM. The Intergroup Rhabdomyosarcoma Study (NIH): objectives and clinical staging classifications. J Pediatr Surg. 1975;10:977–8.
9. Horn RC, Enterline HT. Rhabdomyosarcoma: a clinicopathological study and classification of 39 cases. Cancer. 1958;11:181–99.
10. Shimada H, Newton WA, Soule EH, Beltangady MS, Maurer HM. Pathology of fatal rhabdomyosarcoma. Report from Intergroup Rhabdomyosarcoma Study (IRS-I and IRS-II). Cancer. 1987;59:459–65.
11. Bale PM, Reye RDK. Rhabdomyosarcoma in childhood. Pathology. 1975;7:101–11.
12. Gonzales-Crussi F, Black-Shaffer S. Rhabdomyosarcoma of infancy and childhood. Am J Surg Pathol. 1979;3:157–71.
13. Canale VC, Volpe R, Carbone A, Grigoletto E. Botryoid rhabdomyosarcoma of the nasopharynx. J Laryngol Otol. 1983;97:553–6.
14. Wang-Wuu S, Soukup S, Ballard E, Gotwals B, Lampkin B. Chromosomal analysis of sixteen human rhabdomyosarcomas. Cancer Res. 1988;48:983–7.
15. Hays DM, Newton WJ, Soule EH et al. Mortality among children with rhabdomyosarcoma of the alveolar histologic subtype. J Pediatr Surg. 1983;18:412–17.
16. Gaiger AM, Soule EH, Newton WA. Pathology of rhabdomyosarcoma: experience of the Intergroup Rhabdomyosarcoma Study, 1972–78. Natl Cancer Inst Monogr. 1981;56:19–27.

17. Enterline HG, Horn RC. Alveolar rhabdomyosarcoma: a distinctive tumour type. Cancer. 1958;29:356–66.
18. Tsokos M, Webber BL, Parham DM et al. Rhabdomyosarcoma. A new classification scheme related to prognosis. Arch Pathol Lab Med. 1992;116:847–55.
19. Ruymann FB, Newton WA, Ragab AH, Donaldson MH, Foulkes M. Bone marrow metastases at diagnosis in children and adolescents with rhabdomyosarcoma. A report from the Intergroup Rhabdomyosarcoma Study. Cancer. 1984;53:368–73.
20. Etcubanas E, Peiper S, Stass S, Green A. Rhabdomyosarcoma presenting as disseminated malignancy from an unknown primary site: a retrospective study of ten pediatric cases. Med Pediatr Oncol. 1989;17:39–44.
21. Dehner LP. Soft tissue sarcomas of childhood: the differential diagnostic dilemma of the small blue cell. Natl Cancer Monogr. 1981;56:43–59.
22. Patton RB, Horn RC Jr. Rhabdomyosarcoma: clinical and pathological features and comparison with human fetal and embryonic skeletal muscle. Surgery. 1962;52:572–84.
23. Turc-Carel C, Lizard-Nacol S, Justrabo E, Favrot M, Philip T, Tabone E. Consistent chromosomal translocation in alveolar rhabdomyosarcoma. Cancer Genet Cytogenet. 1986;19:361–2.
24. Rowe D, Gerrard M, Gibbons B, Malpas JS. Two further cases of t(2;13) in alveolar rhabdomyosarcoma indicating a review of the published chromosome breakpoints. Br J Cancer. 1987;56:379–80.
25. Dehner LP. Soft tissue, peritoneum, and retroperitoneum. In: Dehner LP, editor. Pediatric surgical pathology, 2nd edn. Baltimore: Williams & Wilkins; 1987:870.
26. Kodet R, Newton WA, Hamoudi AB, Asmar L. Rhabdomyosarcomas with intermediate-filament inclusions and features of rhabdoid tumors. Light microscopic and immunohistochemical study. Am J Surg Pathol. 1991;15:257–67.
27. Molenaar WM, Oosterhuis JW, Kamps WA. Cytologic 'differentiation' in childhood rhabdomyosarcomas following polychemotherapy. Hum Pathol. 1984;15:973–9.
28. Dickman PS, Triche TJ. Extraosseous Ewing's sarcoma versus primitive rhabdomyosarcoma: diagnostic criteria and clinical correlation. Hum Pathol. 1986;17:881–93.
29. Shimada H, Newton WA, Soule EH, Qualman SJ, Aoyama C, Maurer HM. Pathologic features of extraosseous Ewing's sarcoma: a report from the Intergroup Rhabdomyosarcoma Study. Hum Pathol. 1988;19:442–53.
30. Dito WR, Batsakis JG. Rhabdomyosarcoma of the head and neck. Arch Surg. 1962;84:582–8.
31. Porterfield JF, Zimmerman LE. Rhabdomyosarcoma of the orbit. A clinicopathologic study of 55 cases. Virchows Arch Pathol Anat. 1962;335:329–44.
32. Maurer HM, Beltangady M, Gehan EA et al. The Intergroup Rhabdomyosarcoma Study – 1. A final report. Cancer. 1988;61:209–20.
33. Davis GL, Kissale JM, Ishak KG. Embryonal rhabdomyosarcoma (sarcoma botryoides) of the biliary tree. Cancer. 1969;24:333–42.
34. Loughlin KR, Retik AB, Weinstein HJ et al. Genitourinary rhabdomyosarcoma in children. Cancer. 1989;63:1600–6.
35. Beverley Raney R, Tefft M, Lawrence W et al. Paratesticular sarcoma in childhood and adolescence. A report from the Intergroup Rhabdomyosarcoma Studies I and II, 1973–1983. Cancer. 1987;60:2337–43.
36. Raney RB, Crist W, Hays D et al. Soft tissue sarcoma of the perineal region in childhood. A report from the Intergroup Rhabdomyosarcoma Studies I and II, 1972 through 1984. Cancer. 1990;65:2787–92.
37. Soule EH, Geitz M, Henderson ED. Embryonal rhabdomyosarcoma of the limbs and limb-girdles. A clinicopathologic study of 61 cases. Cancer. 1969;23:1336–46.
38. Crist WM, Raney RB, Tefft M et al. Soft tissue sarcomas arising in the retroperitoneal space in children. A report from the Intergroup Rhabdomyosarcoma Study (IRS) Committee. Cancer. 1985;56:2125–32.
39. Raney RB, Ragab AH, Ruymann FB et al. Soft-tissue sarcoma of the trunk in childhood. Results of the Intergroup Rhabdomyosarcoma Study. Cancer. 1982;49:2612–16.
40. Weeks DA, Beckwith JB, Mierau GW, Zuppan CW. Renal neoplasms mimicking rhabdoid tumor of kidney. A report from the National Wilms' Tumor Pathology Center. Am J Surg Pathol. 1991;15:1042–54.
41. Variend S. Small cell tumours of childhood. A review. J Pathol. 1985;145:1–25.
42. Parham DM, Webber B, Holt H, Williams WK, Maurer H. Immunohistochemical study of childhood rhabdomyosarcomas and related neoplasms. Results of an Intergroup Rhabdomyosarcoma Study Project. Cancer. 1991;67:3072–80.
43. Miettinen M, Lehto VP, Badley RA, Virtanen I. Alveolar rhabdomyosarcoma: demonstration of the muscle type of intermediate filament protein, desmin, as a diagnostic aid. Am J Pathol. 1982;108:246–51.
44. Altmannsberger M, Osborn M, Treuner J et al. Diagnosis of human childhood rhabdomyosarcoma by antibodies to desmin, the structural protein of muscle-specific intermediate filaments. Virchows Arch (Cell Pathol). 1982;39:203–15.
45. Tsokos M, Kouraklis G, Chandra RS, Bhagavan BS, Triche TJ. Malignant rhabdoid tumor of the kidney and soft tissues. Evidence for a diverse morphological and immunocytochemical phenotype. Arch Pathol Lab Med. 1989;113:115–20.
46. Leader M, Patel J, Collins M, Henry K. Myoglobin: an evaluation of its role as a marker of rhabdomyosarcoma. Br J Cancer. 1989;59:106–9.
47. Eusebi V, Bondi A, Rosai J. Immunohistochemical localisation of myoglobin in non-muscular cells. Am J Surg Pathol. 1984;8:51–5.
48. Coindre JM, De Mascarel A, Trojani M, De Mascarel I, Pages A. Immunohistochemical study of rhabdomyosarcoma: unexpected staining with S-100 protein and cytokeratin. J Pathol. 1988;155:127–32.
49. Miettinen M, Rapola J. Immunohistochemical spectrum of rhabdomyosarcoma and rhabdomyosarcoma-like tumors: expression of cytokeratin and the 68-kD neurofilament protein. Am J Surg Pathol. 1989;13:120–32.
50. Carter RL, McCarthy KP, Machin LG, Jameson CF, Philp ER, Pinkerton CR. Expression of desmin and myoglobin in rhabdomyosarcoma and in developing skeletal muscle. Histopathology. 1989;15:585–95.
51. Morales AR, Fine G, Horn RC. Rhabdomyosarcoma; an ultrastructural appraisal. Pathol Annu. 1972;7:81–106.
52. Churg A, Ringus J. Ultrastructural observations on the histogenesis of alveolar rhabdomyosarcoma. Cancer. 1978;41:1355–61.
53. Mierau GW, Favara BE. Rhabdomyosarcoma in children: ultrastructural study of 31 cases. Cancer. 1980;46:2035–40.
54. LaValle Bundtzen J, Norback DH. The ultrastructure of poorly differentiated rhabdomyosarcoma. Hum Pathol. 1982;13:301–13.
55. Ghadially FN. Diagnostic electron microscopy of tumours. London: Butterworths; 1980:123.
56. Garvin AJ, Stanley WS, Bennett DD, Sullivan JL, Sens DA. The in vitro growth, heterotransplantation, and differentiation of a human rhabdomyosarcoma cell line. Am J Pathol. 1986;125:208–17.
57. Dehner LP, Enzinger FM, Font RL. Fetal rhabdomyoma: an analysis of nine cases. Cancer. 1972;30:160–6.
58. Simha M, Doctor V, Dalal S, Manghani DK, Dastur DK. Postauricular fetal rhabdomyoma. Light and electron microscopic study. Hum Pathol. 1982;13:673–7.
59. Albores-Saavedra J, Manivel JC, Essenfeld H et al. Pseudosarcomatous myofibroblastic proliferations in the urinary bladder of children. Cancer. 1990;66:1234–41.
60. Norris HJ, Taylor HB. Polyps of the vagina. A benign lesion resembling sarcoma botryoides. Cancer. 1966;19:227–32.
61. Mills AE. Rhabdomyomatous mesenchymal hamartoma of skin. Am J Dermatopathol. 1989;11:58–63.

Other soft tissue tumours

13

Soft tissue tumours in childhood are histogenetically diverse, comprising a wide range of entities that vary considerably in prevalence, anatomical location and metastatic potential. They have been already discussed to some extent in the preceding chapters, e.g. fibromatosis and rhabdomyosarcoma. This chapter deals essentially with remaining soft tissue entities that are likely to occur in children. Some are seen specifically as childhood tumours while others, occurring more commonly in the older population, are seen from time to time in children, and are therefore also considered here.

BENIGN PERIPHERAL NERVE SHEATH TUMOURS
Neurofibroma

Most neurofibromas occur in children[1] and are usually solitary firm rubbery well-circumscribed non-encapsulated nodules. They are usually located in the dermis or subcutis, but may involve the deep soft tissue. A nerve bundle may be found entering and exiting the nodule. Neurofibromas may be localized or diffuse. Most are of the localized type, showing bland-appearing fusiform cells set in myxocollagenous stroma. Multiple neurofibromas are strongly associated with von Recklinghausen's neurofibromatosis (VRN).

Diffuse neurofibromas occur less commonly and are seen mainly in older children and young adults[1]. Their growth pattern is typically infiltrative. Microscopically, the Schwann cells have a rounder contour and are suspended in fine fibrillary collagen (Figure 13.1). Clusters of Meissner bodies are a characteristic feature (Figure 13.2)[1]. According to Enzinger and Weiss[1], 10% of patients with diffuse neurofibroma also have VRN.

Plexiform neurofibromas are generally deep-seated lesions that involve a major nerve structure[2] and are strongly associated with VRN[2]. Microscopically, there is a tortuous arrangement of expanded nerve bundles, sectioned in different planes (Figure 13.3), and composed of wavy spindle cells set in a myxoid matrix. The neurofibromatous tissue often extends into the adjacent soft tissue.

A cellular variant of neurofibroma or cellular peripheral neural tumour (CPNT) has been reported[3]. In addition to variable degrees of nuclear hyperchromatism and pleomorphism, the lesions often show mitotic figures; these are, however, few in number and none is atypical. Of the nine cases described[3], two recurred postexcision and, after multiple local recurrences, one metastasized.

Neurothekeoma is a name given to a benign tumour of nerve sheath origin, usually affecting individuals in the first and second decades[4]. Girls are predominantly affected. The lesions range in size from 0.4–1.8 cm and tend to occur in the central areas of the face, arms and shoulders, usually involving the dermis. Microscopically, there are nests and cords of large, mostly spindle-shaped, cells set in a variably mucoid matrix. Despite the presence of nuclear atypia and variable mitotic activity the behaviour of the tumour is invariably benign. These tumours are felt to be closely related to neurofibroma[1], but the condition is seemingly unrelated to VRN.

Schwannoma (neurilemmoma)

This is a true neoplasm considered by most to arise from the nerve sheath[5]. Most schwannomas are solitary; when multiple, there is an association with VRN. The tumour arises from spinal sensory, motor and autonomic nerves, as well as cranial nerves. The usual anatomical sites are the head, neck and upper extremity.

Naked eye examination shows that the lesions are encapsulated, round to oval or even fusiform (Figure 13.4). The cut surface is usually solid, firm and white; occasionally it is soft or cystic. An attachment to a nerve may be observed.

Cellular tissue (Antoni type A) and loose tissue (Antoni type B) are the two microscopic patterns usually encountered; they are present in varying proportions. Nuclear regimentation and Verocay bodies form part of Antoni type A tissue and are an important diagnostic feature (Figure 13.5). Congeries of dilated vessels with thickened walls are another characteristic feature, often occurring in association with type B tissue. Malignant change is unusual. A plexiform variant of schwannoma is also recognized[6] but, unlike plexiform neurofibroma, it is not associated with VRN.

MALIGNANT PERIPHERAL NERVE SHEATH TUMOUR (MPNST) (MALIGNANT SCHWANNOMA)

MPNST are the least common sarcomas in children[6]. They are strongly associated with VRN but, in this setting, only rarely arise in patients less than 9 years old.

Tumour size ranges from 2–33 cm[7]. They are usually unencapsulated with a variegate cut surface; cysts, haemorrhage and necrosis are often noted. The majority of tumours show a predominant uniform spindle cell population arranged in fascicles[7]. Other microscopic features are a high degree of cellularity, nuclear pleomorphism and variable mitotic activity (Figure 13.6). Heterologous elements include rhabdomyoblasts (malignant 'Triton tumour') and malignant-appearing glands. Primitive neuroepithelial-like foci and epithelioid patterns may be found. S100-protein positivity is observed in about half of the tumours.

Large tumours, patient age greater than 7 years, microscopic tumour necrosis and the presence of VRN adversely affect prognosis[7].

GRANULAR CELL EPULIS (GINGIVAL GRANULAR CELL TUMOUR)

This is a rare tumour usually limited to the alveolar ridge of newborns; the maxilla is affected twice as often as the mandible[8]. About 10% of the lesions are multiple within the boundary of the gingiva. About 90% of patients are girls.

Microscopically, the lesion is composed of sheets of round-to-polygonal cells with ample granular pink cytoplasm (Figure 13.7). The nucleus is centrally located and there is often a small single nucleolus. The cytoplasmic granularity is accentuated on periodic acid-Schiff staining. Vascularity is prominent.

Immunohistochemically, the cells are reactive for vimentin but negative for S-100 protein[9,10], contrasting

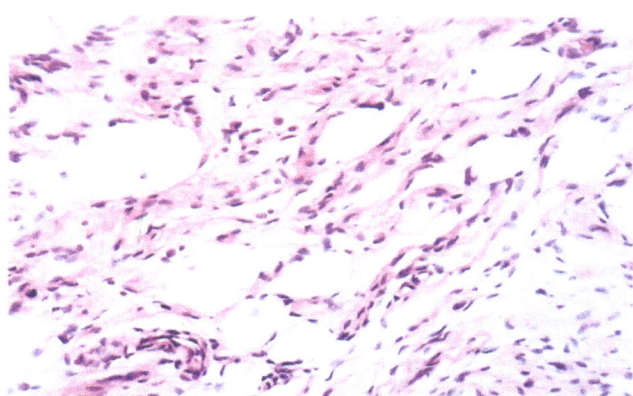

Fig. 13.1 Microscopic field of diffuse neurofibroma shows Schwann cells suspended in a fine fibrillary collagen. The lesion is typically infiltrative and ill-defined. It arose on the sole of the right foot of a 16-year-old girl who suffers from von Recklinghausen's neurofibromatosis. H&E × 185

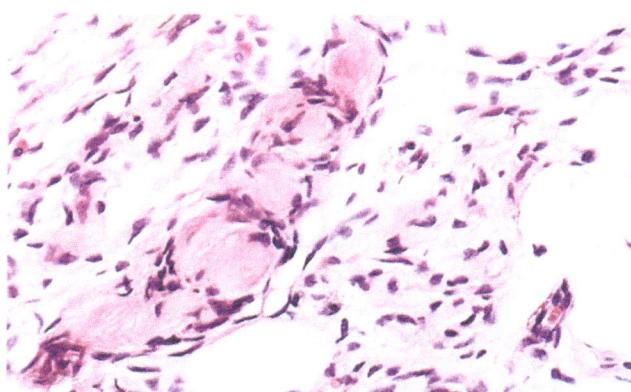

Fig. 13.2 Meissner bodies which are typical of diffuse neurofibroma are demonstrated in this microscopic field (same lesion as shown in preceding figure). H&E × 300

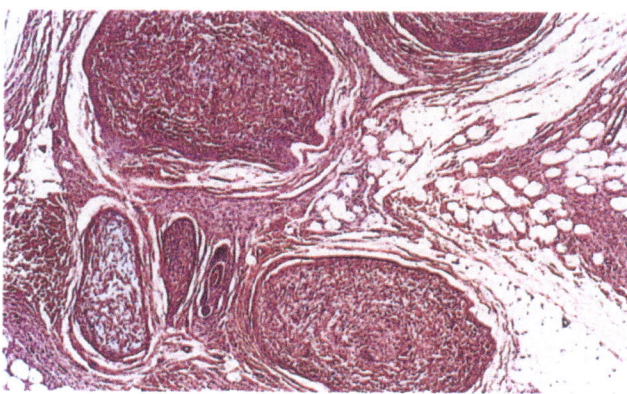

Fig. 13.3 A plexiform neurofibroma is composed of a tortuous arrangement of expanded nerve branches sectioned in various planes with abnormal cells spilled out into the adjacent tissue leading to a background of neurofibroma. The patient was a 10-year-old boy who had a lesion removed from the outer aspect of his left ankle. H&E × 30

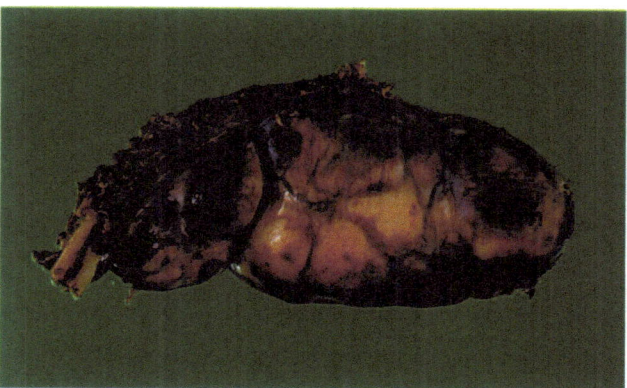

Fig. 13.4 A large posterior mediastinal schwannoma measuring 9 × 5 × 3 cm is attached to inner aspect of the right seventh rib. The lesion is well-circumscribed and capsulated. The patient was an 8-year-old boy who had the lesion discovered incidentally on X-ray

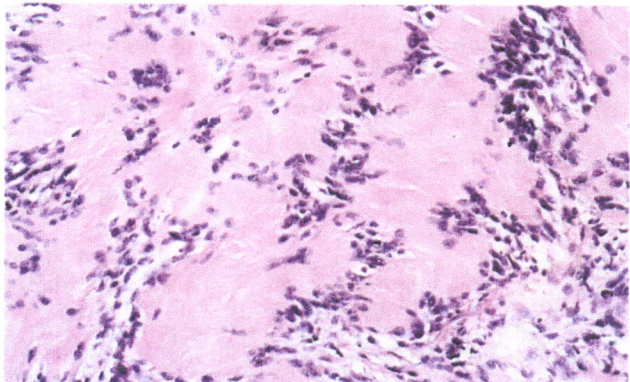

Fig. 13.5 Schwannoma. Same lesion as shown in the preceding figure. Nuclear regimentation and Verocay bodies are demonstrated in Antoni type A tissue. H&E × 300

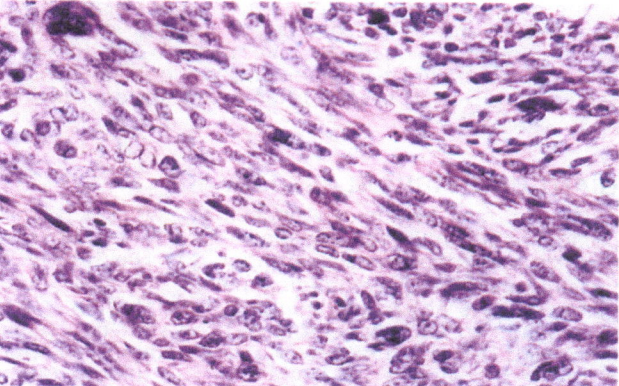

Fig. 13.6 Malignant schwannoma (malignant peripheral nerve sheath tumour) reveals interwoven bundles of spindle cells that display increased cellularity and nuclear pleomorphism. The tumour was resected from the anterior abdominal wall of a 12-year-old girl who had von Recklinghausen's neurofibromatosis. H&E × 300

with the more common granular cell tumours of older individuals.

Cessation of growth after birth, or even regression, argues against a neoplastic process. Local recurrences do not occur, even when excision is incomplete. The histogenesis is uncertain. An unusual instance has been reported of congenital granular cell tumour with systemic involvement[11].

GRANULAR CELL TUMOUR (MYOBLASTOMA)

Granular cell tumours involve all age groups and arise as a small mass in various sites throughout the body[12]. The tongue is most commonly affected. The microscopy is indistinguishable from granular cell tumour of the newborn, apart from less prominent vascularity. The tumour cells regularly express S-100 protein, supporting the proposed derivation from Schwann cells[13], although exceptions occur and argue for alternative cell lineages. A commmon accompaniment is pseudoepitheliomatous hyperplasia of the overlying skin or squamous mucosa.

LIPOBLASTOMA AND LIPOBLASTOMATOSIS

Lipoblastoma is a benign tumour of immature adipose tissue generally diagnosed before the age of 3 years[14,15]. The lesions are slow-growing, painless and non-tender. The growths are usually solitary and the principal sites are the soft tissue of the upper and lower extremities. Occasionally, the mediastinum and the retroperitoneum are involved. Two variants are described[14]. When the tumour is diffuse, poorly circumscribed and deeply located, it is referred to as lipoblastomatosis. When the lesions are circumscribed (or encapsulated) and superficial, they are referred to as lipoblastomas. The latter are more common.

Microscopically, the tumour is composed of lobules of fetal adipose tissue separated by septa of connective tissue (Figure 13.8). The adipose tissue is immature and myxoid along the periphery of the lobule (Figure 13.9), and, near the centres of the lobules, there is a tendency for the adipose tissue to mature (Figure 13.10). Branching thin-walled capillaries course through the lobules, forming a plexiform pattern.

The microscopic resemblance to myxoid liposarcoma may be striking[15]. However, lipoblastomatosis seems to occur exclusively in infants and young children, whereas, at this age, liposarcomas are exceedingly rare. A diagnosis of liposarcoma in patients less than 5 years of age should be made with extreme caution[12].

The prognosis for lipoblastoma and lipoblastomatosis is excellent and simple excision is usually sufficient[14]. Most lipomas in childhood are thought to represent the end-point in maturation of a lipoblastoma, as sections from such lesions often reveal residual foci of lipoblastoma[33].

GIANT CELL FIBROBLASTOMA

This is a rare benign mesenchymal lesion occurring predominantly in the first decade of life[16–18], and showing a notable preponderance among boys. The history is usually one of a slow-growing painless subcutaneous mass. There is no special anatomical distribution[19], and all tumours so far described have been solitary, usually measuring 1–5 cm in diameter. Complete surgical excision is the recommended treatment, but the tumour has a marked tendency to recur. Metastases are not known to occur[16,18].

The tumours occupy the superficial soft tissue (dermis, subcutaneous tissue, occasionally extending into the underlying muscle). The margins are ill-defined and infil-trative. The microscopic picture is distinctive: there are solid and angiectoid areas, present in varying proportions (Figure 13.11). The angiectoid areas vary in size, and may be small and slit-like, or large and gaping, sometimes resembling lymphatic spaces. The solid areas may be poorly cellular or may comprise large numbers of plump fibroblasts (Figure 13.12), although marked hyalinization is seen occasionally. An especially striking feature is the presence of large pleomorphic multinucleate cells with peripherally arranged nuclei, forming a wreath or floret. The giant cells may occupy the solid areas or may be seen to rim the angiectoid spaces (Figures 13.11, 13.12). Mitoses are rare. The spaces sometimes contain pale mucopolysaccharide material. Atrophic adipose tissue may be included.

Immunohistochemically, the lesional cells fail to express factor VIII-related antigen or the lectin *Ulex europaeus*, arguing against a vascular histogenesis[19].

Giant cell fibroblastoma and dermatofibrosarcoma protruberans share clinical and morphological features[20,21], suggesting a histogenetic relationship. Dermatofibrosarcoma protruberans has been reported in the recurrence of an earlier excised giant cell fibroblastoma[22]. Dermatofibrosarcoma protruberans has also been reported to occur *de novo* in infants and children[23]; the histological appearance is no different from that of lesions occurring in later life. Various malignant mesenchymal proliferations should be considered in the differential diagnosis of giant cell fibroblastoma.

PLEXIFORM FIBROHISTIOCYTIC TUMOUR

The clinical and morphological features of this lesion were outlined in 65 patients by Enzinger and Zhang[24]. Children and adolescents are predominantly affected and the female:male ratio is 3:1. Most of the lesions are located in the upper extremity. Clinical presentation is usually a slow-growing solitary small deep-seated nodule in the skin.

The lesions are poorly demarcated and generally measure less than 3 cm in diameter. Microscopically, there is involvement of the mid and lower dermis and the upper part of the subcutis, with sparing of the upper dermis.

Three histological patterns are recognized:

(a)   A predominantly fibrohistiocytic picture with aggregates of histiocyte- or fibroblast-like cells interspersed with multinucleated osteoclast-like giant cells (Figure 13.13). Within the nodular aggregates, small haemorrhages or haemosiderin are seen frequently. Transitional forms are common between the mononuclear histiocyte-like cells and the multinucleate giant cells.

(b)   A mainly fibroblastic picture composed of bundles of spindle-shaped cells (Figure 13.14). The latter pattern may resemble fibromatosis.

(c)   A mixture of the fibrohistiocytic and fibroblastic patterns.

Mitoses are generally rare and there is little cellular pleomorphism. Lymphocytes are scattered throughout, and are seen particularly at the edge of the nodules.

Surgical resection is usually curative but recurrences occur in a third of cases, requiring further surgery. Two of the cases included in the early series of Enzinger and Zhang[24] metastasized to regional lymph nodes.

Hollowood et al.[25] reported immunohistochemical positivity for vimentin and alpha smooth muscle actin, and ultrastructural evidence of myofibroblastic differentiation in the spindle cell component; the osteoclast-like giant cells within the histiocytic nodules showed strong CD68 (KP1) positivity.

ANGIOMATOID MALIGNANT FIBROUS HISTIOCYTOMA

Once considered a variant of malignant fibrous histiocytoma (discussed separately below)[26], there is now a tendency to regard angiomatoid malignant fibrous histiocytoma as a separate and distinct entity[27,28]. This is mainly because of its low-grade malignancy and a propensity to affect patients in the first two decades. A series of 108 cases showed 77% of patients to be aged less than 20 years[27]. The extremities are generally involved, the upper more often than the lower. A slow-growing painless mass in the lower dermis and subcutis is usually seen clinically. Systemic features, such as anaemia, weight loss and pyrexia, may be present. The histogenesis is still debatable.

The gross specimen usually measures 0.7–10 cm; it is generally well circumscribed, rubbery, and grey–tan to red–brown in colour[26]. The cut surface is almost always cystic and the cysts are filled with blood or haemorrhagic fluid. Haemorrhage, on the other hand, may be minimal or absent.

On microscopy, the tumour comprises:

(a) Irregular sheets of round or spindle cells (Figure 13.15);
(b) Focal areas of haemorrhage or cyst-like spaces; and
(c) A dense lymphoplasmacytic infiltrate (Figure 13.16)[26–28].

Mild degrees of nuclear atypia affecting the round/spindle cell component are usually present. Some tumours show large hyperchromatic nuclei, sometimes with multinucleated forms (Figure 13.16). A dense hyaline pseudocapsule is typical. Chronic inflammatory cells aggregate at the periphery and merge with the fibrous pseudocapsule. The cellular and haemorrhagic areas tend to affect the centre of the tumour. Focal haemorrhages are common and many tumour cells contain haemosiderin. The cystic spaces are thought to be secondary to resorption of haemorrhage, or possibly result from dislodgement of blood clot during tissue processing, although some cystic spaces are undoubtedly endothelial-lined. The inflammatory response may be quite marked and there may be accompanying lymphoid follicle formation.

The differential diagnosis includes the aneurysmal (angiomatoid) variant of benign fibrous histiocytoma, histiocytoid haemangioma, cutaneous angiosarcoma and Kaposi's sarcoma.

Recurrences commonly follow surgical excision and usually do so within the first 12 months. Metastases occur only rarely. In the series of Costa and Weiss[27], there were 94 patients with adequate follow-up: 11 patients developed local recurrences and four went on to metastasize locally; all of the latter underwent wide local excision of the metastases and experienced no further problems. Angiomatoid malignant fibrous histiocytoma presenting at birth has been reported[29].

EXTRASKELETAL MYXOID CHONDROSARCOMA

Extraskeletal myxoid chrondrosarcoma is a rare neoplasm with a propensity to affect the extremities[30]. In Enzinger and Shiraki's series[30], the age range was from 13 to 89 years; two of the patients were under 20 years of age. A recent review of the literature disclosed five cases of extraskeletal myxoid chondrosarcoma occurring in children[31], and the authors added two more cases.

Naked eye examination shows an ovoid lobulated soft-to-firm well-circumscribed growth measuring 1.5–23 cm[31]. The cut surface is gelatinous, often cystic and haemorrhage is common.

On microscopic examination[30], the tumour is lobulated or nodular and, in many instances, has a fibrous pseudocapsule. It is composed of small uniform round or elongated cells with a small amount of deeply eosinophilic cytoplasm. The nuclei are small and hyperchromatic and the cytoplasm may reveal spherical hyaline eosinophilic inclusions that compress the nucleus. The cells tend to form cords or nests separated by abundant avascular myxoid stroma rich in reticulin fibres. Overall, there is a resemblance to immature chondroblastic tissue. Many tumour cells contain PAS-positive diastase-labile material (presumably glycogen). Immunohistochemically, the tumour cells express vimentin and S-100 protein[31].

Extraskeletal embryonal chondrosarcoma, which may affect infants, differs from extraskeletal myxoid chondrosarcoma by the presence of microscopic foci of hyaline cartilage, less myxoid material and more primitive tumour cells[32].

The differential diagnosis of extraskeletal myxoid chondrosarcoma includes other myxoid tumours, such as myxoid liposarcoma, nerve sheath myxoma (neurothekeoma), myxoid malignant fibrous histiocytoma and embryonal rhabdomyosarcoma; extrarenal rhabdoid tumour should also be considered because of the possible presence of cytoplasmic eosinophilic inclusions[31]. Extraskeletal myxoid chondrosarcoma in children may behave more aggressively than the adult counterpart[31].

NODULAR FASCIITIS (PSEUDOSARCOMATOUS FASCIITIS)

More than 20% of cases of nodular fasciitis occur in individuals less than 20 years old[33]. Characteristically, the tumour appears suddenly and grows rapidly. There is a predilection for the upper extremity and face, involving the subcutis or deep soft tissue. Colour and consistency of the excised lesion are variable but the majority of the lesions are small, 2 cm or less. A myxoid character is frequent and may impart a slimy consistency. Encapsulation is common, but the lesion may extend into the surrounding tissue.

Microscopically the central portion of the lesion is myxoid and hypocellular (Figure 13.17) while, at the periphery, spindled fibroblasts and mononuclear cells predominate (Figure 13.18). Red blood cells are scattered throughout. The myxoid background is particularly helpful in diagnosis. Multinucleate giant cells are common and are presumably derived from fibroblasts (Figure 13.18); they should be distinguished from multinucleated cells that arise from entrapped skeletal muscle. Mitoses are frequent but rarely atypical.

Bernstein and Lattes[34] recognize four histological types of nodular fasciitis: (a) reactive, (b) densely cellular, (c) lesions with osteoid or cartilaginous metaplasia, and (d) the so-called proliferative fasciitis. The majority of lesions stain for smooth muscle actin, muscle-specific actin, vimentin and KP1 (CD68). Keratin, S-100 protein and desmin are not expressed by the lesional cells[35].

Recurrences are unusual after surgical excision and, in such an event, review of the original diagnosis should be undertaken[34]. The microscopic differential diagnosis includes one of the fibromatoses, neurofibroma, malignant fibrous histiocytoma and inflammatory fibrous histiocytoma.

CRANIAL FASCIITIS OF CHILDHOOD

This is a rare tumour that clinically presents as a rapidly growing mass in the scalp of young children[36]. The usual age range is 3 weeks to 6 years and boys are about twice

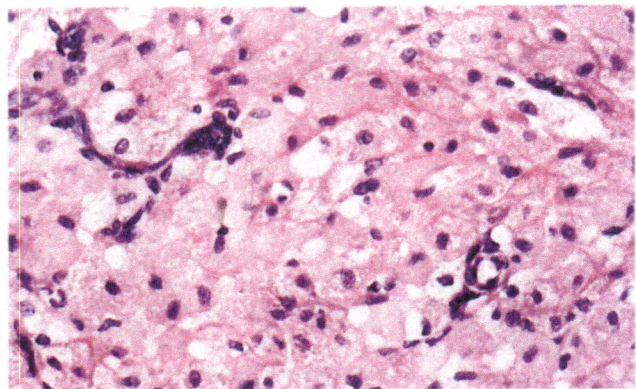

Fig. 13.7 Granular cell tumour of a newborn female. The lesion shows sheets of round to polygonal cells with copious granular pink cytoplasm and small centrally located nuclei. A capillary network is prominent. H&E × 300

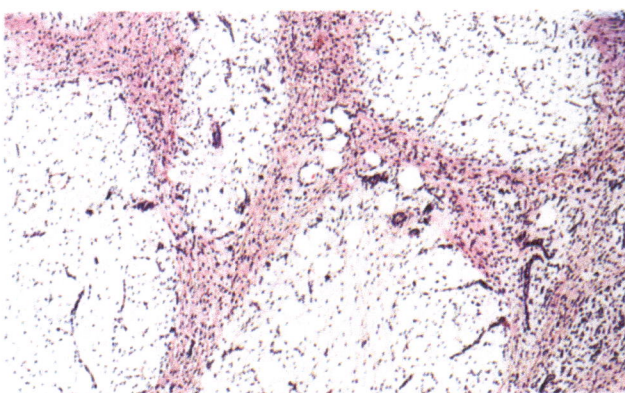

Fig. 13.8 Lipoblastoma composed of lobules of fetal adipose tissue separated by fibrous septa. The adipose tissue tends to be more mature in the centre of the lobules. A rich capillary network is evident within the lobules. The patient was a 1½-year-old boy who had a lump in the soft tissue of the back. The gross specimen measured 4 × 2 × 1 cm. H&E × 48

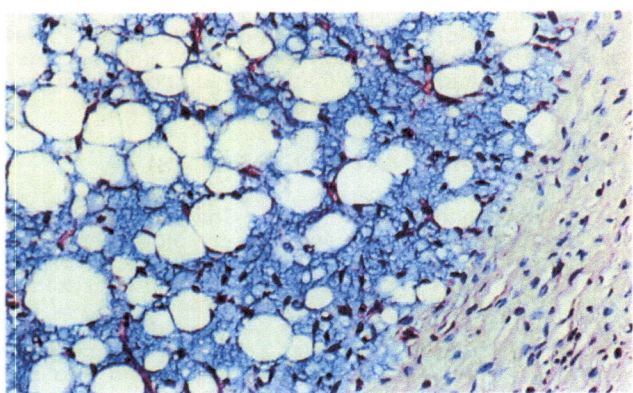

Fig. 13.9 Lipoblastoma. Alcian blue positivity corresponds to the immature component of the tumour that is seen especially at the periphery of the lobules. H&E × 185

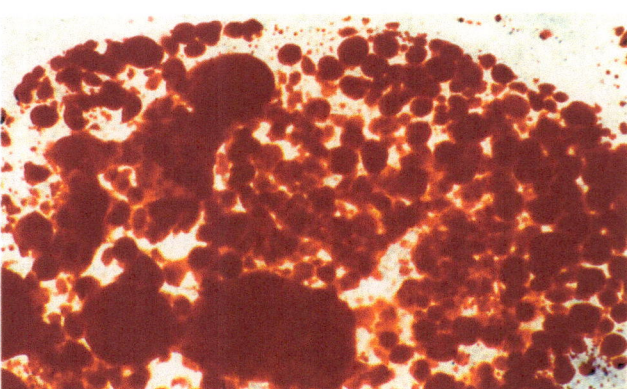

Fig. 13.10 Lipoblastoma. Oil-red-O positivity parallels the degree of mature adipose tissue within the lesion. H&E × 75

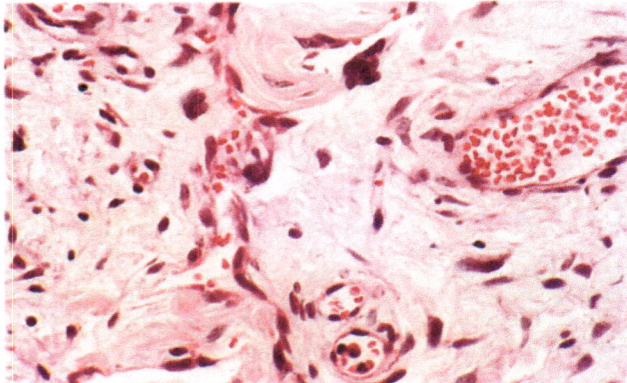

Fig. 13.11 Giant-cell fibroblastoma. Microscopically, there is a mixture of solid and angiectoid areas. Plump fibroblasts, observed in the solid areas, are seen also to line the angiectoid spaces. The lesion was removed from the soft tissue of the left supraclavicular fossa of a 2-year-old girl. H&E × 300

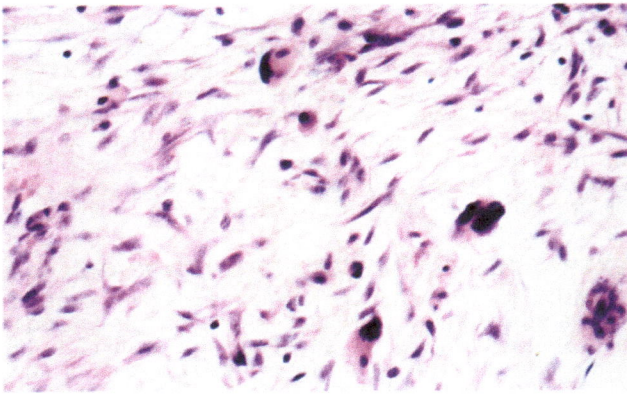

Fig. 13.12 A solid area of giant-cell fibroblastoma reveals fibroblasts and large cells with hyperchromatic nuclei. Same lesion as that shown in preceding figure. H&E × 300

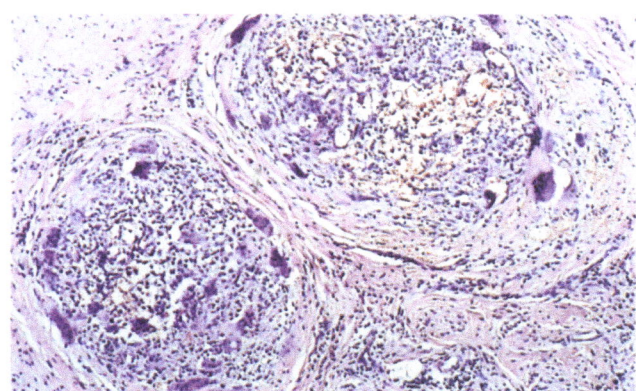

Fig. 13.13 Plexiform fibrohistiocytic tumour with a predominantly fibrohistiocytic pattern. This shows aggregates of histiocyte-like and fibroblast-like cells intermingled with multinucleate osteoclast-like giant cells. Erythrocytes are seen within the nodular aggregates. This was a soft tissue lesion in the neck of a 7-year-old boy. H&E × 75

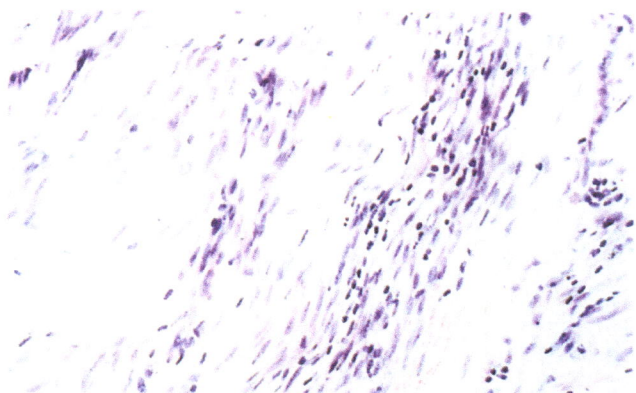

Fig. 13.14 A different field from the same tumour as in Figure 13.13 shows a predominantly fibroblastic microscopic picture composed of bundles of spindle-shaped cells. H&E × 185

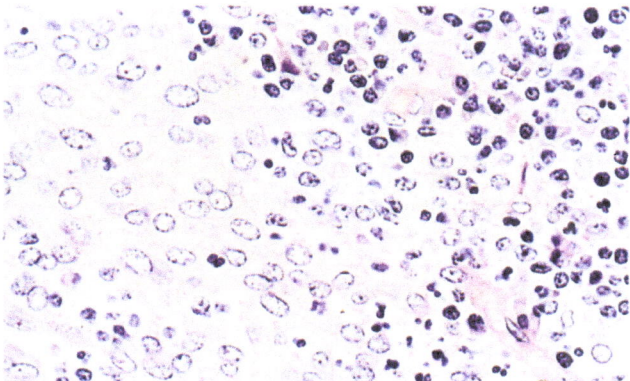

Fig. 13.15 Angiomatoid malignant fibrous histiocytoma shows areas of round to spindle-shaped cells with bland pale nuclei bordered by a dense infiltrate of lymphocytes and plasma cells (right upper field). The lesion was removed from a 5½-year-old girl who presented with a slow-growing mass on the upper part of the right thigh. H&E × 480

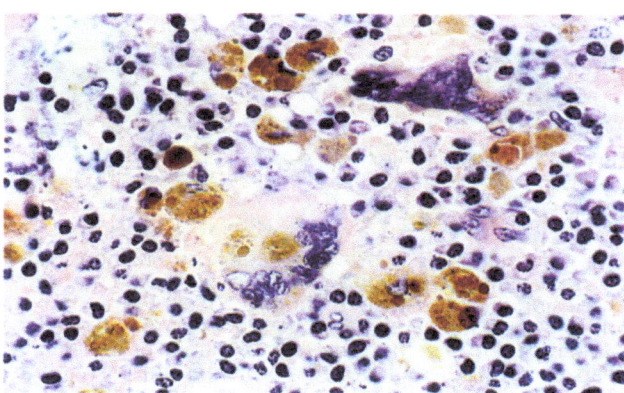

Fig. 13.16 Same tumour as in Figure 13.15 reveals conspicuous haemosiderin deposition in another microscopic field. Several multinucleate cells are also present. H&E × 480

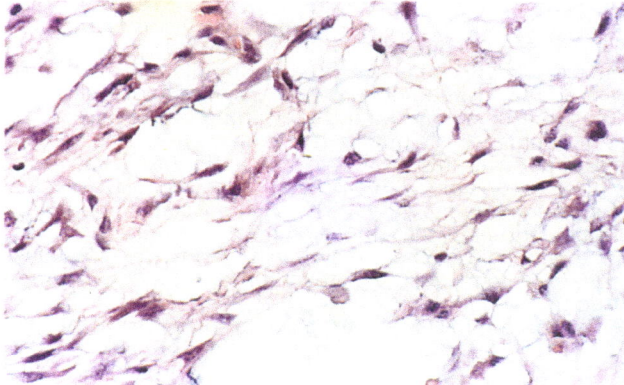

Fig. 13.17 Nodular fasciitis. The lesion is hypocellular with spindle-shaped fibroblasts set in a myxoid stroma. H&E × 300

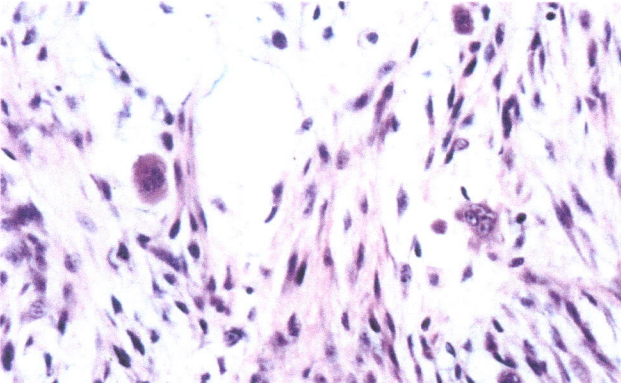

Fig. 13.18 Nodular fasciitis. Multinucleate cells of nodular fasciitis should be distinguished from entrapped skeletal muscle fibres undergoing degeneration. This latter feature is often seen at the edge of the lesion. H&E × 300

as commonly affected as girls. Any region of the scalp may be involved. The lesion is thought to originate from the deep fascia or the periosteum; the underlying bone is often invaded (Figure 13.19), sometimes down to the dura.

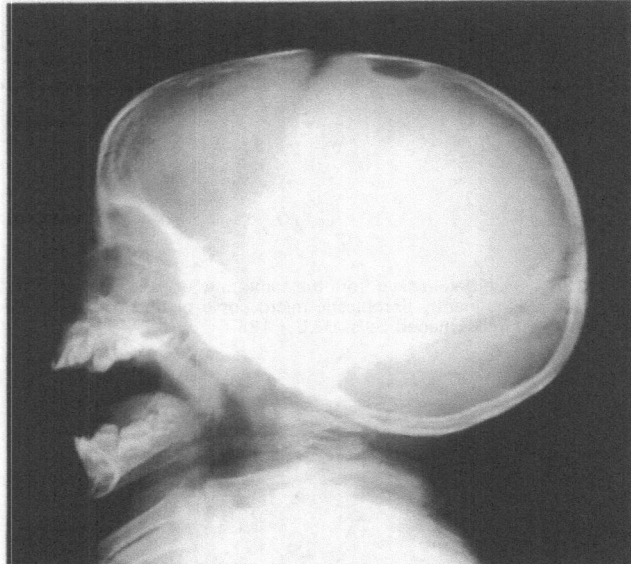

Fig. 13.19 Cranial fasciitis. A 12-month-old male presented with a subcutaneous swelling on the top of his head. Radiologically, this was shown to be associated with a solitary punched-out hole in the underlying skull

In the nine cases reported by Lauer and Enzinger[36], the gross specimen measured 1.5–9 cm in greatest dimension. The lesion is circumscribed (Figure 13.20) with a firm to rubbery consistency and the cut surface is greyish-white.

Microscopically, the picture is variable but generally bears a strong resemblance to nodular fasciitis. A haphazard arrangement of spindle- to stellate-shaped fibroblasts alternates with a vague storiform pattern (Figure 13.21); elsewhere, the picture is more cellular, reminiscent of fibromatosis (Figure 13.22). Mitoses are scarce and, when present, lack atypicality. A sprinkling of chronic inflammatory cells is common and collagenous areas are sometimes seen. Osseous metaplasia may be present (Figure 13.23) and multinucleate giant cells are observed occasionally.

Recurrences are uncommon even after incomplete surgical resection. The differential diagnosis includes myofibromatosis, meningioma and fibrous histiocytoma[12].

HAMARTOMA OF THE SCALP WITH ECTOPIC MENINGOTHELIAL ELEMENTS

This entity, recently reported by Suster and Rosai[37], presents as a solitary well-circumscribed lesion in the scalp, usually occupying the occipital area. All five of their cases, bar one, occurred in children. Histologically, the dermis contains an admixture of mature adipose tissue, small and medium-sized vessels, nerve bundles and fibrous tissue elements. The presence of clusters or strands of plump cuboidal and epithelioid cells is a prominent feature. They often appear to form interanastomosing vessel-like channels lined by plump cells with hyperchromatic ovoid or spindle-shaped nuclei (Figure 13.24). A pseudoinfiltrative growth pattern may be seen in some areas.

Twelve children with the same entity have been reported

under the title of 'sequestrated meningoceles of the scalp (extracranial meningeal heterotopia)'[38].

Histiocytoid haemangioma, epithelioid haemangioendothelioma, spindle-cell haemangioendothelioma, giant-cell fibroblastoma, papillary endothelial hyperplasia and epithelioid sarcoma should be considered in the differential diagnosis[37].

ALVEOLAR SOFT PART SARCOMA

This is an uncommon malignant neoplasm that principally affects adolescents and young adults[39]. However, the growth may arise in children. The lower extremities (especially the anterior portion of the thigh) are the preferred site in adults, while the head and neck (especially the orbit and the tongue) are commonly involved in children.

Grossly, the tumour is poorly circumscribed, soft and friable; haemorrhage and necrosis are often seen. The microscopic picture shows small groups of large round or polygonal tumour cells that are separated by thin-walled vascular channels (Figure 13.25). Tumour cell nuclei are vesicular with a small nucleolus and abundant granular eosinophilic cytoplasm. Mitoses are scarce. Loss of cohesion and degeneration of tumour cells are often present within the centres of the lobules, producing a pattern reminiscent of alveolar rhabdomyosarcoma. Variable amounts of intracellular glycogen are revealed on PAS/diastase reaction. PAS-positive diastase-resistant crystalline material, an important diagnostic feature, is also found in a large proportion of tumours.

The histogenesis is unknown. The lungs, brain and skeleton represent the principal sites for metastases. The prognosis is generally more favourable in children than in adults.

SYNOVIAL SARCOMA

Synovial sarcoma is a neoplasm of uncertain histogenesis and occurs most commonly in the lower extremities of young adults. Of all soft tissue sarcomas in childhood and adolescents, 2–10% are attributable to synovial sarcoma[33]. It has been reported as the third most common soft tissue sarcoma in childhood and adolescence, superseded by rhabdomyosarcoma and peripheral primitive neuroectodermal tumour (PNET)[40]. A painless soft tissue mass in close proximity to articular surfaces, tendons and bursae is the usual clinical presentation.

Grossly, the neoplasm is well circumscribed, firm and lobular with a greyish-white cut surface. Foci of calcification may be present. Microscopically, two patterns are recognized: biphasic and monophasic. The biphasic pattern comprises epithelioid and spindle cells, either of which may predominate. The epithelioid cells are polygonal or columnar and are arranged in solid nests, acini, tubules, cysts or papillary formations[40]. The spindle cell pattern resembles fibrosarcoma (Figure 13.26) and is often associated with calcification and foci reminiscent of haemangiopericytoma. The spindle cell components are analogous to those in the biphasic and monophasic variants. The epithelioid element may be verified by mucin stains, immunohistochemistry (cytokeratin and EMA), or ultrastructurally.

The monophasic variant, which presents a greater diagnostic problem, is composed solely of spindle cells, but small groups of epithelioid cells (transitional cells) are seen frequently (Figure 13.27). Calcifying synovial sarcoma, regarded as a variant of synovial sarcoma, is characterized by extensive calcification and osseous metaplasia. In Schmidt et al.'s series[40] involving children and adolescents, the biphasic pattern was more common.

The differential diagnosis of synovial sarcoma includes most other spindle cell lesions encountered in childhood (see Table 12.1). The influence of histological subtype on prognosis is currently disputed[40]; however, the calcifying synovial sarcoma and small tumours are recognized as carrying a relatively better prognosis. Recurrence and metastases may develop after periods as long as 20 years[41]. The translocation t(X;18)(p11;q11.2) has been reported to be a karyotype abnormality specific for synovial sarcoma[42].

MYOSITIS OSSIFICANS

Patients with this tumour are generally males less than 20 years old[43]. A solitary, rapidly growing, tender or painful mass is the usual symptom and a history of prior trauma is often obtained. The lower extremity, buttock or abdominal wall are the usual anatomical sites. Despite its name, the lesion is not limited to skeletal muscle. Grossly the tumour has a rubbery consistency, and bone is often seen on the cut surface.

A microscopic pattern[43] of zonation is characteristic and comprises fibrin, fibroblasts and histiocytes in the centre of the lesion, and osteoid and immature bone trabeculae along the periphery (Figure 13.28). The edge of the lesion often includes degenerate muscle fibres and chronic inflammatory cells. Cartilage is an uncommon feature.

An excellent prognosis follows surgical excision. Myositis ossificans must be distinguished from other bone-forming tumours of the soft tissue, such as fibrodysplasia ossificans progressiva, osseous metaplasia and extra-osseous osteosarcoma[44]; these entities are rarely encountered in children.

GIANT-CELL TUMOUR OF TENDON SHEATH (LOCALIZED NODULAR TENOSYNOVITIS)

This is a common soft tissue tumour usually affecting adults. Children less than 10 years of age did not occur in a large series of 132 cases[45]. The hand is involved in the great majority of cases, usually the fingers with a predilection for the right side and the volar surface[45]; other sites include wrist, ankle, foot and toes. The antigen profile of the tumour supports a true monocyte/macrophage lineage[46].

The tumours are relatively small, ranging in size from 0.5 to 4 cm[46]. They are firm and lobulated and usually exhibit a yellowish-brown cut surface. Histologically, they are composed of sheets of round or polygonal cells with a vesicular nucleus and faintly eosinophilic cytoplasm (Figure 13.29); other microscopical constituents include foam cells, haemosiderin and multinuclear giant cells (Figure 13.30). The clinical course is invariably benign, but recurrences are not uncommon[47].

The histological findings are similar to those encountered in pigmented villonodular synovitis, which is felt to be part of the same pathological spectrum[45].

FIBROMA OF TENDON SHEATH

This is chiefly a tumour of adults, although most series[48] include a modest number arising in children. The lesion is more common in males and the upper extremity is involved in the majority of cases. Most lesions arise in the fingers, hands and wrist, and a painless nodule is the usual complaint.

Virtually all tumours are attached to tendon and/or tendon sheath and are generally well-circumscribed and lobulated, measuring from 1–2 cm in diameter. The consistency varies from firm to hard, although some of the lesions are soft and cystic.

Scattered spindle-shaped fibroblasts associated with dense fibrous stroma and dilated or slit-like channels form the usual microscopic picture[48]. Some of the channels resemble tenosynovial spaces. Foci of myxoid change are often present and multinucleated giant cells are found occasionally. Electron microscopy shows the lesional cells to be myofibroblasts, or myofibroblasts and fibroblasts[49].

The differential diagnosis includes giant cell tumour of tendon sheath, fibromatosis, nodular fasciitis and fibrous histiocytoma. Absence of foam cells and haemosiderin-laden macrophages usually allows a distinction to be made from giant cell tumour of tendon sheath. Nodular fasciitis rarely involves the hands and feet, and it usually appears suddenly and grows rapidly, features that contrast with fibroma of tendon sheath[49]. Surgical excision is the treatment of choice in fibroma of tendon sheath. The recurrence rate is about 24%.

FOCAL MYOSITIS

This is a benign inflammatory pseudotumour of skeletal muscle. The youngest patient in a reported series of 16 cases was 10 years old[50]. An enlarging, often painful, mass in muscle is the usual clinical presentation. The histological picture discloses variation of myofibre diameter with features of necrosis and regeneration, large numbers of internal nuclei, and increase in endomysial connective tissue with variable inflammatory infiltrate. The aetiology is unknown. Surgical resection is curative.

NEUROMUSCULAR HAMARTOMA (NEUROMUSCULAR CHORISTOMA; BENIGN 'TRITON TUMOUR')

This is an exceedingly rare tumour which usually arises in close proximity to a large nerve trunk (e.g. brachial plexus and sciatic nerve)[51]. Most tumours are solitary and they occur with equal frequency in boys and girls. They are multinodular growths, generally 1–4 cm in diameter. Microscopically, there is a disorganized proliferation of mature skeletal muscle fibres intermixed with small nerve fibres. Recurrences are uncommon after excision, and the clinical course is always benign. The histogenesis is unknown, although an origin from the muscle spindle has been suggested[51].

EXTRARENAL RHABDOID TUMOUR (ERRT)

Tumours with cytological features similar to those of rhabdoid tumour of the kidney (RTK) (see Chapter 3) are reported also to arise primarily outside the kidney (ERRT)[52]. Unlike RTK, ERRT involves a wide age range, including adults[53,54]. In their review of such tumours entered into the Intergroup Rhabdomyosarcoma Studies I–III (1972–1989), Kodet et al.[55] were able to identify 26 patients, in whom the mean age was 5.5 years; 11 were less than 1 year of age. The proximal extremity and the axial soft tissues were preferentially involved. As with the renal counterpart, tumour behaviour is typically aggressive, accompanied by poor survival[55]. ERRT is reported to occur less commonly in parenchymal organs, such as the thymus, liver, heart and central nervous system[56]. Understandably, a primary ERRT of the central nervous system may be difficult to distinguish from one that has metastasized from a subclinical RTK. The histogenesis of the ERRT is unclear, as is its relationship with RTK[54,55]. Ultrastructural and immunohistochemical studies have been reported[53].

Rhabdomyosarcoma, epithelioid sarcoma, 'intra-abdominal desmoplastic small round-cell tumour', large cell lymphoma, synovial sarcoma and extraskeletal myxoid

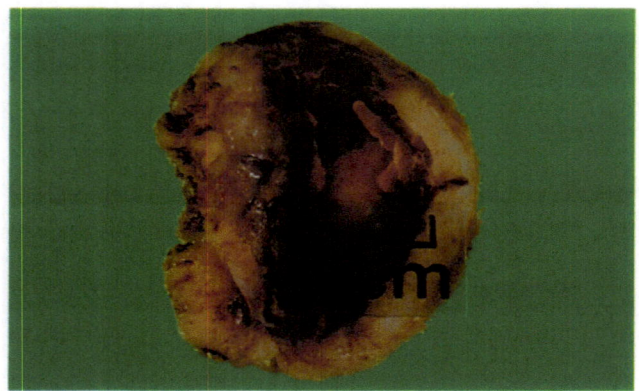

Fig. 13.20   Cranial fasciitis. Gross specimen was discoid and measured 3 cm in diameter and 1.1 cm deep

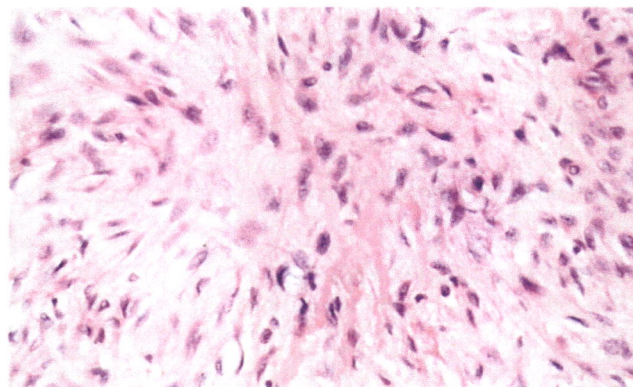

Fig. 13.21   Cranial fasciitis. Microscopy shows a spindle-cell lesion which in some areas demonstrates a storiform pattern. H&E × 112

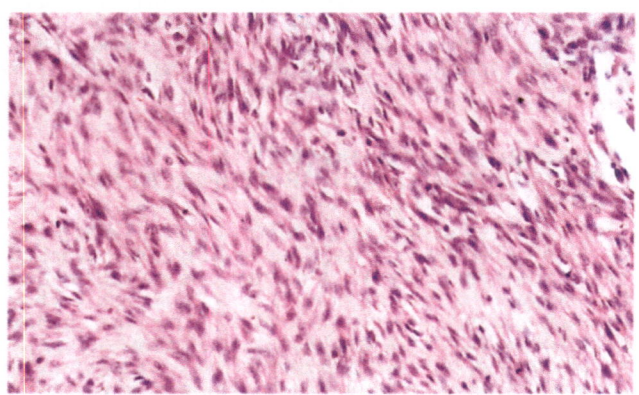

Fig. 13.22   Cranial fasciitis. This microscopic field shows a fascicular arrangement of closely packed spindle-shaped fibroblasts, resembling fibromatosis. H&E × 185

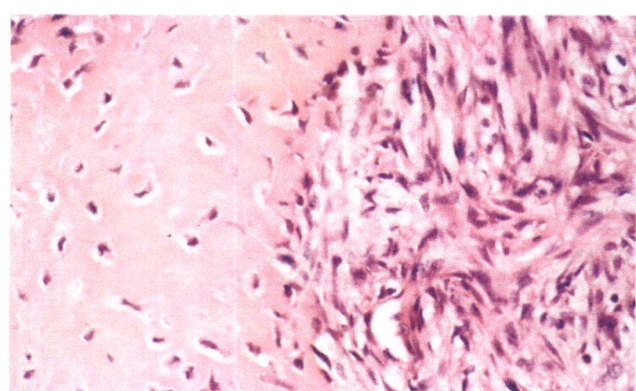

Fig. 13.23   Cranial fasciitis. In addition to a vague storiforn pattern, there is metaplastic bone, a common feature of the lesion. H&E × 300

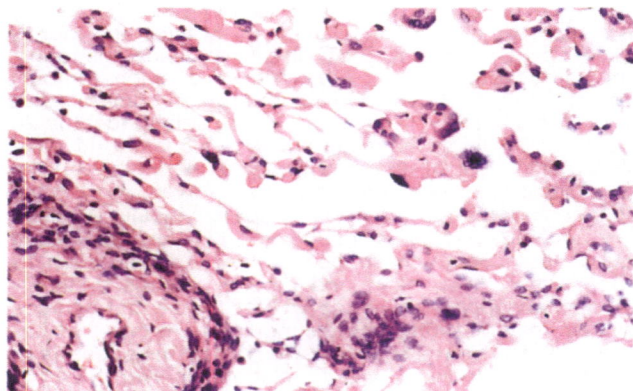

Fig. 13.24   Sequestrated meningocele of the scalp in an 8-month-old boy shows vascular-like channels that are often lined by plump hyperchromatic cells. This may give a false impression of malignancy. H&E × 185

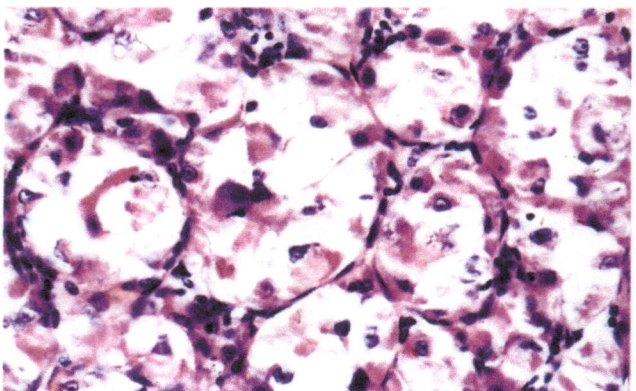

Fig. 13.25   Microscopy of alveolar soft-part sarcoma resected from the right thigh of a 17-year-old boy. There are small clusters of large polygonal cells that are separated by thin-walled vascular channels. The nuclei are vesicular and the cytoplasm is abundant, eosinophilic and granular. The groups of cells have lost cohesion centrally, producing a picture somewhat reminiscent of alveolar rhabdomyosarcoma. H&E × 300

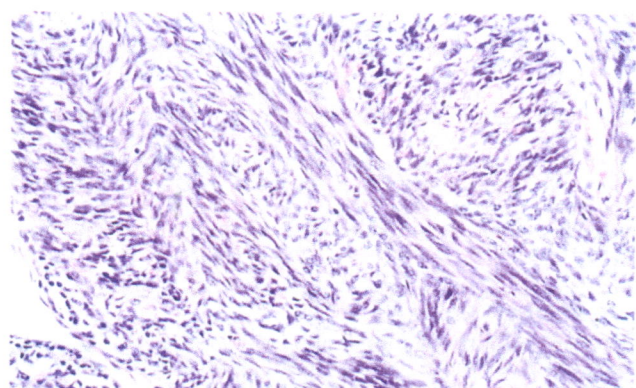

Fig. 13.26 A monophasic variant of synovial sarcoma is composed solely of spindle cells. The tumour cells were positive focally for keratin on immunohistochemistry, and electron microscopy showed focal epithelial differentiation. The tumour was removed from the left upper arm of a 13-year-old boy. H&E × 185

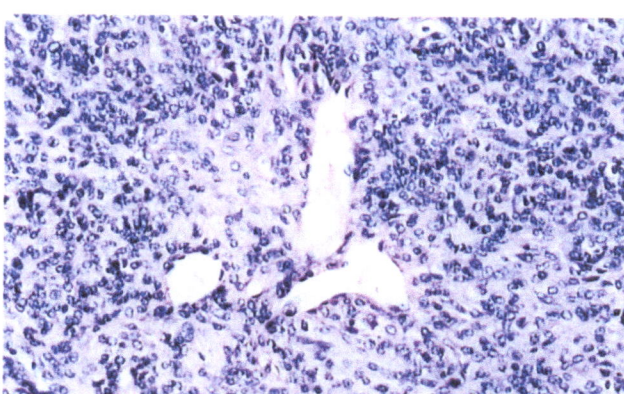

Fig. 13.27 Synovial sarcoma from the right forearm of a 10-year-old boy comprises an area of epithelioid cells and a haemangiopericytoma-like focus. Electron microscopy of the tumour confirmed focal epithelial differentiation. H&E × 185

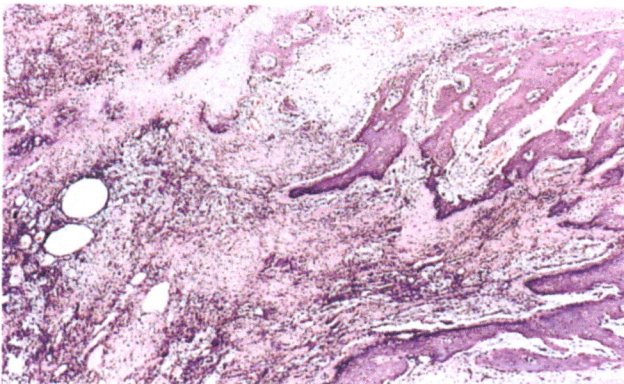

Fig. 13.28 Myositis ossificans. The tumour was located in the subcutaneous tissue of the right thigh and measured 2.5 cm across. The microscopic picture is characterized by zonation; fibroblasts and histiocytes occur centrally, and osteoid and mature bone are arranged peripherally. H&E × 30

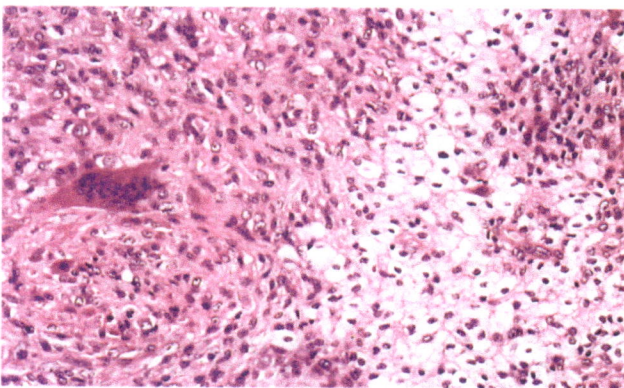

Fig. 13.29 Giant-cell tumour of tendon sheath. The lesion was excised from around the right knee of a 13-year-old girl. Microscopically, there is a mixture of round to polygonal mononuclear cells and foam cells; a multinucleate giant cell is also shown. H&E × 185

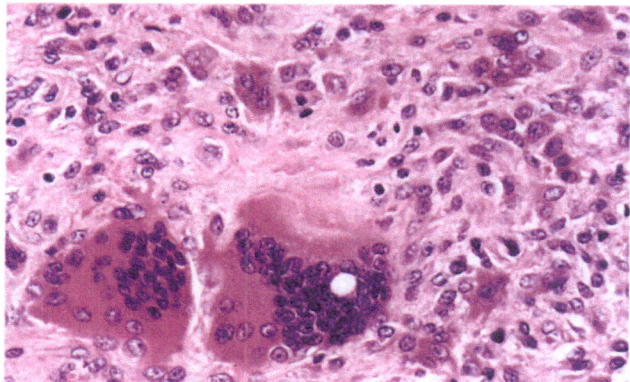

Fig. 13.30 Giant-cell tumour of tendon sheath. A higher-power view of the same tumour as in Figure 13.29 shows two large multinucleate giant cells set in a background of round cells with vesicular nuclei and eosinophilic cytoplasm. H&E × 300

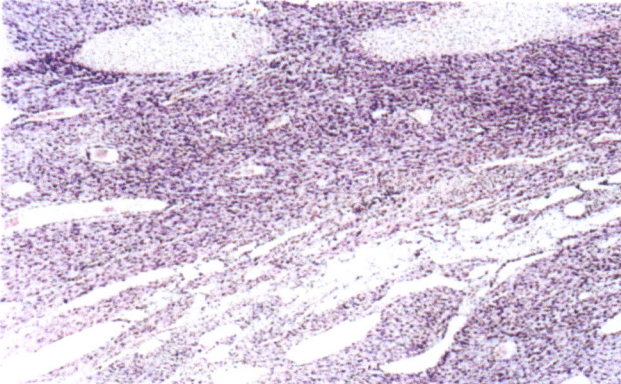

Fig. 13.31 Benign mesenchymoma. Swelling of the upper two thirds of the right lower leg was noted at birth. Microscopically, the tumour contained a variety of tissues including haemangiomatous elements, haemangiopericytomatous tissue, immature adipose tissue and cartilage. H&E × 30

chondrosarcoma should be considered in the differential diagnosis. On purely cytological grounds, the distinction between ERRT and epithelioid sarcoma may present difficulties[53-55].

EPITHELIOID SARCOMA

This is a malignant tumour of uncertain histogenesis arising predominantly in the distal extremities of young adults[57]. The tumour usually occurs in the skin, subcutis or deeper soft tissues, often presenting a firm to hard mass in close association with tendon sheaths, fascial planes or aponeuroses. Among the 241 cases reported by Chase and Enzinger[57], 5% were in their first decade and 27% in their second decade. The youngest patient in this series was 4 years old. The clinical course tends to be protracted with frequent recurrences. In children, the prognosis seems to be considerably better[57].

A nodular proliferation of plump polygonal cells is seen microscopically, the latter merging gradually with spindle cell areas[57,58]. The polygonal cells appear epithelioid with copious deeply eosinophilic cytoplasm. Necrosis is common, usually involves the centres of nodules, and may be confluent. Other features include intracytoplasmic vacuolation, storiform pattern, multinucleate cells and calcification. Intracytoplasmic glycogen (PAS-positivity/diastase lability) is found in a large proportion of neoplasms.

According to Schmidt and Harms[59] epithelioid sarcoma affecting children tends to occupy a more central anatomical location and more often shows multinucleated cells, compared with the adult tumour.

Tumour cells are frequently immunoreactive for vimentin and epithelial markers (cytokeratin and EMA)[60]. A similar antigenic phenotype is shared by synovial sarcoma and extrarenal rhabdoid tumour (see above), and they should be considered in the differential diagnosis. Necrobiotic granulomas may mimic epithelioid sarcoma.

INFLAMMATORY MYOFIBROBLASTIC TUMOUR (INFLAMMATORY PSEUDOTUMOUR; PLASMA CELL GRANULOMA; MYOFIBROBLASTOMA; OMENTAL–MESENTERIC MYXOID HAMARTOMA)

These are rare solid tumours that predominate in the lung. Of 20 patients with pulmonary lesions reported by Pettinato et al.[61], 10 were aged between 2 and 17 years. A preceding history of pulmonary disease may be present. Extrapulmonary growths also occur and affect a variety of sites[62]. Constitutional features, such as fever, anaemia, hypergammaglobulinaemia and thrombocytosis, are common[61,62].

Grossly the masses are large and measure from 6–13 cm in diameter. Most lesions are circumscribed, but lack a true capsule. The surfaces are smooth and glistening with a yellow–tan to greyish–white cut surface.

Microscopy shows a proliferation of mesenchymal spindled cells with an inflammatory infiltrate composed of mature plasma cells, lymphocytes or neutrophils. Mitoses are observed occasionally in the spindle cell component. The plasma cells may be multinucleate and Russell's bodies are common. Electron microscopy and immunohistochemistry of the spindle cells reveal features of myofibroblasts[61].

The pathogenesis of the lesion is unclear, although a reactive proliferation is the most likely. Rarely are adjacent structures infiltrated, and surgical excision is usually curative. Recurrences are documented but metastases do not occur. Spontaneous regression of the tumour has been reported[63,64].

Within this category of tumours, Meis and Enzinger[65] recently identified a group with similar histological features, involving specifically the mesentery and retroperitoneum. They emphasized the local aggressiveness and potential for metastases, and believed that these lesions were fibrosarcomas containing a prominent inflammatory component. The term 'inflammatory fibrosarcoma of the mesentery and peritoneum' was proposed for this entity. Of the 38 cases reported, the ages ranged from 2 months to 74 years; forty-seven per cent were 5 years old or younger. Their data indicate that children with this tumour may have a better prognosis than adults.

MESENCHYMOMA

This is a rare tumour comprising two or more mesenchymal tissue derivatives[66]. Fibrous tissue, which is present in all mesenchymal tumours, is excluded. The great majority of tumours are solitary, circumscribed and unencapsulated. Adipose tissue, blood vessels and smooth muscle are the most common mesenchymal constituents; other elements include myxomatous tissue, lymphoid tissue, haemangiopericytoma, benign haemangioendothelioma, cartilage (Figure 13.31) and skeletal muscle[66,67].

Le Ber and Stout[66] included in this category angiomyolipoma of the kidney in patients with tuberous sclerosis. A review of benign mesenchymomas of the head and neck showed that half the patients were less than 1 year old, and 31% were between 1 and 25 years old[67]. Benign mesenchymoma may infiltrate locally, a feature not to be construed as ominous. A 20% local recurrence rate has been reported[66]. Recurrent tumours may exhibit only one of the mesenchymal components of the original tumour[67].

The most common components of malignant mesenchymomas are rhabdomyosarcoma, liposarcoma and osteo/chondrosarcoma[68]. The retroperitoneum and the thigh are the common sites and most of the patients are adults. Newman and Fletcher[68] suggest that the tumour is not as aggressive as is usually inferred by the histological composition; they make a plea for the utilization of strict criteria in the diagnosis[69].

LIPOSARCOMA

Of 2500 cases of liposarcoma identified in the files of the Armed Forces Institute of Pathology in the United States of America, 17 tumours were from children between the ages of 8 months and 15 years[70]. Only two patients were younger than 10 years. Juvenile liposarcoma showed a distinct female preponderance and there was a predilection for the lower extremity, especially the thigh. Myxoid liposarcoma was the most common histological type. None of the tumours metastasized and only three patients experienced local recurrence; there was only one fatality. Liposarcoma should not be confused with lipoblastomatosis (see above), an entity which occurs exclusively in the first few years after birth.

MALIGNANT FIBROUS HISTIOCYTOMA (MFH)

MFH arises predominantly in middle to late adult life and is uncommon in children[71]. Of the 200 cases analysed by the latter authors, three (1%) affected children between 0 and 10 years of age. Zuppan et al.[72] found 27 well-documented cases in children (16 years of age or less) in their review of the English literature, to which they added two cases. Three children were less than 12 months old; the youngest affected was a newborn. MFH may arise as a postirradiation tumour[71].

The precise histogenesis is unknown. Involvement of the deep structures, large size of the tumour and lack of a significant inflammatory component are features that appear to correlate with metastatic potential[71].

Immunohistochemically, factor XIIIa, a subunit of factor XIII present in the 'fixed mesenchymal cell', is expressed by numerous cells throughout the tumour[73].

REFERENCES

1. Enzinger FM, Weiss SW. Neurofibromatosis (von Recklinghausen's disease). In: Enzinger FM, Weiss SW, editors. Soft tissue tumors. St Louis, Toronto, London: CV Mosby; 1983:606–15.
2. Raffensperger J, Cohen R. Plexiform neurofibromas in childhood. J Pediatr Surg. 1972;7:144–51.
3. Coffin CM, Dehner LP. Cellular peripheral neural tumors (neurofibromas) in children and adolescents: a clinicopathological and immunohistochemical study. Pediatr Pathol. 1990;10:351–61.
4. Gallager RL, Helwig EB. Neurothekeoma – a benign cutaneous tumor of neural origin. Am J Clin Pathol. 1980;74:759–64.
5. Abell MA, Hart WR, Olson JR. Tumors of the peripheral nervous system. Hum Pathol. 1970;1:503–51.
6. Fletcher CDM. Peripheral nerve sheath tumors. Pathol Annu. 1990;2:53–74.
7. Meis JM, Enzinger FM, Martz KL, Neal JA. Malignant peripheral nerve sheath tumors (malignant schwannomas) in children. Am J Surg Pathol. 1992;16:694–707.
8. Lack EE, Worsham GF, Callihan MD, Crawford BE, Vawter GF. Gingival granular cell tumors of the newborn (congenital 'epulis'): a clinical and pathologic study of 21 patients. Am J Surg Pathol. 1981;5:37–46.
9. Lifshitz MS, Flotte TJ, Greco MA. Congenital granular cell epulis. Immunohistochemical and ultrastructural observations. Cancer. 1984;53:1845–8.
10. Tucker MC, Rusnock EJ, Azumi N, Hoy GR, Lack EE. Gingival granular cell tumors of the newborn. An ultrastructural and immunohistochemical study. Arch Pathol Lab Med. 1990;114:895–8.
11. Park SH, Kim TJ, Chi Je G. Congenital granular cell tumor with systemic involvement. Immunohistochemical and ultrastructural study. Arch Pathol Lab Med. 1991;115:934–8.
12. Chung EB. Pitfalls in diagnosing benign soft tissue tumors in infancy and childhood. Pathol Annu. 1985;20:323–86.
13. Regezi JA, Zarbo RJ, Courtney RM, Crissman JD. Imunoreactivity of granular cell lesions of skin, mucosa, and jaw. Cancer. 1989;64:1455–60.
14. Chung EB, Enzinger FM. Benign lipoblastomatosis. An analysis of 35 cases. Cancer. 1973;32:482–92.
15. Chaudhuri B, Ronan SG, Ghosh L. Benign lipoblastoma. A case report. Cancer. 1980;46:611–14.
16. Abdul-Karim FW, Evans HL, Silva EG. Giant cell fibroblastoma: a report of three cases. Am J Clin Pathol. 1985;83:165–70.
17. Dymock RB, Allen PW, Sterling JW, Gilbert EF, Thornbery JM. Giant cell fibroblastoma. A distinctive, recurrent tumor of childhood. Am J Surg Pathol. 1987;11:263–71.
18. Chou P, Gonzalez-Crussi F. Mangkornkanok M. Giant cell fibroblastoma. Cancer. 1989;63:756–62.
19. Fletcher CDM. Giant cell fibroblastoma of soft tissue: a clinicopathological and immunohistochemical study. Histopathology. 1988;13:499–508.
20. Shmookler BM, Enzinger FM, Weiss WW. Giant cell fibroblastoma. A juvenile form of dermatofibrosarcoma protruberans. Cancer. 1989;64:2154–61.
21. Beham A, Fletcher CDM. Dermatofibrosarcoma protruberans with areas resembling giant cell fibroblastoma: a report of two cases. Histopathology. 1990;17:165–7.
22. Alguacil-Garcia A. Giant cell fibroblastoma recurring as dermatofibrosarcoma protruberans. Am J Surg Pathol. 1991;15:798–801.
23. McKee PH, Fletcher CDM. Dermatofibrosarcoma protruberans presenting in infancy and childhood. J Cutan Pathol. 1991;18:241–6.
24. Enzinger FM, Zhang R. Plexiform fibrohistiocytic tumor in children and young adults. An analysis of 65 cases. Am J Surg Pathol. 1988;12:818–26.
25. Hollowood K, Holley MP, Fletcher CDM. Plexiform fibrohistiocytic tumour: clinicopathological, immunohistochemical and ultrastructural analysis in favour of a myofibroblastic lesion. Histopathology. 1991;19:503–13.
26. Enzinger FM. Angiomatoid malignant fibrous histiocytoma. A distinctive fibrohistiocytic tumor of children and young adults simulating a vascular neoplasm. Cancer. 1979;44:2147–57.
27. Costa MJ, Weiss SW. Angiomatoid malignant fibrous histiocytoma. A follow-up study of 108 cases with evaluation of possible histological predictors of outcome. Am J Surg Pathol. 1990;14:1126–32.
28. Fletcher CDM. Angiomatoid 'malignant fibrous histiocytoma'. An immunohistochemical study indicative of myoid differentiation. Hum Pathol. 1991;22:563–8.
29. Argenyi ZB, Van Rybroek JJ, Kemp JD, Soper RT. Congenital angiomatoid malignant fibrous histiocytoma. A light-microscopic, immunopathologic, and electron-microscopic study. Am J Dermatopathol. 1988;10:59–67.
30. Enzinger FM, Shiraki M. Extraskeletal myxoid chondrosarcoma. An analysis of 34 cases. Hum Pathol. 1972;3:421–35.
31. Hachitanda Y, Tsuneyoshi M, Daimaru Y et al. Extraskeletal myxoid chondrosarcoma in young children. Cancer. 1988;61:2521–6.
32. Jessurun J, Rojas ME, Albores-Saavedra J. Congenital extraskeletal chondrosarcoma. J Bone Jt Surg. 1982;64:293–6.
33. Coffin CM, Dehner LP. Soft tissue neoplasms in childhood: a clinicopatholic overview. In: Finegold M, editor. Pathology of neoplasia in children and adolescents. Philadelphia: WB Saunders; 1986:223–55.
34. Bernstein KE, Lattes R. Nodular (pseudosarcomatous) fasciitis, a nonrecurrent lesion: clinicopathological study of 134 cases. Cancer. 1982;49:1668–78.
35. Montgomery EA, Meis JM. Nodular fasciitis. Its morphological spectrum and immunohistochemical profile. Am J Surg Pathol. 1991;15:942–8.
36. Lauer DH, Enzinger FM. Cranial fasciitis of childhood. Cancer. 1980;45:401–6.
37. Suster S, Rosai J. Hamartoma of the scalp with ectopic meningothelial elements. A distinctive benign soft tissue lesion that may simulate angiosarcoma. Am J Surg Pathol. 1990;14:1–11.
38. Bale PM, Hughes L, de Silva M. Sequestrated meningoceles of scalp: extracranial meningeal heterotopia. Hum Pathol. 1990;21:1156–63.
39. Enzinger FM, Weiss SW. Alveolar soft part sarcoma. In: Enzinger FM, Weiss SW, editors. Soft tissue tumors. St. Louis, Toronto, London: CV Mosby; 1983:780–87.
40. Schmidt D, Thum P, Harms D, Treuner J. Synovial sarcoma in children and adolescents. A report from the Kiel Pediatric Tumor Registry. Cancer. 1991;67:1667–72.
41. Enzinger FM, Weiss SW. Synovial sarcoma. In: Enzinger FM, Weiss SW, editors. Soft tissue tumors. St Louis, Toronto, London: CV Mosby; 1983:519–49.
42. Smith S, Reeves BR, Wong L, Fisher C. A consistent chromosome translocation in synovial sarcoma. Cancer Genet Cytogenet. 1987;26:179–80.
43. Enzinger FM, Weiss SW. Myositis ossificans. In: Enziger FM, Weiss SW, editors. Soft tissue tumors. St Louis, Toronto, London: CV Mosby; 1983:720–9.
44. Cramer SF, Ruehl A, Mandel MA. Fibrodysplasia ossificans progressiva. A distinctive bone-forming lesion of the soft tissue. Cancer. 1981;48:1016–21.
45. Myers BW, Masi AT, Feigenbaum SL. Pigmented villonodular synovitis and tenosynovitis: a clinical epidemiologic study of 166 cases and review of the literature. Medicine. 1980;59:223–38.
46. Wood GS, Beckstead JH, Medeiros LJ, Kempson RL, Warnke RA. The cells of giant cell tumour of tendon sheath resemble osteoclasts. Am J Surg Pathol. 1988;12:444–52.
47. Enzinger FM, Weiss SW. Fibroma of tendon sheath. In: Enzinger FM, Weiss SW, editors. Soft tissue tumors. St Louis, Toronto, London: CV Mosby; 1983:31–3.
48. Chung EB, Enzinger FM. Fibroma of tendon sheath. Cancer. 1979;44:1945–54.
49. Pulitzer DR, Martin PC, Reed RJ. Fibroma of tendon sheath. A clinicopathologic study of 32 cases. Am J Surg Pathol. 1989;13:472–9.
50. Heffner RR, Armbrustmacher VW, Earle KM. Focal myositis. Cancer. 1977;40:301–6.
51. Markel SF, Enzinger FM. Neuromuscular hamartoma – a benign 'Triton tumor' composed of mature neural and striated muscle elements. Cancer. 1982;49:140–4.
52. Gonzalez-Crussi F, Goldschmidt RA, Hsueh W et al. Infantile sarcoma with intracytoplasmic filamentous inclusions. Cancer. 1982;49:2365–75.
53. Tsuneyoshi M, Daimaru Y, Hashimoto H, Enjoji M. Malignant soft tissue neoplasms with the histologic features of renal rhabdoid tumors: an ultrastructural and immunohistochemical study. Hum Pathol. 1985;16:1235–42.
54. Perrone T, Swanson PE, Twiggs L, Ulbright TM, Dehner LP. Malignant rhabdoid tumour of the vulva: is distinction from epithelioid sarcoma possible? A pathologic and immunohistochemical study. Am J Surg Pathol. 1989;13:848–58.
55. Kodet R, Newton WA, Sachs N et al. Rhabdoid tumors of soft tissues: a clinicopathologic study of 26 cases enrolled on the Intergroup Rhabdo-

myosarcoma Study. Hum Pathol. 1991;22:674–84.
56. Berry PJ, Vujanic GM. Commentary: Malignant rhabdoid tumour. Histopathology. 1992;20:189–93.
57. Chase DR, Enzinger FM. Epithelioid sarcoma. Diagnosis, prognostic indicators, and treatment. Am J Surg Pathol. 1985;9:241–63.
58. Enzinger FM. Epithelioid sarcoma. A sarcoma simulating a granuloma or a carcinoma. Cancer. 1970;26:1029–41.
59. Schmidt D, Harms D. Epithelioid sarcoma in children and adolescents. An immunohistochemical study. Virchows Arch. A. 1987;410:423–31.
60. Fisher C. Epithelioid sarcoma: the spectrum of ultrastructural differentiation in seven immunohistochemically defined cases. Hum Pathol. 1988;19:255–75.
61. Pettinato G, Manivel JC, De Rosa N, Dehner LP. Inflammatory myofibroblastic tumor (plasma cell granuloma). Clinicopathologic study of 20 cases with immunohistochemical and ultrastructural observations. Am J Clin Pathol. 1990;94:538–46.
62. Scott L, Blair G, Taylor G, Dimmick J, Fraser G. Inflammatory pseudotumors in children. J Pediatr Surg. 1988;23:755–8.
63. Berardi RS, Lee SS, Chen HP, Stines GJ. Inflammatory pseudotumor of the lung. Surg Gynecol Obstet. 1983;156:89–96.
64. Chen KT. Inflammatory pseudotumour of the liver. Hum Pathol. 1984;15:694–6.
65. Meis JM, Enzinger FM. Inflammatory fibrosarcoma of the mesentery and retroperitoneum. A tumor closely simulating inflammatory pseudotumor. Am J Surg Pathol. 1991;15:1146–56.
66. Le Ber MS, Stout AP. Benign mesenchymomas in children. Cancer. 1962;15:598–605.
67. Bures C, Barnes L. Benign mesenchymomas of the head and neck. Arch Pathol Lab Med. 1978;102:237–41.
68. Newman PL, Fletcher CDM. Malignant mesenchymoma. Clinicopathologic analysis of a series with evidence of low-grade behavior. Am J Surg Pathol. 1991;15:607–14.
69. Enzinger FM, Weiss SW. Malignant mesenchymoma. In: Enzinger FM, Weiss SW, editors. Soft tissue tumours. St Louis, Toronto, London: CV Mosby; 1983:808–10.
70. Shmookler BM, Enzinger FM. Liposarcoma occurring in children. An analysis of 17 cases and review of the literature. Cancer. 1983;52:567–74.
71. Weiss SW, Enzinger FM. Malignant fibrous histiocytoma. An analysis of 200 cases. Cancer. 1978;41:2250–66.
72. Zuppan CW, Mierau GW, Wilson HL. Malignant fibrous histiocytoma in childhood: a report of two cases and review of the literature. Pediatr Pathol. 1987;7:303–18.
73. Nemes Z, Thomazy V. Factor XIIIa and the classic histiocytic markers in malignant fibrous histiocytoma: a comparative immunohistochemical study. Hum Pathol. 1988;19:822–9.

Index

References to figure legends are in *italic* type